2013
YEAR BOOK OF
HAND AND UPPER
LIMB SURGERY®

The 2013 Year Book Series

Year Book of Critical Care Medicine®: Drs Dries, Zanotti-Cavazzoni, Latenser, Martinez, Rincon, and Zwank

Year Book of Emergency Medicine®: Drs Hamilton, Bruno, Handly, Minczak, Quintana, and Ramoska

Year Book of Endocrinology®: Drs Schott, Apovian, Clarke, Eugster, Meikle, Oetgen, Ovalle, Schteingart, and Toth

Year Book of Hand and Upper Limb Surgery®: Drs Yao, Adams, Isaacs, and Rizzo

Year Book of Medicine®: Drs Barker, Garrick, Gersh, Khardori, LeRoith, Panush, Talley, and Thigpen

Year Book of Neonatal and Perinatal Medicine®: Drs Fanaroff, Benitz, Donn, Neu, Papile, and Van Marter

Year Book of Neurology and Neurosurgery®: Drs Klimo, Minagar, Gandhi, Liu, Panagariya, Rezania, Riel-Romero, Riesenburger, Robottom, Schwendimann, Shafazand, and Yang

Year Book of Obstetrics, Gynecology, and Women's Health®: Drs Dungan and Shulman

Year Book of Oncology®: Drs Arceci, Bauer, Chiorean, Gordon, Lawton, Murphy, Thigpen, and Tsao

Year Book of Ophthalmology®: Drs Rapuano, Cohen, Flanders, Hammersmith, Milman, Myers, Nagra, Nelson, Penne, Pyfer, Sergott, Shields, Talekar, and Vander

Year Book of Orthopedics®: Drs Morrey, Huddleston, Rose, Swiontkowski, and Trigg

Year Book of Otolaryngology-Head and Neck Surgery®: Drs Sindwani, Balough, Franco, Gapany, and Mitchell

Year Book of Pathology and Laboratory Medicine®: Drs Raab and Bissell

Year Book of Pediatrics®: Dr Stockman

Year Book of Plastic and Aesthetic Surgery™: Drs Miller, Boehmler, Gosman, Gutowski, Ruberg, Salisbury, and Smith

Year Book of Psychiatry and Applied Mental Health®: Drs Talbott, Ballenger, Buckley, Frances, Krupnick, and Mack

Year Book of Pulmonary Disease®: Drs Barker, Jones, Maurer, Spradley, Tanoue, and Willsie

Year Book of Sports Medicine®: Drs Shephard, Cantu, Feldman, Galea, Jankowski, Janssen, Lebrun, and Nieman

Year Book of Surgery®: Drs Behrns, Daly, Fahey, Hines, Howe, Huber, Klodell, Mozingo, and Pruett

Year Book of Urology®: Drs Andriole and Coplen

Year Book of Vascular Surgery®: Drs Gillespie, Bush, Passman, Starnes, and Watkins

2013

The Year Book of HAND AND UPPER LIMB SURGERY®

Editor-in-Chief
Jeffrey Yao, MD
Associate Professor of Orthopaedic Surgery, Robert A. Chase Hand and Upper Limb Center, Stanford, California

Associate Editors
Julie Adams, MD
Assistant Professor of Orthopedic Surgery, University of Minnesota, Minneapolis, Minnesota

Jonathan Isaacs, MD
Chair, Division of Hand Surgery, Associate Professor, Department of Orthopedic Surgery, VCU Medical Center, Richmond, Virginia

Marco Rizzo, MD
Associate Professor, Department of Orthopedic Surgery, Mayo Clinic College of Medicine, Rochester, Minnesota

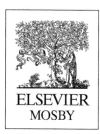

ELSEVIER
MOSBY

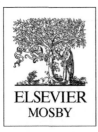

ELSEVIER
MOSBY

Senior Vice President, Content: Linda Belfus
Developmental Editor: Jennifer Flynn-Briggs
Production Supervisor, Electronic Year Books: Donna M. Skelton
Electronic Article Manager: Mike Rainey
Illustrations and Permissions Coordinator: Dawn Vohsen

Composition by TNQ Books and Journals Pvt Ltd, India

Printed and bound by CPI Group (UK) Ltd, Croydon, CR0 4YY

Transferred to digital print 2012

Editorial Office:
Elsevier
Suite 1800
1600 John F. Kennedy Blvd.
Philadelphia, PA 19103-2899

International Standard Serial Number: 1551-7977
International Standard Book Number: 978-1-4557-7276-6

Contributing Editors

Julie E. Adams, MD
Assistant Professor, Orthopaedic Surgery, University of Minnesota, Minneapolis, Minnesota

Peter Amadio, MD
Lloyd and Barbara Amundson Professor, Department of Orthopedic Surgery, Mayo Clinic, Rochester, Minnesota

Keith Bengtson, MD
Assistant Professor, Department of Physical Medicine and Rehabilitation, Mayo Clinic, Rochester, Minnesota

Philip Blazar, MD
Assistant Professor, Department of Orthopaedic Surgery, Brigham and Women's Hospital, Boston, Massachusetts

Jeff Brault, MD
Assistant Professor, Department of Physical Medicine and Rehabilitation, Mayo Clinic, Rochester, Minnesota

Lance M. Brunton, MD
Excela Health Orthopaedics and Sports Medicine, Latrobe, Pennsylvania

John Capo, MD
Professor, Department of Orthopaedic Surgery, New York University Hospital for Joint Diseases, New York, New York

Charles Carroll IV, MD
Associate Professor of Clinical Orthopedic Surgery, Feinberg School of Medicine, Northwestern University, Chicago, Illinois

R. Chris Chadderdon, MD
OrthoCarolina, Charlotte, North Carolina

Neal C. Chen, MD
Assistant Professor in Orthopaedic Surgery, Thomas Jefferson University Hospital, The Philadelphia Hand Center, P.C., Philadelphia, Pennsylvania

Emilie Cheung, MD
Assistant Professor, Robert A. Chase Hand & Upper Limb Center, Department of Orthopaedic Surgery, Redwood City, California

Matthew Seung Suk Choi, MD
Associate Professor, Chief, Department of Plastic and Reconstructive Surgery, Hanyang University Guri Hospital, Guri, Gyunggi-do, Korea

Alphonsus KS Chong, MD
Head and Senior Consultant, Department of Hand and Reconstructive Microsurgery, National University Hospital, Singapore

Susan J. Clark, OTR/L, CHT
Certified Hand Therapist, Stanford University Medical Center, Redwood City, California

Catherine Curtin, MD
Assistant Professor, Robert A. Chase Hand & Upper Limb Center, Division of Plastic Surgery Stanford University Medical Center, Stanford, California

Bassem Elhassan, MD
Associate Professor, Department of Orthopedic Surgery, Mayo Clinic, Rochester, Minnesota

Felicity G. Fishman, MD
Assistant Professor, Department of Orthopaedics and Rehabilitation, Yale University School of Medicine, New Haven, Connecticut

Jessica Frankenhoff, MD
Assistant Professor, Division of Hand Surgery, Department of Orthopedics, Virginia Commonwealth University, Richmond, Virginia

Jeffrey B. Frederick, MD, FACS
Associate Professor of Surgery and Orthopedics, Division of Plastic Surgery, University of Washington, Seattle, Washington

John M. Froelich, MD
Assistant Professor, Department of Orthopaedics, University of Colorado, School of Medicine, Aurora, Colorado

R. Glenn Gaston, MD
OrthoCarolina, Chief of Hand Surgery, Carolinas Medical Center, Department Orthopedic Surgery, Charlotte, North Carolina

Ruby Grewal, MD MSc FRCS
Assistant Professor, The Hand and Upper Limb Centre, St Joseph's Health Centre, London, Ontario, Canada

Rohan Habbu, MS (Orthopedics)
Consultant Orthopaedic Surgeon, Arthroscopy & Sports Surgery, Hand, Nerve & Upper Extremity Surgeon, Habbu Orthopaedic Care, Vile Parle East, Mumbai, India

Warren C. Hammert, MD
University of Rochester Medical Center, Department of Orthopaedic Surgery, Rochester, New York

Alicia K. Harrison, MD
Assistant Professor, Orthopaedic Surgery, University of Minnesota, Minneapolis, Minnesota

Vincent R. Hentz, MD
Professor of Surgery, Robert A. Chase Hand & Upper Limb Center, Division of Plastic Surgery Stanford University Medical Center, Stanford, California

Thomas Hughes, MD
Assistant Professor, AGH Department of Orthopedics, Allegheny Orthopedics Associates, Pittsburgh, Pennsylvania

Jonathan Isaacs, MD
Chair, Division of Hand Surgery, Associate Professor, Department Of Orthopedic Surgery, Virginia Commonwealth University Medical Center, Hand & Wrist, Orthopedic Microsurgical Reconstruction, Richmond, Virginia

Sidney M. Jacoby, MD
Assistant Professor in Orthopaedic Surgery, Thomas Jefferson University Hospital, The Philadelphia Hand Center, P.C., Philadelphia, Pennsylvania

Sanjeev Kakar, MD
Associate Professor, Department of Orthopedic Surgery Mayo Clinic, Rochester, Minnesota

Ryosuke Kakinoki, MD, PhD
Associate Professor, Chief, Hand Surgery and Microsurgery, Department of Orthopedic Surgery and Rehabilitation Medicine, Graduate School of Medicine, Kyoto University, Kyoto, Japan

F. Thomas D. Kaplan, MD
Indiana Hand to Shoulder Center, Indianapolis, Indiana

Sonja Kranz, OTL/R, CHT
Hand Therapist, Department of Physical Medicine and Rehabilitation, Mayo Clinic, Rochester, Minnesota

Amy L. Ladd, MD
Editor-in-Chief, Emeritus, Yearbook of Hand & Upper Limb Surgery, Professor of Orthopaedic Surgery & Plastic Surgery, Robert A. Chase Hand & Upper Limb Center at Stanford University, Palo Alto, California

Jeffrey Macalena, MD
Assistant Professor, Orthopaedic Surgery, University of Minnesota, Minneapolis, Minnesota

Dan Mastella, MD
Assistant Clinical Professor, Department of Orthopaedic Surgery, University of Connecticut, Hartford, Connecticut

Kai Megerle, MD
Assistant Professor, Department of Plastic Surgery and Hand Surgery, Technical University of Munich, Munich, Germany

Peter Murray, MD
Professor, Department of Orthopedic Surgery, Mayo Clinic, Jacksonville, Florida

Virginia H. O'Brien, OTD, OTR/L, CHT
Supervisor, Hand and Physical Therapy, Fairview Hand Center, University Orthopaedics Therapy Center, University of Minnesota Medical Center, Fairview, Minneapolis, Minnesota

Rick F. Papendrea, MD
Assistant Clinical Professor, Department of Orthopaedic Surgery, Medical College of Wisconsin, Orthopedic Associates of Wisconsin, Waukesha, Wisconsin

Marco Rizzo, MD
Professor, Department of Orthopedic Surgery, Mayo Clinic, Rochester, Minnesota

Tamara Rozental, MD
Assistant Professor of Orthopaedic Surgery, Harvard Medical School, Beth Israel Deaconess Medical Center, Carl J. Shapiro Department of Orthopaedics, Boston, Massachusetts

Joaquin Sanchez-Sotelo, MD
Associate Professor, Department of Orthopedic Surgery, Mayo Clinic, Rochester, Minnesota

Eon K. Shin, MD
Assistant Professor in Orthopaedic Surgery, Thomas Jefferson University Hospital, The Philadelphia Hand Center, P.C., Philadelphia, Pennsylvania

Steven Shin, MD
Chief of Hand Surgery, Kerlan-Jobe Orthopaedic Clinic, Los Angeles, California

John Sperling, MD
Professor, Department of Orthopedic Surgery, Mayo Clinic, Rochester, Minnesota

Jin Bo Tang, MD
Professor and Chair, Department of Hand Surgery, Affiliated Hospital of Nantong University, Chair, Hand Surgery Research Center, Nantong University, Jiangsu, China

Christopher J. Tuohy, MD
Assistant Professor, Department of Orthopaedic Surgery, Wake Forest University, Winston-Salem, North Carolina

Christina M. Ward, MD
Assistant Professor, Orthopaedic Surgery, University of Minnesota, Regions Hospital, St Paul, Minnesota

Jeffrey Yao, MD
Associate Professor, Robert A. Chase Hand & Upper Limb Center, Department of Orthopaedic Surgery, Redwood City, California

David Zelouf, MD
Assistant Clinical Professor, Department of Orthopaedic Surgery, Thomas Jefferson University Hospital and The Philadelphia Hand Center, King of Prussia, Pennsylvania

Dan Zlotolow, MD
Associate Professor, Department of Orthopaedic Surgery, Shriner's Children's Hospital, Philadelphia, Pennsylvania

Table of Contents

Journals Represented

Journals represented in this YEAR BOOK are listed below.

American Journal of Sports Medicine
Anaesthesia
Annals of Plastic Surgery
Arthroscopy
Clinical Neurology and Neurosurgery
Clinical Orthopaedics and Related Research
European Journal of Plastic Surgery
European Journal of Radiology
Injury
Journal of Bone and Joint Surgery (American)
Journal of Bone and Joint Surgery (British)
Journal of Hand Surgery
Journal of Hand Therapy
Journal of Manipulative and Physiological Therapeutics
Journal of Neurosurgery
Journal of Oral and Maxillofacial Surgery
Journal of Orthopaedic Research
Journal of Orthopaedic Trauma
Journal of Pediatric Orthopedics
Journal of Plastic, Reconstructive & Aesthetic Surgery
Journal of Surgical Research
Journal of Trauma and Acute Care Surgery
Microsurgery
Neurosurgery
Orthopedics
Plastic and Reconstructive Surgery
Skeletal Radiology

STANDARD ABBREVIATIONS

The following terms are abbreviated in this edition: acquired immunodeficiency syndrome (AIDS), cardiopulmonary resuscitation (CPR), central nervous system (CNS), cerebrospinal fluid (CSF), computed tomography (CT), deoxyribonucleic acid (DNA), electrocardiography (ECG), health maintenance organization (HMO), human immunodeficiency virus (HIV), intensive care unit (ICU), intramuscular (IM), intravenous (IV), magnetic resonance (MR) imaging (MRI), ribonucleic acid (RNA), and ultrasound (US).

NOTE

To facilitate the use of the YEAR BOOK OF HAND AND UPPER LIMB SURGERY® as a reference tool, all illustrations and tables included in this publication are now identified as they appear in the original article. This change is meant to help the reader recognize that any illustration or table appearing in the YEAR BOOK OF HAND AND UPPER LIMB SURGERY® may be only one of many in the original article. For this reason, figure and table numbers will often appear to be out of sequence within the YEAR BOOK OF HAND AND UPPER LIMB SURGERY®.

Introduction

We are proud to present the 29th edition of the YEAR BOOK OF HAND AND UPPER LIMB SURGERY. It is our honor to continue a Mayo Clinic and Stanford University collaborative editorial tradition begun by Drs James Dobyns and Robert Chase and continued by Drs Peter Amadio and Vincent Hentz and, most recently, by Drs Richard Berger, Amy Ladd, James Chang, and Scott Steinmann.

This is the second year the YEAR BOOK has enlisted an editorial board, with associate editors chosen for their expertise in the field of upper limb surgery, as well as for their geographic diversity around the United States. Dr Jeffrey Yao remains the editor-in-chief and is indebted to the editorial board (Drs Julie Adams, Jonathan Isaacs, and Marco Rizzo) for their contributions.

As the number of available sources of information regarding upper limb surgery or the busy surgeon increases, the goal of the YEAR BOOK is to distill the previous year's most salient journal articles into a shorter, more digestible form, all in one place. Upper limb surgeons continue to express interest in pathology of the entire limb, including the shoulder, elbow, wrist, and hand. The content of this year's YEAR BOOK OF HAND AND UPPER LIMB SURGERY continues to reflect this trend. The literature surveyed by this year's YEAR BOOK covers a diverse subject matter, stretching from the brachial plexus to the fingertip. Many articles have addressed current concepts and the cutting edge regarding topics ranging from arthroplasty, reconstruction, trauma, arthroscopy, and congenital conditions of the entire upper limb.

We are deep within the Internet generation, with information readily at a surgeon's fingertips. As a result, the YEAR BOOK OF HAND AND UPPER LIMB SURGERY strives to evolve as well. Moving forward, we hope to embrace a real time electronic eClips Consult format (www.eclips.consult. com), which keeps us even more up to date and makes the information from the YEAR BOOK more accessible and current throughout the year. Ultimately, the goal of the editorial board will be to have year-long continuous updating of the YEAR BOOK with the most current and salient articles uploaded online shortly after they are published. This format will allow the subscribing physician to access the YEAR BOOK electronically throughout the year to obtain the most up-to-date reviews and commentaries available.

As with every year, we would like to acknowledge the immense effort of the contributing editors to the YEAR BOOK, without whom this edition would not be possible. All of the contributing editors have been personally selected for their national and international expertise in particular areas of the upper limb. The contributing editors have been enlisted from around the world and we are indebted to them for their commentary printed on these pages.

Finally, we would like to thank David Parsons and Jennifer Flynn-Briggs from Elsevier for their stewardship in helping guide us through this edition, and into the future.

Jeffrey Yao, MD

1 Hand and Wrist Arthritis

Influence of Index Finger Proximal Interphalangeal Joint Arthrodesis on Precision Pinch Kinematics

Domalain M, Evans PJ, Seitz WH Jr, et al (Cleveland Clinic, OH)

J Hand Surg 36A:1944-1949, 2011

Purpose.—To evaluate the impact of proximal interphalangeal (PIP) joint arthrodesis on the kinematics of precision pinch.

Methods.—Eleven healthy subjects performed index finger–thumb pinch motions under 4 conditions: unrestricted thumb and index finger (CONTROL) and fusion of the PIP joint of the index finger in flexion of 30° (PIP30), 40° (PIP40), and 50° (PIP50). Fusion was simulated with metallic splints. Kinematics of the thumb and index finger were recorded with a motion capture system.

Results.—Proximal interphalangeal joint fusion at 30°, 40°, and 50° restricted maximal pinch span between the thumb tip and index finger tip by 6%, 10%, and 14%, respectively. At the time of pulp contact, PIP fusion led to an increase in index metacarpophalangeal joint flexion angle for the PIP30 condition and an increase in variability of thumb tip location for the PIP50 condition. Furthermore, the dynamic coordination between joint angles throughout the movement was affected by PIP fusion.

Conclusions.—This study reports impairment in the kinematics of precision pinch associated with index finger PIP joint fusion. A PIP joint fusion at 40° to 50° leads to a more natural precision pinch posture, but it restricts the aperture and reduces pinch precision.

▶ The prescribed position for proximal interphalangeal (PIP) joint has traditionally been established as the resting position of the digit. In this study, Domalain et al provide objective evidence that alterations in PIP joint arthrodesis angle may affect pinch aperture and pinch kinematics. In this well-designed and controlled study, the authors simulated index finger PIP joint arthrodesis at 30°, 40°, and 50°. They identified that with increasing PIP joint arthrodesis angle, the aperture or span of the thumb and the index finger diminishes, likely compromising pinch ability. Furthermore, they observed that compensatory motion of the metacarpophalangeal (MCP) and PIP joints was greatest at the 30° PIP joint arthrodesis angle, whereas little, if any, compensatory MCP or PIP joint motion occurred at the 40° or 50° PIP joint arthrodesis angle. According to the authors, the natural pinch angle for the index PIP joint is 44°, which would explain the lack of compensatory MCP and PIP joint movements in those PIP arthrodesis positions.

Arthrodesis of the PIP joint currently remains the preferred treatment for advanced degenerative disease of that joint. The findings of the article call into question the traditional position of 30° of flexion as the desired position for PIP arthrodesis of the index finger. More practically, however, establishing a precise position for arthrodesis at the time of surgery may not be technically achievable, and the surgeon should be made aware of the potential limitations created by PIP joint arthrodesis of the index finger.

P. Murray, MD

Lunatocapitate and Triquetrohamate Arthrodeses for Degenerative Arthritis of the Wrist

Wang ML, Bednar JM (Thomas Jefferson Univ Hosp, Philadelphia, PA; The Philadelphia and South Jersey Hand Ctrs, Cherry Hill, NJ)
J Hand Surg 37A:1136-1141, 2012

Purpose.—Proximal row carpectomy and 4-corner arthrodesis are 2 well-established motion-preserving treatment strategies for scapholunate advanced collapse. In this study, we present an arthrodesis technique involving the capitolunate and triquetrohamate joints as another potential treatment option.

Methods.—From 2000 to 2009, 27 consecutive patients with degenerative scapholunate advanced collapse and scaphoid nonunion advanced collapse were evaluated prospectively and treated with scaphoid excision and intercarpal arthrodesis between the capitate and lunate and between the hamate and triquetrum. This cohort consisted of 18 men and 9 women, involving dominant-sided surgery in 20 of 27 patients. Two patients were active smokers, and 3 cases were work related. Average age at time of surgery was 55 ± 3 years, and average follow-up was 51 ± 7 months. Preoperative and postoperative range of motion, grip strength, and radiographic evidence of osseous union were documented. Standardized Patient-Rated Wrist Evaluation scores for both pain and function were collected.

Results.—Wrist extension and flexion were decreased after surgery by 17% and 25% respectively, yielding a 21% decrease in mean flexion–extension arc. There was no significant difference with regard to postoperative radial and ulnar deviation or mean coronal plane arc compared to preoperative values. Compared to the contralateral side, preoperative and postoperative grip strength were 53% and 70%, respectively. The average operative-sided grip strength increased by 27%. The mean Patient-Rated Wrist Evaluation pain score was 11 ± 3 (of 50). The mean Patient-Rated Wrist Evaluation functional score was 17 ± 5 (of 100). Complications included 1 nonunion (yielding a 96% fusion rate), 1 median neuropathy (which resolved), and 2 superficial wound infections (treated successfully with oral antibiotics).

Conclusions.—Arthrodesis of the capitolunate and triquetrohamate joints offers a motion-preserving strategy with a high union rate and good clinical function and pain outcomes for the treatment for scapholunate advanced collapse and scaphoid nonunion advanced collapse.

Type of Study/Level of Evidence.—Therapeutic IV.

▶ The authors present the results of their clinical experience using a particular surgical technique for scapholunate advanced collapse (SLAC) or scaphoid nonunion advanced collapse (SNAC) wrists. This technique consists of scaphoid excision with arthrodeses of the lunatocapitate and triquetrohamate joints using headless compression screws and autograft from the scaphoid. This article provides clinical evidence that this technique can produce results similar to those of the conventional 4-corner arthrodesis.

This was a well-designed and well-executed study with very good follow-up data.

The authors present a useful technique for addressing the difficult problem of SLAC or SNAC wrist. It has advantages over other arthrodesis techniques, and I believe this technique will continue to grow in popularity.

I have personally performed a large number of salvage procedures for SNAC and SLAC wrists, including limited intercarpal fusions with scaphoid excision, and have been very pleased with the technique described in this article. Regarding the implant used, I have tried various types of circular plates, Kirschner wires, staples, and headless compression screws, and the technique described here is my preferred technique. Advantages are: less time needed removing cartilage (only from lunatocapitate and triquetrohamate joints), no need to remove bone for hardware placement (as seen when reaming for a circular plate), ease of placement and insertion with complete burial of only 3 screws (no risk of impingement with the dorsal lip of the distal radius, as can sometimes be seen with a circular plate), excellent compression provided by these compression screws, and no need to remove hardware (as with K-wires) unless absolutely necessary (eg, screw backing out, conversion to total wrist arthrodesis).

S. Shin, MD, MMSc

Results After Radioscapholunate Arthrodesis With or Without Resection of the Distal Scaphoid Pole
Mühldorfer-Fodor M, Ha HP, Hohendorff B, et al (Clinic for Hand Surgery, Bad Neustadt/Saale, Germany)
J Hand Surg 37A:2233-2239, 2012

Purpose.—To evaluate the differences between radioscapholunate (RSL) arthrodesis alone versus RSL arthrodesis with additional distal scaphoidectomy.

Methods.—We retrospectively evaluated 61 patients who were treated with RSL arthrodesis for painful posttraumatic osteoarthritis. Thirty patients had an RSL arthrodesis with additional resection of the distal scaphoid pole (group A), and 31 had RSL arthrodesis alone (group B). Six patients in group A and 8 in group B had the RSL arthrodesis converted to a complete wrist arthrodesis during follow-up. Those patients were excluded from the survey. Of the remaining 47 patients, 35 (20 from group A, 15 from group B) returned for a clinical and radiological examination at an average of 28 (range, 10–47) months after the index surgery. The results were rated by the Disabilities of the Arm, Shoulder, and Hand score and the modified Mayo Wrist Score. The patients' outcomes after RSL arthrodesis with or without distal scaphoidectomy were compared for pain, wrist motion, grip strength, nonunion rate, osteoarthritis of the adjacent joints, the Disabilities of the Arm, Shoulder, and Hand score and the modified Mayo Wrist Score.

Results.—Three patients with RSL arthrodesis alone showed a radioscaphoid nonunion. All arthrodeses in group A healed. In the clinical evaluation, there was no significant difference between groups A and B in the Disabilities of the Arm, Shoulder, and Hand score, the modified Mayo Wrist Score, grip strength, pain, or wrist motion. Assuming that wrist motion might be better in patients with a nonunion, the average wrist motion was recalculated after eliminating 3 patients with a radioscaphoid nonunion from group B. Radial deviation was then found to be significantly better in group A.

Conclusions.—Additional distal scaphoidectomy with RSL arthrodesis seems to improve postoperative radial deviation of the wrist. The radioscaphoid nonunion rate is high with RSL arthrodesis alone. Distal scaphoidectomy appeared to increase the successful fusion rate of RSL arthrodeses. No significant effect on wrist extension, flexion, ulnar deviation, pain level, restriction in activities of daily living, or grip strength was noted.

▶ Radioscapholunate (RSL) fusion is useful in cases of posttraumatic arthritis, rheumatoid arthritis, and Kienböck's disease. This study tries to answer the question whether resection of the distal pole of the scaphoid at the time of RSL fusion improves postoperative motion, pain, or function. Pervaiz et al[1] found, in a biomechanical study, improved flexion, extension, and radial and ulnar deviation after distal pole scaphoid and triquetrum excision; however, clinical results have been conflicting.

In this study, the authors retrospectively assessed the outcome in patients who underwent RSL fusion with or without distal scaphoid excision. They identified 61 patients, 30 with concomitant distal scaphoid excision, who had surgery at one institution between 2002 and 2007. The authors do not state the rationale behind choosing to add the distal scaphoid excision for some patients and not others other than to mention that it was performed inconsistently, although when performed it was hoped the patients would have improved outcomes. Despite the weakness of the study's retrospective nature and the failure to have patients randomly selected for procedures, the authors were able to evaluate more than half of the patients (35) at an average of 28 months after surgery.

Although the authors found no difference between groups in Disabilities of the Arm, Shoulder, and Hand score; modified Mayo wrist score; grip strength; pain; or motion, they did find that there were 3 scaphoid nonunions in the group without distal pole excision compared with none in the excision group. Hypothesizing that these patients likely had motion at the nonunion site, they re-evaluated the results after eliminating these nonunions and found a significantly increased radial deviation in the distal scaphoid resection group, with all other motions similar.

Although a prospective study is still needed, this study supports the routine addition of distal scaphoid excision when performing RSL fusion to increase postoperative radial deviation and possibly reduce scaphoid nonunion.

F. T. D. Kaplan, MD

Reference

1. Pervaiz K, Bowers WH, Isaacs JE, Owen JR, Wayne JS. Range of motion effects of distal pole scaphoid excision and triquetral excision after radioscapholunate fusion: a cadaver study. *J Hand Surg Am*. 2009;34:832-837.

Proximal interphalangeal joint replacement in patients with arthritis of the hand: A meta-analysis

Adams J, Ryall C, Pandyan A, et al (Univ of Southampton, UK)
J Bone Joint Surg Br 94-B:1305-1312, 2012

We systematically reviewed all the evidence published in the English language on proximal interphalangeal joint (PIPJ) replacement, to determine its effectiveness on the function of the hand and the associated postoperative complications.

Original studies were selected if they reported clinical outcome with a minimum of one year's follow-up. Quality was assessed using the Cowley systematic review criteria modified for finger-joint replacements. Of 319 articles identified, only five were adequately reported according to our quality criteria; there were no randomised controlled trials. PIPJ replacements had a substantial effect size on hand pain of -23.2 (95% confidence interval (CI) -27.3 to -19.1) and grip strength 1.2 (95% CI -10.7 to 13.1), and a small effect on range of movement 0.2 (95% CI -0.4 to 0.8). A dorsal approach was most successful. Post-operative loosening occurred in 10% (95% CI 3 to 30) of ceramic and 12.5% (95% CI 7 to 21) of pyrocarbon replacements. Post-operative complications occurred in 27.8% (95% CI 20 to 37).

We conclude that the effectiveness of PIPJ replacement has not been established. Small observational case studies and short-term follow-up, together with insufficient reporting of patient data, functional outcomes and complications, limit the value of current evidence.

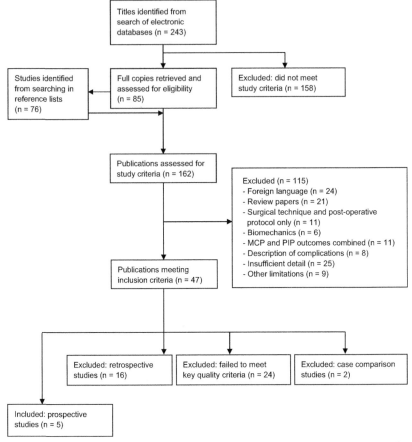

FIGURE 1.—Flow of papers through the study. (Reproduced with permission. Adams J, Ryall C, Pandyan A, et al. Proximal interphalangeal joint replacement in patients with arthritis of the hand: a meta-analysis. *J Bone Joint Surg Br.* 2012;94-B:1305-1312, © 2012, of the British Editorial Society of Bone and Joint Surgery.)

We recommend that a defined core set of patients, surgical and outcome data for this intervention be routinely and systematically collected within the framework of a joint registry (Fig 1).

▶ The degenerated proximal interphalangeal joint (PIPJ) is far from a solved problem. Fusion can provide reliable pain relief, but it can be functionally limiting, particularly for the ulnar-sided digits. Silicone spacers can also provide pain relief and retain some motion, but they are typically used for very low demand patients. There has been increasing interest in joint replacements for the PIPJ, and this meta-analysis attempts to characterize the best evidence available for the use of these prostheses.

The authors completed a rigorous literature review using both literature databases and references from prior papers. Their evaluation progression is detailed in Fig 1. In the end, only 5 papers, using either pyrocarbon or ceramic, met the criteria for the analysis, which is a testament to the lack of rigor in many of the studies on PIPJ's. Many papers did not document long-term follow-up (at least 1 year) or adequate inclusion or exclusion criteria, and some were lost to follow-up, among other factors.

On examining the 5 articles that did meet the criteria, the authors found that most patients experienced improvement in hand pain and grip (power and key) strength, but that range of motion gains were small and likely not significant. Most worrisome is the complication rate, which was 28% overall. At the outset of the article, the authors discuss a prior analysis that noted a 20% complication rate for PIPJ's, and they state that orthopedists would not accept this complication rate for knees or hips. This is a very telling observation about our willingness to overlook these problems in the hand.

This is a well-done and compelling study that should cause all of us to take a hard look at PIPJ replacement procedures. The authors ultimate conclusion is that a joint registry is needed to provide robust data that allow for rigorous analysis of this technique, and it is difficult not to agree with this contention.

J. B. Friedrich, MD, FACS

Results After Radioscapholunate Arthrodesis With or Without Resection of the Distal Scaphoid Pole
Mühldorfer-Fodor M, Ha HP, Hohendorff B, et al (Clinic for Hand Surgery, Bad Neustadt/Saale, Germany)
J Hand Surg 37A:2233-2239, 2012

Purpose.—To evaluate the differences between radioscapholunate (RSL) arthrodesis alone versus RSL arthrodesis with additional distal scaphoidectomy.

Methods.—We retrospectively evaluated 61 patients who were treated with RSL arthrodesis for painful posttraumatic osteoarthritis. Thirty patients had an RSL arthrodesis with additional resection of the distal scaphoid pole (group A), and 31 had RSL arthrodesis alone (group B). Six patients in group A and 8 in group B had the RSL arthrodesis converted to a complete wrist arthrodesis during follow-up. Those patients were excluded from the survey. Of the remaining 47 patients, 35 (20 from group A, 15 from group B) returned for a clinical and radiological examination at an average of 28 (range, 10—47) months after the index surgery. The results were rated by the Disabilities of the Arm, Shoulder, and Hand score and the modified Mayo Wrist Score. The patients' outcomes after RSL arthrodesis with or without distal scaphoidectomy were compared for pain, wrist motion, grip strength, nonunion rate, osteoarthritis of the adjacent joints, the Disabilities of the Arm, Shoulder, and Hand score and the modified Mayo Wrist Score.

Results.—Three patients with RSL arthrodesis alone showed a radioscaphoid nonunion. All arthrodeses in group A healed. In the clinical evaluation, there was no significant difference between groups A and B in the Disabilities

TABLE 3.—Wrist Motion and Grip Strength in Absolute Values (Median, Range, SD) and Percentage in Comparison to the Opposite Hand for Group A and Group B

	Group A (n = 20)	Group B (n = 12)	P Value
Extension	28° (30, 0–50, SD 12.0), 55%	28° (30, 0–40, SD 11.2), 55%	.95
Flexion	25° (28, 5–50, SD 11.0), 40%	20° (20, 0–45, SD 12.0), 29%	.25
Ulnar deviation	17° (15, 5–35, SD 8.2), 51%	16° (18, 0–30, SD 7.9), 47%	.76
Radial deviation	12° (15, 0–25, SD 7.0), 63%	7° (8, 0–15, SD 4.9), 47%	.02
Grip strength (kg)	23 (22, 4–47, SD 10.0), 56%	27 (25, 4–56, SD 15.5), 66%	.32

Three patients were disqualified because of a nonunion.

of the Arm, Shoulder, and Hand score, the modified Mayo Wrist Score, grip strength, pain, or wrist motion. Assuming that wrist motion might be better in patients with a nonunion, the average wrist motion was recalculated after eliminating 3 patients with a radioscaphoid nonunion from group B. Radial deviation was then found to be significantly better in group A.

Conclusions.—Additional distal scaphoidectomy with RSL arthrodesis seems to improve postoperative radial deviation of the wrist. The radioscaphoid nonunion rate is high with RSL arthrodesis alone. Distal scaphoidectomy appeared to increase the successful fusion rate of RSL arthrodeses. No significant effect on wrist extension, flexion, ulnar deviation, pain level, restriction in activities of daily living, or grip strength was noted (Table 3).

▶ This is a relatively large series for a procedure (radioscapholunate fusion) that is not done very frequently. The authors showed better union rates with distal pole scaphoidectomy but not the expected increase in wrist flexion. They did note significant improvement in radial deviation (Table 3). When I first began performing the operation, I was uncertain of the benefit of distal scaphoidectomy. Therefore, I would fixate the fusion and then resect the distal pole secondarily. Direct observation intraoperatively of improved motion has convinced me to continue this practice. It definitely unlocks the midcarpal joint. I have been tempted to resect the triquetrum as well (as reported by Bain)[1] but have been concerned about having too much midcarpal instability. As the authors state, more study of triquetrectomy is necessary before I would proceed with this procedure. There are certainly limitations to the study. I am most concerned about the significant difference in patients with Bower's hemisection of the distal ulna. There were far more in the scaphoidectomy group who underwent this procedure, indicating a more complex set of pathologies and reflecting less on the benefits of scaphoidectomy alone. Finally, I agree that distal scaphoidectomy would alleviate a lot of stress on the fusion construct, which may contribute to the higher fusion rate in this group. However, with newer implants and modes of fixation (locking plates), scaphoidectomy may not affect union rates as much as when k-wires alone are used for fixation.

T. Hughes, MD

Reference

1. Bain GI, Ondimu P, Hallam P, et al. Radioscapholunate arthrodesis - a prospective study. *Hand Surg.* 2009;14(2-3):73-82.

An Exercise Program for Carpometacarpal Osteoarthritis Based on Biomechanical Principles

Valdes K, von der Heyde R (Hand Works Therapy, Sarasota, FL; Maryville Univ, St Louis, MO)
J Hand Ther 25:251-263, 2012

A review of the literature was performed to design a hand exercise regimen based on biomechanical principles of the carpometacarpal (CMC) joint and the forces that act upon the joint. Sixteen biomechanical studies were included in the review: four studies developed a mathematical model of the thumb and 12 performed cadaveric dissections to study the CMC joint. Clinical application of the biomechanical findings from the studies was synthesized into specific recommendations for a hand exercise program to preserve CMC joint range of motion and increase the strength of the stabilizing muscles of the thumb. The exercise regimen was developed in accordance with recommendations of the American College of Sports

TABLE 1.—Causes of CMC Instability

Author, Year	Theory	Consequence
Ligamentous Laxity theory		
Imaeda et al. (1999)[16]	Changes in length of the anterior oblique ligament and the ulnar collateral ligament	Small changes in ligament length affect thumb stability and alter the path of circumduction
Moulton et al. (2001)[17]	The beak ligament becomes lax, OA initially occurs in the palmar compartment, directly adjacent to the beak ligament insertion where the joint surfaces of the first metacarpal and trapezium primarily contact each other during functional activities	OA then progresses along the joint in a dorsoradial direction
Bettinger et al. (2000)[15]	The dorsoradial ligament primarily affords CMC joint stability. If this ligament should fail, the primary and preceding site for degeneration is the dorsoradial aspect of the trapezium	As the deterioration progresses within the first CMC joint, the volar region will become affected
Joint Impingement theory		
Ateshian et al. (1995)[18]	Excessive contact occurs on the volareulnar and dorsaleradial regions of the trapezium during lateral pinch in the presence of metacarpal pronation	
Koff et al. (2003)[19]	Found cartilage wear patterns occur on both the volareulnar and dorsaleradial quadrants of the CMC joint during pronation of the metacarpal (lateral pinch)	Considerable wear on articular surface regions identifies as high load bearing supporting the evidence to the theory that abnormally high stresses may initiate or exacerbate OA progression in articular cartilage
Kovler et al. (2004)[12]	The dorsoradial trapezial region was found to be significantly more degenerated than other quadrants in both males and females	CMC OA is likely to be promoted by joint impingement resulting from thumb pronation (lateral pinch)

Editor's Note: Please refer to original journal article for full references.
CMC = carpometacarpal; OA = osteoarthritis.

Medicine guidelines for the development of individualized exercise prescriptions.
Level of Evidence.—4 (Table 1).

▶ This is a must-read article for all practicing hand therapists working with the thumb carpometacarpal (CMC) osteoarthritis (OA) population. The authors have put together one of the most relevant, practical articles in recent journal history. Not only did they fully research and review the cause of CMC instability (Table 1) in 16 studies, but they also applied this to the appropriate use of stretch and exercise for the thumb with degenerative CMC changes. Taking into consideration the causes of thumb CMC instability, the forces acting on the thumb during activity, and the American College of Sports Medicine guidelines for exercise programs, the authors were able to formulate a specific step-by-step exercise program for the client to adhere to. The exercise program is printed as an appendix and is a wonderful adjunct to our therapy treatments. Attention is placed on exercises that strengthen the wrist extensors, thumb abductors, and thumb extensors. Pinch strengthening is only advised for those who do not have advanced OA or thumb instability. Because a large percentage of the patients seen in our clinic have a primary or secondary diagnosis of CMC OA, having access to this research and exercise regime is invaluable.

The authors do note that the efficacy of this CMC exercise program has not yet been established through clinical research. This would be a good future endeavor, although it might be limited by the ability to determine patient adherence to the specifics of the exercise program.

S. J. Clark, OTR/L, CHT

A Prospective, Randomized Comparison of 3 Types of Proximal Interphalangeal Joint Arthroplasty
Daecke W, Kaszap B, Martini AK, et al (Klinikum Frankfurt Hoechst, Germany; Heidelberg Univ Hosp, Germany; Seegarten Clinic Heidelberg, Germany; et al)
J Hand Surg 37A:1770-1779.e3, 2012

Purpose.—For surface replacement arthroplasty in proximal interphalangeal joint osteoarthritis, titanium-polyethylene (TI) and pyrocarbon (PY) implants are frequently used. However, their superiority in comparison to the silicone (SI) spacer has not been established. The purpose of this study was to compare these 3 types of implants with regard to outcome.

Methods.—A prospective, randomized, multicenter trial was performed. A total of 43 patients (62 proximal interphalangeal joints) had surgery in the 3 participating centers, and each patient was randomly allocated to one of the 3 groups (TI, PY, SI). Range of motion (ROM) and strength were measured before surgery; pain and disability self-assessment and radiographic analysis were also completed. The same examination protocol was planned for 3 months, 6 months, and 1, 2, and 3 years after surgery, but some follow-up visits did not take place due to patient death or poor compliance.

Results.—The mean follow-up time at the final follow-up was 35 ± 3 months (range, 30–41 mo). All implant types led to significant pain reduction at rest and at load. Tip pinch strength was slightly improved by all 3 devices at the 3-year follow-up. No significant improvement in ROM for silicone or resurfacing implants was found. However, when comparing the highest ROM values reached after surgery, the resurfacing devices tended to show superior joint motility compared to silicone spacers, albeit only temporarily and not significantly. Sixteen explantations were necessary: 2 of 18 SI (11%), 7 of 26 TI (27%) and 7 of 18 PY (39%) implants had to be removed. An additional 4 secondary surgical procedures were performed in group TI.

Conclusions.—Surface replacement arthroplasty devices showed a tendency for a temporarily superior maximum postoperative ROM, but markedly higher postoperative complication and explantation rates were observed compared to the silicone spacer implantation.

▶ Arthroplasty of the proximal interphalangeal (PIP) joint remains an unsolved problem in hand surgery. Although arthrodesis provides a painless, stable result, many patients are unwilling to sacrifice their remaining motion. Arthroplasty, while preserving motion, is compromised by its higher complication rate and limited lifespan. In an attempt to improve the results of silicone PIP arthroplasty, surface replacement arthroplasty designs have become available in the past decade.

The authors present a prospective, randomized trial comparing the outcomes at 3 years, in patients with osteoarthritis, of silicone and 2 surface replacement prostheses—pyrocarbon and titanium-polyethylene in an attempt to determine whether the newer designs are superior to the silicone design. The study is somewhat limited because of its small sample size and found no significant difference among the 3 prostheses in regard to implant survival, range of motion, pain at rest, or pain with gripping. Of note, though, is the trend toward decreased implant survival in both the titanium and pyrocarbon groups, which may have become significant with a longer follow-up period.

Based on the results of this study, there is no superiority at 3 years to the newer, surface replacement designs. All implants preserved preoperative range of motion and strength while decreasing pain. The risk of failure of the prostheses ranged from 11% for the silicone at 3 years, to 27% for the titanium, and 39% for the pyrocarbon. Patients with osteoarthritis should be educated on potential for limited longevity with any of the PIP arthroplasty options when deciding between treatment options.

F. T. D. Kaplan, MD

Dorsoradial Capsulodesis for Trapeziometacarpal Joint Instability

Rayan G, Do V (INTEGRIS Baptist Med Ctr, Oklahoma City, OK; Univ of Oklahoma Health Sciences Ctr, Oklahoma City)
J Hand Surg 38A:382-387, 2013

We describe an alternative method for treating chronic trapeziometacarpal (TM) joint instability after acute injury or chronic repetitive use of the thumb by performing a dorsoradial capsulodesis procedure. The procedure is done by imbricating the redundant TM joint dorsoradial ligament and capsule after reducing the joint by pronating the thumb. The dorsoradial capsulodesis is a reasonable reconstructive option for chronic TM joint instability and subluxation.

▶ The authors report on a novel method of stabilizing the unstable thumb carpometacarpal (CMC) joint with a capsular plication of the dorsal radial aspect of the trapeziometacarpal joint. It is a simple method of affording stability to the thumb base. The authors offer advice on recommended overlap of the capsule of approximately 1 cm to tension it appropriately and to avoid too tight plication that may limit motion or a "not tight enough" plication that may result in continued instability.

They go on to share 5 case reports as examples. Most fared well. One case, while pain improved, had some degree of persistent pain. Grip and pinch strengths did not improve compared with the contralateral side; however, three cases were treated on the nondominant side.

Overall, I think the technique is creative and I applaud its simplicity. I have concerns regarding efficacy in patients with systemic ligament laxity such as Marfan or Ehler-Danlos syndromes. I also agree that the procedure must include the dorsal-radial ligament (not just the capsule), because this ligament is one of the primary stabilizers of the thumb CMC joint.

It is helpful to have this option when considering techniques to stabilize the thumb base.

M. Rizzo, MD

The Scaphotrapezial Joint After Partial Trapeziectomy for Trapeziometacarpal Joint Arthritis: Long-term Follow-up

Noland SS, Saber S, Endress R, et al (Stanford Univ Hosp, CA)
J Hand Surg 37A:1125-1129, 2012

Purpose.—Partial trapeziectomy addresses trapeziometacarpal (TM) joint arthritis without the risk of destabilizing the scaphotrapezial (ST) joint. However, partial trapeziectomy has been criticized because of concern that ST joint arthritis will develop, requiring additional surgery. We hypothesized that partial trapeziectomy is a durable treatment for TM joint arthritis, even in patients with radiographically abnormal but asymptomatic ST joints.

Methods.—We evaluated 13 patients (16 thumbs) who underwent a partial trapeziectomy between 1995 and 2005. Assessment included grip strength, pinch strength, ST joint direct palpation, and ST joint stress testing. We classified standardized radiographs of the ST joint using a simple scoring system. Subjective data included the Disabilities of the Arm, Shoulder, and Hand questionnaire, a pain scale, and a satisfaction survey.

Results.—The length of follow-up averaged 9 years (range, 5−13 y). No patient had pain at the ST joint with direct palpation or stress testing. Radiographs demonstrated a mean ST joint arthritis score of 1, indicating mild arthritic changes. Mean grip strength was 28 kg on the operated hand and 28 kg on the nonoperated hand. Mean pinch strength was 5 kg on the operated hand and 5 kg on the nonoperated hand. Scores on the pain scale averaged 6 (range, 0−100; 100 = worst). Average Disabilities of the Arm, Shoulder, and Hand score was 11 (range, 0−100; 100 = worst). Of 13 patients, 12 were very satisfied or extremely satisfied, and 1 was not satisfied.

Conclusions.—Partial trapeziectomy for TM joint arthritis provides long-lasting relief of symptoms in patients with radiographically abnormal but clinically insignificant ST joint degeneration. Satisfaction is equivalent to other published series. The radiographic appearance of the ST joint did not correlate with symptoms at this joint. Unless the patient has symptomatic ST joint arthritis, the ST joint may be retained.

Type of Study/Level of Evidence.—Therapeutic IV.

▶ There are several options for the treatment of trapeziometacarpal (TM) joint arthritis, including total trapeziectomy followed by interposition of tendons or artificial materials, partial trapeziectomy arthroscopically and nonarthroscopically with or without interpositional materials, artificial joint replacement, and arthrodesis of the TM joint. Total trapeziectomy is indicated for patients having arthritis involving not only the TM but also scaphotrapezial (ST) joints. Previous investigators have mentioned that patients having TM joint arthritis involving the scaphotrapezoid joint were not relieved from the symptoms even after total trapeziectomy.[1] In addition, total trapeziectomy is often followed by proximal migration of the first metacarpal resulting in swan-neck deformity of the thumb. Partial trapeziectomy is beneficial in terms of less invasiveness and less chance of the proximal migration of the thumb metacarpal. Although it is not clearly understood why removal of the TM joint cartilage can deteriorate pain of the joint, there are several reports of good outcomes after partial trapeziectomy for the treatment of TM joint arthritis.[2,3] Removal of the TM joint cartilage may restrict joint motion, resulting in pain relief of the joint. I am afraid that restricted motion of the TM joint would predispose patients to an increase in the mechanical stress loads of the ST joint, which would help develop and promote ST arthritis. The weakness of this article was the low follow-up rate (only 13 of 47 patients), although the average follow-up length was quite long (average 9 years). The authors should have performed this study on a larger cohort to draw a definitive conclusion that partial trapeziectomy was not followed by the development of significant ST joint degeneration.

R. Kakinoki, MD

References

1. Tomaino MM, Vogt M, Weiser R. Scaphotrapezoid arthritis: prevalence in thumbs undergoing trapezium excision arthroplasty and efficacy of proximal trapezoid excision. *J Hand Surg Am.* 1999;24:1220-1224.
2. Menon J. Arthroscopic management of trapeziometacarpal joint arthritis of the thumb. *Arthroscopy.* 1996;12:581-587.
3. Menon J. Partial trapeziectomy and interpositional arthroplasty for trapeziometacarpal osteoarthritis of the thumb. *J Hand Surg Br.* 1995;20:700-706.

Macroscopic and Microscopic Analysis of the Thumb Carpometacarpal Ligaments: A Cadaveric Study of Ligament Anatomy and Histology

Ladd AL, Lee J, Hagert E (Stanford Univ, CA)
J Bone Joint Surg Am 94:1468-1477, 2012

Background.—Stability and mobility represent the paradoxical demands of the human thumb carpometacarpal joint, yet the structural origin of each functional demand is poorly defined. As many as sixteen and as few as four ligaments have been described as primary stabilizers, but controversy exists as to which ligaments are most important. We hypothesized that a comparative macroscopic and microscopic analysis of the ligaments of the thumb carpometacarpal joint would further define their role in joint stability.

Methods.—Thirty cadaveric hands (ten fresh-frozen and twenty embalmed) from nineteen cadavers (eight female and eleven male; average age at the time of death, seventy-six years) were dissected, and the supporting ligaments of the thumb carpometacarpal joint were identified. Ligament width, length, and thickness were recorded for morphometric analysis and were compared with use of the Student t test. The dorsal and volar ligaments were excised from the fresh-frozen specimens and were stained with use of a triple-staining immunofluorescent technique and underwent semiquantitative analysis of sensory innervation; half of these specimens were additionally analyzed for histomorphometric data. Mixed-effects linear regression was used to estimate differences between ligaments.

Results.—Seven principal ligaments of the thumb carpometacarpal joint were identified: three dorsal deltoid-shaped ligaments (dorsal radial, dorsal central, posterior oblique), two volar ligaments (anterior oblique and ulnar collateral), and two ulnar ligaments (dorsal trapeziometacarpal and intermetacarpal). The dorsal ligaments were significantly thicker ($p < 0.001$) than the volar ligaments, with a significantly greater cellularity and greater sensory innervation compared with the anterior oblique ligament ($p < 0.001$). The anterior oblique ligament was consistently a thin structure with a histologic appearance of capsular tissue with low cellularity.

Conclusions.—The dorsal deltoid ligament complex is uniformly stout and robust; this ligament complex is the thickest morphometrically, has the highest cellularity histologically, and shows the greatest degree of sensory nerve endings. The hypocellular anterior oblique ligament is thin, is variable in its location, and is more structurally consistent with a capsular structure than a proper ligament.

▶ The authors of this article provide a detailed anatomic and histologic overview of the ligamentous anatomy of the thumb carpometacarpal (CMC) joint. They should be commended on their findings and for challenging the controversy that exists regarding primary thumb trapeziometacarpal stabilizers.

Seven principal ligaments of the thumb were consistently identified, including 2 volar ligaments (anterior oblique and ulnar collateral), 2 ulnar ligaments (dorsal trapeziometacarpal and intermetacarpal), and 3 dorsal ligaments (dorsal radial, posterior oblique, and dorsal central). The authors draw attention to the fact that the dorsal central ligament has not been previously described, and this was found to be the shortest and stoutest ligament stabilizing the thumb CMC joint. In keeping with the findings of others,[1] they note the importance of the dorsal radial ligamentous complex to CMC stability. Interestingly, the anterior oblique ligament was found to be a thin thickening of the volar capsule rather than a true ligament affording static joint stability.

Using histologic and immunofluorescent staining techniques, the authors noted that the dorsal ligaments had a more organized collagen fiber orientation, greater cellularity, and distribution of nerve endings compared with the volar ligaments. A greater number of mechanoreceptors and nerve fibers were found in the ligament epifascicular layers and at the ligament insertion site, thereby providing a target for possible denervation procedures of the thumb CMC joint.

As reported by the authors, there are a few methodological concerns with the study. The average age range of the cadavers was from 43 to 99 years. Although the authors excluded joints with "global eburnation and joint dysmorphology," the quality of the ligaments examined may have already undergone degeneration, given the age of the cadavers. This is especially poignant with respect to measures of cellularity and collagen orientation. This was recognized by the authors, in addition to the higher number of male vs female donors. The functionality of the ligaments was primarily assessed by nonstandardized biomechanical tests within embalmed cadavers.

Despite these limitations, I believe the authors should be congratulated on their macro- and microscopic study of thumb CMC joint ligament anatomy. They have described the importance of the dorsal central ligament and the varied distribution of mechanoreceptors within the CMC ligamentous complex, thereby paving the way for further studies, for example, in the development of improved denervation procedures for basilar thumb joint pathology.

M. Rizzo, MD

Reference

1. Bettinger PC, Linscheid RL, Berger RA, Cooney WP 3rd, An KN. An anatomic study of the stabilizing ligaments of the trapezium and trapeziometacarpal joint. *J Hand Surg Am.* 1999;24:786-798.

A Prospective, Randomized Comparison of 3 Types of Proximal Interphalangeal Joint Arthroplasty

Daecke W, Kaszap B, Martini AK, et al (Klinikum Frankfurt Hoechst, Hessen, Germany; Heidelberg Univ Hosp, Germany; Seegarten Clinic Heidelberg, Germany; et al)
J Hand Surg 37A:1770-1779.e3, 2012

Purpose.—For surface replacement arthroplasty in proximal interphalangeal joint osteoarthritis, titanium-polyethylene (TI) and pyrocarbon (PY) implants are frequently used. However, their superiority in comparison to the silicone (SI) spacer has not been established. The purpose of this study was to compare these 3 types of implants with regard to outcome.

Methods.—A prospective, randomized, multicenter trial was performed. A total of 43 patients (62 proximal interphalangeal joints) had surgery in the 3 participating centers, and each patient was randomly allocated to one of the 3 groups (TI, PY, SI). Range of motion (ROM) and strength were measured before surgery; pain and disability self-assessment and radiographic analysis were also completed. The same examination protocol was planned for 3 months, 6 months, and 1, 2, and 3 years after surgery, but some follow-up visits did not take place due to patient death or poor compliance.

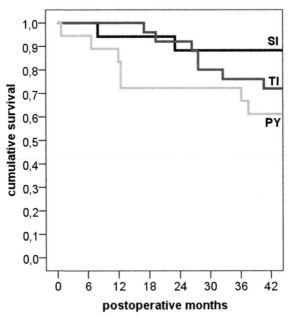

FIGURE 8.—Kaplan-Meyer curves of implant survival. Each explantation is indicated by one step fall of the relevant curve. The fourth steps of PY and TI indicate double explantations. (Reprinted from The Journal of Hand Surgery. Daecke W, Kaszap B, Martini AK, et al. A prospective, randomized comparison of 3 types of proximal interphalangeal joint arthroplasty. *J Hand Surg.* 2012;37A:1770-1779.e3, Copyright 2012, with permission from the American Society for Surgery of the Hand.)

Results.—The mean follow-up time at the final follow-up was 35 ± 3 months (range, 30—41 mo). All implant types led to significant pain reduction at rest and at load. Tip pinch strength was slightly improved by all 3 devices at the 3-year follow-up. No significant improvement in ROM for silicone or resurfacing implants was found. However, when comparing the highest ROM values reached after surgery, the resurfacing devices tended to show superior joint motility compared to silicone spacers, albeit only temporarily and not significantly. Sixteen explantations were necessary: 2 of 18 SI (11%), 7 of 26 TI (27%) and 7 of 18 PY (39%) implants had to be removed. An additional 4 secondary surgical procedures were performed in group TI.

Conclusions.—Surface replacement arthroplasty devices showed a tendency for a temporarily superior maximum postoperative ROM, but markedly higher postoperative complication and explantation rates were observed compared to the silicone spacer implantation (Fig 8).

▶ This is an excellent prospective, randomized study with postoperative evaluations by independent examiners (although it's not clear from the article if these evaluators were blinded). Not many studies can live up to these strict standards, so this is definitely an article worth reading.

As for the results, there are a few significant things to note. Pyrocarbon surface replacement arthroplasties were significantly more disabled than silicone arthroplasties. There was no difference in pain at rest or with motion among the 3 groups. However, there was significantly less pain with activity in silicone implants than in titanium surface replacement. There was no improvement in pinch in any group or between groups. There was a significantly higher complication rate and explantation rate with surface replacement arthroplasties (Fig 8) These findings need to be examined carefully but tend to suggest few benefits of surface replacement arthroplasty over silicone, whereas silicone may have some advantages.

My only criticism of the study is that the authors choose to include the following in the abstract and conclusions: "The resurfacing devices tended to show superior joint mobility compared to silicone spacers, albeit only temporarily and not significantly." The authors seem to be stretching to find an advantage of surface replacement over silicone when none seems to exist. There is never a statistically significant finding showing surface replacement to be superior to silicone, and even the trending data fade with follow-up. This seems to demonstrate a bias of the authors for surface replacement.

This article shows, in a well-designed study, that with primary osteoarthritis, silicone arthroplasty may be superior to surface replacement arthroplasty in some respects with a lower level of complications and explantation.

T. Hughes, MD

Influence of Index Finger Proximal Interphalangeal Joint Arthrodesis on Precision Pinch Kinematics

Domalain M, Evans PJ, Seitz WH Jr, et al (Cleveland Clinic, OH)
J Hand Surg 36A:1944-1949, 2011

Purpose.—To evaluate the impact of proximal interphalangeal (PIP) joint arthrodesis on the kinematics of precision pinch.

Methods.—Eleven healthy subjects performed index finger—thumb pinch motions under 4 conditions: unrestricted thumb and index finger (CONTROL) and fusion of the PIP joint of the index finger in flexion of 30° (PIP30), 40° (PIP40), and 50° (PIP50). Fusion was simulated with metallic splints. Kinematics of the thumb and index finger were recorded with a motion capture system.

Results.—Proximal interphalangeal joint fusion at 30°, 40°, and 50° restricted maximal pinch span between the thumb tip and index finger tip by 6%, 10%, and 14%, respectively. At the time of pulp contact, PIP fusion led to an increase in index metacarpophalangeal joint flexion angle for the PIP30 condition and an increase in variability of thumb tip location for the PIP50 condition. Furthermore, the dynamic coordination between joint angles throughout the movement was affected by PIP fusion.

Conclusions.—This study reports impairment in the kinematics of precision pinch associated with index finger PIP joint fusion. A PIP joint fusion at 40° to 50° leads to a more natural precision pinch posture, but it restricts the aperture and reduces pinch precision.

▶ Clinically, loss of full proximal interphalangeal (PIP) joint motion is quite frequent, and these patients usually have compensatory hyperextension of the distal interphalangeal joint when making a pinch, and pinch power is often decreased. This is a report based on measurements using healthy individuals. The findings validate a general impression of clinicians that the maximal pinch span is decreased by loss of PIP joint motion. The analytic approaches in this report are complex and may not be understood by most practitioners. The pinch investigated by the authors should be tip pinch, rather than key pinch (lateral pinch). The hands examined in this study are healthy, and the functionality of the intrinsic muscles is normal as well. This is in contrast to the usually weaker power of intrinsic muscles that develops with joint problems of the hand in symptomatic patients. Clinically, pinch power can be affected by losses of both finger joint motion and muscle power. Loss of PIP joint motion is usually accompanied by losses of both grip and pinch power.

The authors suggest that PIP joint fusion at 40° to 50° maximizes the natural precision pinch posture. However, fusion is a last resort for the PIP joint problem. Currently, PIP joint arthrosplasty (by means of pyrocarbon implant, silicone implant, surface replacement, or hemihamate arthroplasty) has been a more sensible choice before proceeding to arthrodesis. As for PIP joint arthrodesis, my experience indicates that it provides reliable pain relief and reasonably good functionality of the hand. As shown in the data of this report, the loss of the pinch span after PIP joint fusion is actually not large (6%, 10%, and 14%, after fusion of the joint at 30°, 40°, and 50°, respectively). Interpreted in another way, the results show that PIP joint arthrodesis still maintains a reasonably large pinch span and are in agreement with what we see clinically with PIP joint fusion.

The findings of this study provide information helpful in deciding the functional position of the PIP joint arthrodesis. Functional pinch may remain after PIP joint arthrodesis if the position of fusion is carefully planned. Judging by the patients I have seen, recovery of pinch and grip strength after PIP fusion can be expected, and hand function is acceptable when the PIP joint requires an arthrodesis and the surgery keeps the PIP joint moderately flexed (40°—50°) with consideration of finger flexion cascade.

J. B. Tang, MD

Promising one- to six-year results with the Motec wrist arthroplasty in patients with post-traumatic osteoarthritis
Reigstad O, Lütken T, Grimsgaard C, et al (OUS-Rikshospitalet, Oslo, Norway)
J Bone Joint Surg Br 94:1540-1545, 2012

The Motec cementless modular metal-on-metal ball-and-socket wrist arthroplasty was implanted in 16 wrists with scaphoid nonunion advanced collapse (SNAC; grades 3 or 4) and 14 wrists with scapholunate advanced collapse (SLAC) in 30 patients (20 men) with severe (grades 3 or 4) post-traumatic osteoarthritis of the wrist. The mean age of the patients was 52 years (31 to 71). All prostheses integrated well radiologically. At a mean follow-up of 3.2 years (1.1 to 6.1) no luxation or implant breakage occurred. Two wrists were converted to an arthrodesis for persistent pain. Loosening occurred in one further wrist at five years post-operatively. The remainder demonstrated close bone—implant contact. The clinical results were good, with markedly decreased Disabilities of the Arm Shoulder and Hand (DASH) and pain scores, and increased movement and grip strength. No patient used analgesics and most had returned to work.

Good short-term function was achieved using this wrist arthroplasty in a high-demand group of patients with post-traumatic osteoarthritis.

▶ The authors reviewed their experience with the Motec (cementless ball and socket) total wrist arthroplasty. Sixteen wrists were treated and followed for a mean 3.2 years. All were nonrheumatoid (14 scapholunate advanced collapse and 2 scaphoid nonunion advanced collapse).

The Motec is a cementless design with threaded stems that effectively join the radius and third metacarpal. Secondary bony ingrowth is afforded with a hydroxy-apatite or Bonit coating. The hope is that (especially distally) a 1 bone capitate-third metacarpal can be achieved and provide longer survivorship. The ball-socket articulation allows for a maximum degree of freedom and movement.

The results demonstrated good overall pain relief. Range of motion improved and was maintained over 5 years postoperatively. Although better in years 2 and 3 following surgery, grip strength did not significantly improve at the most recent measurement (5 years). The Disabilities of the Arm, Shoulder, and Hand scores were improved. Reoperations included 2 for persistent pain despite well-fixed implant (1 of which was infected) that were revised to fusion. Five additional surgeries were performed secondary to painful distal radioulnar joints: One underwent a Darrach, and the others underwent partial ulnar head resection to alleviate impingement. One patient had loosening at 4 to 5 years postoperatively, with minor symptoms and no further intervention to date. Focal osteolysis of the radius was seen in 3 cases, and distally periprosthetic lucent lines appeared in 2 wrists. All are clinically irrelevant to date. Estimated survivorship at 6 years was 93.3%.

The authors shared their experience with the Motec total wrist arthroplasty from nonrheumatoid reconstruction. Overall, the follow-up was brief, but their results are encouraging. These patients tend to be higher demand than those with rheumatoid arthritis. Good clinical results were achieved. Longer-term follow-up will better validate this implant both radiographically and clinically.

M. Rizzo, MD

Macroscopic and Microscopic Analysis of the Thumb Carpometacarpal Ligaments: A Cadaveric Study of Ligament Anatomy and Histology
Ladd AL, Lee J, Hagert E (Stanford Univ, CA)
J Bone Joint Surg Am 94:1468-1477, 2012

Background.—Stability and mobility represent the paradoxical demands of the human thumb carpometacarpal joint, yet the structural origin of each functional demand is poorly defined. As many as sixteen and as few as four ligaments have been described as primary stabilizers, but controversy exists as to which ligaments are most important. We hypothesized that a comparative macroscopic and microscopic analysis of the ligaments of the thumb carpometacarpal joint would further define their role in joint stability.

Methods.—Thirty cadaveric hands (ten fresh-frozen and twenty embalmed) from nineteen cadavers (eight female and eleven male; average age at the time of death, seventy-six years) were dissected, and the supporting ligaments of the thumb carpometacarpal joint were identified. Ligament width, length, and thickness were recorded for morphometric analysis and were compared with use of the Student t test. The dorsal and volar ligaments were excised from the freshfrozen specimens and were stained with use of a triple-staining immunofluorescent technique and underwent semi-quantitative analysis of sensory innervation; half of these specimens were additionally analyzed for histomorphometric data. Mixed-effects linear regression was used to estimate differences between ligaments.

Results.—Seven principal ligaments of the thumb carpometacarpal joint were identified: three dorsal deltoid-shaped ligaments (dorsal radial, dorsal central, posterior oblique), two volar ligaments (anterior oblique and ulnar collateral), and two ulnar ligaments (dorsal trapeziometacarpal and intermetacarpal). The dorsal ligaments were significantly thicker ($p < 0.001$) than the volar ligaments, with a significantly greater cellularity and greater sensory innervation compared with the anterior oblique ligament ($p < 0.001$). The anterior oblique ligament was consistently a thin structure with a histologic appearance of capsular tissue with low cellularity.

Conclusions.—The dorsal deltoid ligament complex is uniformly stout and robust; this ligament complex is the thickest morphometrically, has the highest cellularity histologically, and shows the greatest degree of sensory nerve endings. The hypocellular anterior oblique ligament is thin, is variable in its location, and is more structurally consistent with a capsular structure than a proper ligament.

Clinical Relevance.—Delineation of the structural and microscopic anatomy of the ligaments of the thumb carpometacarpal joint provides further evidence regarding the stability and mobility of this joint that is often affected by osteoarthritis.

▶ This anatomical study of 30 cadaveric hands by Ladd et al uses dissection, histology, immunohistology, and immunofluorescent staining to characterize the gross morphology, collagen orientation, cellularity, and innervation of the thumb carpometacarpal ligaments. Contrary to traditional teaching, this study reports that the dorsal ligamentous complex is consistently thicker, has more organized collagen, is more cellular, and possesses more dense innervation than the volar ligamentous complex. The average donor age of 76 prevents definitive inference of clinical implications from these results because the volar incompetency may be the result of age-related changes. However, these results do challenge conventional concepts regarding thumb carpometacarpal (CMC) stability. This well-done anatomical study supports the concept that the dorsal thumb CMC ligaments are more important than the volar oblique ligament. It would be interesting to perform a similar study comparing older donor limbs to younger donor limbs.

D. Zelouf, MD

Arthroscopic Versus Open Distal Clavicle Excision: A Comparative Assessment at Intermediate-Term Follow-up
Robertson WJ, Griffith MH, Carroll K, et al (UT Southwestern Med Ctr at Dallas, TX; Reston Hosp Ctr, VA; Massachusetts General Hosp, Boston)
Am J Sports Med 39:2415-2420, 2011

Background.—While few comparative studies exist, it has been suggested that open distal clavicle excisions (DCEs) provide inferior results when compared with the all-arthroscopic technique.

Purpose.—The purpose of this study was to compare the intermediate-term (5-year follow-up) results of patients undergoing arthroscopic versus open DCE for the treatment of recalcitrant acromioclavicular joint pain.

Study Design.—Cohort study; Level of evidence, 3.

Methods.—All patients who underwent an arthroscopic or open DCE between January 1999 and September 2006 were reviewed. Forty-eight patients (49 shoulders; 32 arthroscopic, 17 open) following DCE without significant glenohumeral pathologic changes were included. The mean follow-up for group I (open) and group II (arthroscopic) was 5.3 years and 4.2 years, respectively. The American Shoulder and Elbow Surgeons (ASES) score, visual analog scale (VAS) pain score, surgical time, and minimum radiographic acromioclavicular joint distance were calculated. Each patient completed a questionnaire assessing their scar satisfaction, percentage of normal shoulder function, and willingness to have the surgery again. Risk factors for poor outcomes were analyzed.

Results.—Arthroscopic patients had significantly less pain ($P = .035$) by VAS (0.61 ± 1.02) compared with open (1.59 ± 2.15) at final follow-up. There was no significant difference between group I and group II with regard to ASES (87.5 ± 17.6 vs 94.6 ± 8.6), percentage of normal shoulder function ($89.7\% \pm 12.5$ vs $92.9\% \pm 8.6$), average operative time (53.1 minutes vs 48 minutes), or radiographic resection distance (12.8 ± 2.1 mm vs 9.5 ± 2.9 mm). In the open group, patients with 16 of 17 shoulders were satisfied with their scar and 100% would do it again. In the arthroscopic group, patients with 31 of 32 shoulders (97%) were both satisfied and would have the surgery again.

Conclusion.—Open and arthroscopic DCE are both effective surgeries to treat recalcitrant acromioclavicular joint pain. At intermediate-term follow-up, they provide similarly good to excellent results with regard to patient satisfaction and shoulder function. Although both are effective treatments, less residual pain was found using the arthroscopic technique.

▶ A single surgeon's distal clavicle excisions with average follow-up of 4 to 5 years were retrospectively reviewed. This was a nonrandomized study in which the patients decided if they had open or arthroscopic distal clavicle excisions.

Appropriate exclusion criteria were used and the glenohumeral joint was examined arthroscopically in both groups. Cost of procedure was not measured.

Both techniques resulted in excellent outcomes with all open and 31 of 32 (97%) arthroscopic patients stating they would undergo the surgery again. American Shoulder and Elbow Surgeons scores were statistically similar, with a trend toward higher scores in the arthroscopic group. Visual analog scale scores were statistically lower in the arthroscopic group, averaging 0.6 compared with 1.6 in the open group.

Although not level 1 evidence, this study demonstrates excellent outcomes in both open and arthroscopic techniques, with a slight edge to the arthroscopic intervention.

R. F. Papandrea, MD

2 Wrist Arthroscopy

An All-Inside Technique for Arthroscopic Suturing of the Volar Scapholunate Ligament

del Piñal F, Studer A, Thams C, et al (Private Practice and Hosp Mutua Montañesa, Santander, Spain)
J Hand Surg 36A:2044-2046, 2011

Repair of the volar scapholunate ligament has not been performed arthroscopically. We present an all-inside technique that presents closure of the anterior scapholunate interval. A Tuohy needle and a resorbable suture are all that is required.

▶ This strictly technique-based presentation is interesting in concept but lacking in clinical relevance. For this technique to have merit, the authors should have developed an argument against focusing on the dorsal portion of the scapholunate ligament in the setting of dissociative carpal instability. Given the inferior role of the volar portion of the scapholunate ligament, I am left to wonder how patients are selected for this procedure. Unfortunately, there is no guiding information as to how the patients presented or what clues may be found from physical examination. Furthermore, the overall value of advanced imaging in characterizing injuries of the scapholunate ligament has been questionable at best, and arthroscopic findings do not always correlate. Because objective postoperative data are noticeably absent in this report, one must question the ultimate impact of this procedure on wrist extension. The technical ability to repair such a precise anatomic structure through a narrow window of safety can only be praised when the clinical decision-making process to undergo such an endeavor is sound and justified. This procedure cannot be endorsed without learning more about the problem it is trying to address and without honest appraisal of the potential consequences of performing a volar-based capsulodesis. This does not appear to be an appropriate technique for the novice wrist arthroscopist.

L. M. Brunton, MD

Prognosis and Prognostic Factors for Patients with Persistent Wrist Pain Who Proceed to Wrist Arthroscopy
Prosser R, Hancock MJ, Nicholson LL, et al (Sydney Hand Therapy and Rehabilitation Centre, Australia; Univ of Sydney, Australia; et al)
J Hand Ther 25:264-270, 2012

Wrist pain is common. People with persistent pain commonly undergo arthroscopic investigation. Little is known about the prognosis or prognostic factors for these patients. The purpose of the study was to evaluate prognosis and prognostic factors for pain and functional disability in patients with persistent wrist pain who proceed to arthroscopic investigation. The study design used was a prospective cohort study. One hundred and five consecutive participants who underwent arthroscopic investigation for undiagnosed wrist pain for at least four-week duration were recruited. Patient-rated wrist and hand evaluation (PRWHE) scores were determined at baseline (before arthroscopy) and one year after arthroscopy. One-year follow-up data were obtained for 97 (92%) of 105 participants. Mean PRWHE total score declined from 49 of 100 (standard deviation [SD] 18.5) at baseline to 26 of 100 (SD 20.4) at one year. Two prognostic factors were identified: baseline PRWHE and duration of symptoms. These factors explained 19% and 5% of the variability in the final PRWHE score, respectively. Results of provocative wrist tests and arthroscopic findings did not significantly contribute to prognosis in this cohort. This study provides the first robust evidence of the prognosis of persistent wrist pain. Participants who underwent arthroscopic investigation for persistent wrist pain improved on average by approximately 50% at one year; however, most continued to have some pain and disability. Duration of pain and PRWHE at baseline explained 24% of the one-year PRWHE score.
Level of Evidence.—Level 2.

▶ This study had a good objective: to find out prognostic indicators for persistent pain and disability in those who underwent a wrist arthroscopy for undiagnosed wrist pain. Unfortunately, although the study was prospective and had more than 100 participants, it was poorly designed.

Inclusion criteria are unclearly defined. Those with a fracture, inflammatory arthropathy, complex regional pain syndrome, or prior surgery were excluded. Apparently, any other patients that failed treatment as defined as a lack of improvement following rest, an orthosis or splint, an exercise program, or soft-tissue massage were candidates for the study.

A high percentage of patients referred for hand surgery after failing conservative treatment were not offered arthroscopy, although this distinction is not explained.

Additionally, prior workup—such as magnetic resonance imaging or steroid shots—is not included in the analysis. Many pathologies were found at surgery, including complete scapholunate tears and triangular fibrocartilage tears. Some patients underwent concomitant ligament reconstruction and/or ulnar shortening.

All of these various surgeries were included in their results for wrist arthroscopy as well as patients who did not undergo specific surgical manipulation.

In summary, all patients with undefined wrist pain of at least a month's duration who ultimately went on to have wrist arthroscopy did improve, though it is not clear why. The authors conclude that the longer the presence of preoperative symptoms and the worse the preoperative patient rated wrist and hand evaluation, the less improvement in pain relief and function is seen postoperatively.

It is hard to see why information gathered from this study will change current management of idiopathic wrist pain.

J. Frankenhoff, MD

Ganglions of the Wrist and Associated Triangular Fibrocartilage Lesions: A Prospective Study in Arthroscopically-treated Patients

Langner I, Krueger PC, Merk HR, et al (Universitymedicine Greifswald, Germany)
J Hand Surg 37A:1561-1567, 2012

Purpose.—Wrist ganglions are the most common soft tissue tumors of the hand and wrist and can occur at any age. Their etiology remains controversial. A high prevalence of associated intrinsic ligamentous lesions has been described. We hypothesized that painful wrist ganglions are an indicator of an underlying joint abnormality, particularly of lesions of the triangular fibrocartilage complex (TFCC). The aim of our study was to prospectively determine the prevalence of associated TFCC lesions in patients with painful wrist ganglions.

Methods.—Forty-six patients (35 women, 11 men; mean age, 36 ± 11 y; range, 18−57 y) with painful wrist ganglions (20 radiopalmar and 26 dorsal) had surgery from January 2008 to June 2010. There were 18 primary and 28 recurrent ganglions. Clinical examinations, pain score evaluations, disabilities in daily life evaluations, plain radiographs, and magnetic resonance imaging were obtained before arthroscopic resection. Concomitant intrinsic lesions of the wrist were assessed with magnetic resonance imaging and re-evaluated by arthroscopy.

Results.—All ganglions were successfully resected. Overall, arthroscopy identified 22 TFCC lesions (48%) and 2 intracarpal ligament lesions. The TFCC perforations were more commonly associated with radiopalmar ganglions with a positive ulnocarpal stress test result and with recurrent radiopalmar ganglions. At 1-year follow-up, all patients were meaningfully improved in terms of pain and disabilities in daily life.

Conclusions.—Arthroscopy allows for the simultaneous treatment of ganglions and other pathologies. Therefore, arthroscopy should be contemplated as the primary treatment option for patients with painful ganglions of the wrist if they are in a radiopalmar location with a positive ulnocarpal stress test and for patients with recurrent radiopalmar ganglions, which are also highly associated with TFCC abnormalities.

Type of Study/Level of Evidence.—Therapeutic IV.

▶ The authors investigate the incidence of wrist ganglia and concurrent lesions of the triangular fibrocartilage complex (TFCC). In 46 patients who were treated for wrist ganglia, 22 demonstrated (asymptomatic) lesions of the TFCC. The authors conclude that arthroscopy should be considered as primary treatment modality for patients with wrist ganglia.

This is a well-designed prospective study that provides data that may be interesting for the treatment of both wrist ganglia and TFCC lesions. The incidence of TFCC lesions in this cohort seems indeed higher than in the average population, although I am not sure whether a correct classification of the lesions as traumatic and degenerative is always possible. It is, however, interesting to notice that, despite treatment of the potentially underlying cause, the recurrence rate of wrist ganglia is similar to previous studies (17%). This makes a true causal relationship between the 2 conditions rather unlikely. The high sensitivity and specificity of preoperative examinations seems worth mentioning and may partially be attributed to the use of 3 Tesla magnetic resonance imaging scans. Personally, I still prefer open surgery to arthroscopic treatment for most cases because I think that a certain amount of scarring occurring after opening of the joint capsule may help reduce recurrence rates at the operative site, and the skin usually heals nicely.

K. Megerle, MD

Sonography-guided Arthroscopy for Wrist Ganglion
Yamamoto M, Kurimoto S, Okui N, et al (Nagoya Univ Graduate School of Medicine, Showa-ku, Japan)
J Hand Surg 37A:1411-1415, 2012

Purpose.—To describe how to combine the complementary features of sonography and arthroscopy to make the arthroscopic resection of wrist ganglions a safer and more reliable surgery.

Methods.—A total of 22 patients with wrist ganglions had sonography-assisted arthroscopic resection. Sonographic visualization of ganglions, adjacent structures (ie, vessels, nerves, and tendons), and the cycling tip of the arthroscopic shaver was assessed. Arthroscopic visualization of the ganglions or ganglion stalk was also assessed. Clinical outcome measures included wrist range of motion, grip strength, and our patient-rated Hand 20 questionnaire.

Results.—Sonographic visualization of the ganglion stalk, adjacent structures, and the cycling tip of the arthroscopic shaver was possible in all 22 cases. However, ganglion stalks were visualized by arthroscopy in only 4 cases. The mean range of motion and grip strength were not significantly changed following surgery. However, the mean Hand 20 score was significantly improved from 17 to 6 at final follow-up. Ganglion recurrence was seen in 2 cases at 6 and 8 months after surgery.

Conclusions.—Sonography-guided wrist arthroscopy provides several advantages for surgeons, including visualization of the ganglions and ganglion stalk, as well as of the arthroscopic shaver and adjacent structures such as nerves, vessels, and tendons to perform surgery safely.

▶ In my experience, the visualization of an actual stalk during arthroscopically assisted resection of dorsal ganglion cysts is an irregular endeavor at best. It seems that redundant dorsal capsular tissues are more frequently encountered and are best treated by aggressive resection with a full-radius resector or shaver of choice. The use of arthroscopy for dorsal ganglion cyst excisions is my preferred approach for its minimally invasive nature and relatively low recurrence rate.

I commend the authors for combining the technologies of arthroscopy and conography in an attempt to achieve better results for their patients. Interestingly, ganglions were located dorsally in 16 patients, volarly in 5 patients, and radially in 1 patient. They concluded that the use of sonography may decrease the risk of injury to nerves, vessels, and tendons. However, 2 recurrences were noted in their cohort of 22 patients, which does not represent an improvement over recurrence rates seen in previously reported series. With a relatively small patient cohort and the lack of a control group, it may be difficult to reach definitive conclusions regarding the efficacy and utility of sonography during wrist arthroscopy. Although this article will not necessarily alter my surgical technique or sway me toward use of sonography intraoperatively, it highlights an interesting adjunct that may hold limited appeal, at least for now.

E. Shin, MD

Prognosis and Prognostic Factors for Patients with Persistent Wrist Pain Who Proceed to Wrist Arthroscopy
Prosser R, Hancock MJ, Nicholson LL, et al (Sydney Hand Therapy & Rehabilitation Centre, Sydney, Australia; Univ of Sydney, Australia; et al)
J Hand Ther 25:264-270, 2012

Wrist pain is common. People with persistent pain commonly undergo arthroscopic investigation. Little is known about the prognosis or prognostic factors for these patients. The purpose of the study was to evaluate prognosis and prognostic factors for pain and functional disability in patients with persistent wrist pain who proceed to arthroscopic investigation. The study design used was a prospective cohort study. One hundred and five consecutive participants who underwent arthroscopic investigation for undiagnosed wrist pain for at least four-week duration were recruited. Patient-rated wrist and hand evaluation (PRWHE) scores were determined at baseline (before arthroscopy) and one year after arthroscopy. One-year follow-up data were obtained for 97 (92%) of 105 participants. Mean PRWHE total score declined from 49 of 100 (standard deviation [SD] 18.5) at baseline to 26 of 100 (SD 20.4) at one year. Two prognostic factors were identified: baseline PRWHE and duration of symptoms. These factors

TABLE 3.—PRWHE Data for Participants

PRWHE	Baseline Mean (SD) (n = 105)	One-Year Mean (SD) (n = 97)	Change Mean (SD) (n = 97)
Pain/50	28.0 (9.5)	16.6 (11.9)	−11.4 (11.4)
Function/50	21.1 (10.3)	9.4 (9.5)	−11.7 (10.9)
Total/100	49.1 (18.5)	26.0 (20.4)	−23.1 (20.7)

PRWHE = patient-rated wrist and hand evaluation; SD = standard deviation.

explained 19% and 5% of the variability in the final PRWHE score, respectively. Results of provocative wrist tests and arthroscopic findings did not significantly contribute to prognosis in this cohort. This study provides the first robust evidence of the prognosis of persistent wrist pain. Participants who underwent arthroscopic investigation for persistent wrist pain improved on average by approximately 50% at one year; however, most continued to have some pain and disability. Duration of pain and PRWHE at baseline explained 24% of the one-year PRWHE score.

Level of Evidence.—Level 2 (Table 3).

▶ The authors of this article found that no previous studies have been reported on prognosis of patients who undergo arthroscopy for persistent wrist pain, and they were determined to research this. They carried out a prospective cohort study using a large group of patients that had been studied for an earlier report on diagnostic accuracy of common wrist tests. Each of the 105 participants had a primary complaint of wrist pain longer than 4 weeks in duration that did not respond to conservative management. Baseline prognostic factors evaluated before or during arthroscopic intervention included: duration of symptoms, physical demand of work, the Patient Related Wrist/Hand Evaluation (PRWHE), 6 clinical provocative wrist tests, and 6 arthroscopic findings correlating with the wrist structures clinically tested. The PRWHE was then administered to each participant at 1 year after diagnostic arthroscopy procedure. It is noted that at the time of the arthroscopy, debridement of synovitis, torn ligaments, and/or cartilage was performed at the surgeon's discretion. Those with full ruptures went on to have some type of repair or reconstructive surgery.

The authors were able to obtain 1-year follow-up data from 97 of the 105 participants. Their outcome studies were impressive with pain reduced on average by 11.4 points and disability reduced on average by 11.7 points on the PRWHE (Table 3). Of note, only the duration of symptoms and the baseline PRWHE were significant in predicting the total PRWHE at the 1-year follow-up. None of the clinical tests or arthroscopic findings significantly predicted the PRWHE outcomes.

The most significant result of this study is that those who underwent arthroscopy improved by 50% over the year's time. Thus, the prognosis for patients with persistent wrist pain who undergo arthroscopy is reasonably good. One can now cite this study when guiding patients in selecting treatment options for persistent wrist pain that has not responded to our traditional conservative measures. The authors do note that some participants typically reported continued low levels of pain and disability and that their disability score at the 1-year follow-up improved more that their pain score at 1 year on the PRWHE. Higher levels of pain and disability prior to intervention correlated with higher levels of pain and disability at the 1-year follow-up.

Unfortunately, this study only reviewed participants who underwent arthroscopic intervention and did not have a nonarthroscopy population for comparison. It is possible that time (1 year) was a factor in healing as well as the arthroscopy. The authors do suggest that future studies that include both groups would add to their findings, and I agree.

S. J. Clark, OTR/L, CHT

3   Carpus

Long-term results of dorsal intercarpal ligament capsulodesis for the treatment of chronic scapholunate instability
Megerle K, Bertel D, Germann G, et al (BG Trauma Ctr Ludwigshafen, Germany)
J Bone Joint Surg Br 94-B:1660-1665, 2012

The purpose of this study was to assess the clinical and radiological outcomes of dorsal intercarpal ligament capsulodesis for the treatment of static scapholunate instability at a minimum follow-up of four years. A total of 59 patients who underwent capsulodesis for this condition were included in a retrospective analysis after a mean of 8.25 years (4.3 to 12). A total of eight patients underwent a salvage procedure at a mean of 2.33 years (0.67 to 7.6) and were excluded. The mean range of extension/flexion was 88° (15° to 135°) and of ulnar/radial deviation was 38° (0° to 75°) at final follow-up. The mean Disabilities of the Arm Shoulder and Hand (DASH) score and Mayo wrist scores were 28 (0 to 85) and 61 (0 to 90), respectively. After significant improvement immediately post-operatively ($p < 0.001$ and $p = 0.001$, respectively), the mean scapholunate and radiolunate angles deteriorated to 70° (40° to 90°) and 8° (−15° to 25°), respectively, at final follow-up, which were not significantly different from their pre-operative values ($p = 0.6$ and $p = 0.4$, respectively). The mean carpal height index decreased significantly from 1.53 (1.38 to 1.65) to 1.48 (1.29 to 1.65) indicating progressive carpal collapse ($p < 0.001$); 40 patients (78%) had radiological evidence of degenerative arthritis. Capsulodesis did not maintain carpal reduction over time. Although the consequent ongoing scapholunate instability resulted in early arthritic degeneration, most patients had acceptable long-term function of the wrist.

▶ Regardless of the topic, studies that report the long-term results of treatment for a relatively common condition have tremendous value. The authors provide data on a moderately sized cohort of patients treated by dorsal intercarpal ligament capsulodesis for static but reducible scapholunate instability. This, of course, remains an unsolved problem in hand surgery, with a multitude of procedures described but none that has proven superior in maintaining carpal alignment and preventing the progression of posttraumatic wrist osteoarthrosis. Lending credence to the orthopedic axiom, "we don't treat x-rays, we treat patients," short-term symptom relief and long-term patient satisfaction were paradoxically favorable despite progressive carpal collapse and degenerative changes seen radiographically. Yet again, the contribution of wrist denervation is debatable within this report. All of these procedures raise similar questions for future inquiry: What is the natural course of scapholunate ligament injury? What creates the best substitute for the torn dorsal portion? What constitutes a satisfactory initial reduction of the scapholunate interval? How long should the patient be immobilized after reconstruction? Is there a chance that treatment accelerates osteoarthrosis rather than preventing it? Like many other colleagues, I have attempted many variations on the same theme for treatment of this clinical entity. The seemingly triumphant feat of preliminary reduction and reconstruction has consistently been followed by a steady regression of radiographic findings in virtually every case. Novel techniques will continue to emerge and entice all of us to give each a chance to supplant our current method of choice for scapholunate instability.

L. M. Brunton, MD

Osteotomy of the Radius Without Shortening for Kienböck Disease: A 10-Year Follow-Up
Blanco RH, Blanco FR (Universidad Católica de Córdoba, Argentina)
J Hand Surg 37A:2221-2225, 2012

Purpose.—To determine the long-term effect of distal radius osteotomy without modifying the radial length or inclination for Kienböck disease.

Methods.—Over 9 years, 14 patients underwent osteotomy of the distal radius without altering radial length or inclination. A total of 11 of these patients were available for follow-up after 10 or more years. We assessed pain, range of wrist motion, and grip strength preoperatively and postoperatively in all cases, as well as preoperative and postoperative posteroanterior and lateral x-rays.

Results.—The osteotomy healed in all cases. All 11 patients had decreased pain and showed improvement in wrist motion and grip strength. Radiographically, there were no measurable changes in ulnar variance and there was minimal loss of carpal height. In some patients, the lunate showed increased sclerosis or fragmentation.

Conclusions.—An osteotomy of the distal radius without altering radial length or inclination was effective in decreasing pain and improving grip strength and wrist motion regardless of ulnar variance.

▶ This article is significant for its honesty in looking at distal radius osteotomy with no change in length or inclination. There is a significant question as to the cause of Kienböck's disease and the mechanism of improvement in Kienböck's disease after surgical treatment. Strengths of the study are long-term follow-up of a novel operative intervention for a difficult wrist problem and the novelty of the approach. Weaknesses are that it is a retrospective case review of a small number of patients. No significant controls were used, and the study is largely observational. Additional information that would have made a contribution to the case study would have been to follow each of the cases through to show which Lichtman classification stages progressed and which patients reported significant pain postoperatively. One confounder is that the patients were all immobilized despite plating of what would be a stable osteotomy. They were all immobilized for 4 to 5 weeks. This confounds the results because simple immobilization can be an effective treatment for Kienböck's disease.

The findings of the study are important for future treatment as we try to elucidate both the etiology and pathomechanics of Kienböck's disease and design a treatment that will address the pathology effectively with a positive impact on a patient's function.

In our treatment of Kienböck's disease, we utilize a distal radius osteotomy, as suggested by the author in early-stage disease that has not responded to immobilization. For stage 3B, scaphotrapeziotrapezoid fusion is the preferred treatment. This operative intervention will produce the vascular improvement through response to injury similar to that of distal radius osteotomy but will have the benefit of physically unloading the lunate, which is showing anatomic change. We feel unloading the lunate is an important goal of surgery, as further progression of Kienböck's disease through stage 3B may render the wrist unsalvageable.

D. Mastella, MD

Ulnar-sided Wrist Pain: Evaluation and Treatment of Triangular Fibrocartilage Complex Tears, Ulnocarpal Impaction Syndrome, and Lunotriquetral Ligament Tears
Sachar K (Hand Surgery Associates, Denver, CO)
J Hand Surg 37A:1489-1500, 2012

Ulnar-sided wrist pain is a common cause of upper extremity disability. Presentation can vary from acute traumatic injuries to chronic degenerative conditions. Because of its overlapping anatomy, complex differential diagnosis, and varied treatment outcomes, the ulnar side of the wrist has been referred to as the "black box" of the wrist, and its pathology has been compared with low back pain. Common causes of ulnar-sided wrist pain include triangular fibrocartilaginous complex injuries, lunotriquetrial ligament injuries, and ulnar impaction syndrome.

▶ Ulnar-sided wrist pain is often a black box in hand surgery. Dr Sachar did a great job of trying to give us a glimpse into this complex problem. This is a well-written review article that highlights the issues of lunotriquetral ligament injuries, ulnar impaction, extensor carpi ulnaris pain, and triangular fibrocartilage complex injuries. The author did well by starting off with an excellent review of ulnar-sided anatomy at a level that is not often seen in review articles. He then went through a systematic approach to investigating and diagnosing these oftentimes unclear issues. This article also serves as a nice review of classic articles related to ulnar-sided wrist pain. The author astutely balanced what was pertinent from previous publications, while not allowing the article to get too bogged down by simply recapping previously published works. The level of detail covered in this article for ulnar-sided wrist pain allows this to be a nice go-to review article for all residents, fellows, and practicing physicians. In closing, this is a great review article that is superior to most review articles, especially when considering such a complex issue as ulnar-sided wrist pain.

J. M. Froelich, MD

Idiopathic Multicentric Osteolysis: Upper Extremity Manifestations and Surgical Considerations During Childhood
Goldfarb CA, Steffen JA, Whyte MP (Washington Univ School of Medicine, St Louis, MO; Shriners Hosp for Children, St Louis, MO)
J Hand Surg 37A:1677-1683, 2012

Purpose.—Idiopathic multicentric osteolysis (IMO) is an uncommon disease presenting during childhood with resorption of the carpus and tarsus with nephropathy. The few case reports and literature reviews do not focus on the upper extremity disease manifestations or surgical treatment options. We review our experience with the upper extremity in IMO.

Methods.—We evaluated 8 affected children, specifically assessing early disease manifestations, misdiagnoses, radiographic progression, and surgical treatments rendered.

Results.—Wrist pain and swelling are typically the first manifestations of IMO. Characteristic upper extremity findings, once the disease has progressed, include metacarpophalangeal joint hyperextension, wrist ulnar deviation and flexion, and loss of elbow extension. Radiographically, there is osteolysis of the carpus and proximal metacarpals with resorption of the elbow joint in some patients. Surgical treatments, including soft tissue release with pinning or joint arthrodesis, may offer pain relief and improve alignment, but outcomes are inconsistent.

Conclusions.—Children with IMO are almost always misdiagnosed initially, and the correct diagnosis may be delayed by years. The hand surgeon is ideally suited to provide an accurate diagnosis of IMO, because wrist pain and swelling and thumb interphalangeal joint contracture are common early manifestations.

Type of Study/Level of Evidence.—Prognostic IV.

▶ Goldfarb et al present the largest reported series of patients with idiopathic multicentric osteolysis (IMO). This unusual disease typically includes a triad of carpal destruction, tarsal destruction, and proteinuria. In the 8 patients in this series, most presented with swelling and pain in the wrists and ankles between 6 and 36 months of age. There were an equal number of girls and boys, and all patients had bilateral upper extremity involvement. Over time, patients had loss of wrist motion and ulnar deviation deformity. Many patients also had thumb or digit interphalangeal (IP) joint contractures and metacarpophalangeal (MP) hyperextension.

There was progressive osteolysis of the carpus on serial radiographs, but this was initially difficult to discern because of the cartilaginous nature of the carpus in toddlers. However, the authors noted that, "ossification of the capitate and hamate, typically apparent by age 1 year, did not occur in most patients." Most patients also suffered resorption of the proximal metacarpals. Elbow osteolysis and dislocation occurred at an average age of 7 years. A previously described heterozygous mutation in the *MAFB* gene was identified in all 6 patients who underwent DNA testing.

Although this series is too small to draw any definitive conclusions, MP capsulectomies and IP joint pinning offered some improvement in hand posture in several patients. There is no accepted medical treatment for IMO.

The authors noted that initial misdiagnosis is common, with 7 of 8 patients undergoing treatment for juvenile rheumatoid arthritis before the correct diagnosis was made (after an average delay of 30 months). The constellation of wrist and ankle involvement, thumb IP contracture, MP hyperextension, and wrist flexion and ulnar deviation should raise suspicion of IMO. Although many surgeons may never see a single case of IMO, this case series will help raise awareness of this unusual problem.

C. M. Ward, MD

Functional Outcome of Open Reduction of Chronic Perilunate Injuries
Massoud AHA, Naam NH (Al Azhar Univ, Cairo, Egypt; Southern Illinois Univ and Southern Illinois Hand Ctr, Effingham)
J Hand Surg 37A:1852-1860, 2012

Purpose.—Perilunate injuries are complex and occasionally go unrecognized acutely. Open reduction and internal fixation is a valid treatment option for these injuries. The purpose of this study was to evaluate the functional outcome of treating chronic perilunate injuries with open reduction and internal fixation.

Methods.—Between 1998 and 2007, we treated 24 patients for chronic perilunate injuries. We excluded 5 patients from this study because they underwent proximal row carpectomy or limited wrist arthrodesis. We treated the remaining 19 patients with open reduction and internal fixation. Mean time from injury to surgery was 29 weeks. All patients were men, with a mean age of 27 years. A total of 13 patients had fracture dislocations (group 1); of these, 11 were transscaphoid and 2 were transscaphoid transcapitate fracture dislocations. Six patients had perilunate dislocations (group 2).

Results.—Postoperative follow-up averaged 58 months. All carpal fractures healed at an average of 18 weeks. At final evaluation, the average pain scores during rest, daily activities, and manual work on a 20-point visual analog scale were 0, 2, and 3, respectively, with no significant difference between groups. The active extension and flexion of the wrist averaged 39% and 52% of the uninjured side, respectively. Grip strength averaged 87% of the uninvolved extremity. According to the Mayo wrist scoring system, 58% of all patients (69% of group 1 and 33% of group 2) achieved good to excellent results. A total of 18 patients returned to their original work activities; 14 patients (74%) were very satisfied. No patients required secondary procedures.

Conclusions.—Despite late presentation, patients with chronic perilunate injuries can be treated with open reduction internal fixation, with satisfactory results. Patients with lesser arc injuries have less successful outcome. Patients with irreducible dislocations or major articular damage may require wrist salvage procedures.

▶ Chronic perilunate injuries are not frequent and represent a significant challenge to all who treat wrist and hand injuries. This study, although small, reflects the epidemiology and relative frequency over a 7-year period. The time from injury to fixation at 29 weeks may seem long or may reflect the referral pattern of the authors. Although the study was small and retrospective, the authors offer a reasonable prognosis to those who treat the problems in terms of ultimate outcomes. The results were perhaps better than what one might expect. Motion was diminished, as may be expected. A good return of grip strength was also noted. For the future care of these injuries, the study reflects the efficacy of careful fracture fixation and reconstruction of these badly traumatized wrists. In my practice and for others, this study offers a relative benchmark to consider when providing care to patients with similar problems.

My clinical approach is to carefully consider the plain films and consider a computed tomography scan to look for occult fractures. A closed reduction will follow with consideration of multiple Kirschner wire fixations. If open surgery is necessary, I consider a volar and dorsal approach with ligament reconstruction with suture anchors and multiple Kirschner wire fixations. I will leave wires in place for 3 months and then follow with rehabilitation for 3 to 6 months. I anticipate changes in alignment over time and follow the clinical recovery and return to activity. My experience and outcomes are consistent with reported data.

C. Carroll, MD

The clinical and radiological outcome of pulsed electromagnetic field treatment for acute scaphoid fractures: a randomised double-blind placebo-controlled multicentre trial
Hannemann PFW, Göttgens KWA, van Wely BJ, et al (Maastricht Univ Med Centre, The Netherlands)
J Bone Joint Surg Br 94-B:1403-1408, 2012

The use of pulsed electromagnetic fields (PEMF) to stimulate bone growth has been recommended as an alternative to the surgical treatment of ununited scaphoid fractures, but has never been examined in acute fractures. We hypothesised that the use of PEMF in acute scaphoid fractures would accelerate the time to union by 30% in a randomised, double-blind, placebo-controlled, multicentre trial. A total of 53 patients in three different medical centres with a unilateral undisplaced acute scaphoid fracture were randomly assigned to receive either treatment with PEMF (n = 24) or a placebo (n = 29). The clinical and radiological outcomes were assessed at four, six, nine, 12, 24 and 52 weeks.

A log-rank analysis showed that neither time to clinical and radiological union nor the functional outcome differed significantly between the groups. The clinical assessment of union indicated that at six weeks tenderness in the anatomic snuffbox ($p = 0.03$) as well as tenderness on longitudinal compression of the scaphoid ($p = 0.008$) differed significantly in favour of the placebo group.

We conclude that stimulation of bone growth by PEMF has no additional value in the conservative treatment of acute scaphoid fractures.

▶ This study investigates the influence of pulsed electromagnetic fields (PEMF) on the healing rate of acute scaphoid fractures. The authors conclude that PEMF has no additional value in the treatment of acute scaphoid fractures.

This is a well designed randomized, placebo-controlled, multicenter trial; the use of nonfunctional PEMF devices in the placebo group seems especially remarkable. The authors demonstrate solid evidence in terms of clinical symptoms, range of motion, and grip strength. However, I feel that they should have used additional computed tomography (CT) scans to better characterize the fractures and follow the radiographic course of treatment. Because of its complex 3-dimensional form, the scaphoid is very difficult to assess on plain x-ray studies, and displaced fractures are frequently misjudged. The same is true for the assessment of osseous union, which is one major outcome parameter in the present study. Radiographic changes in the healing scaphoid may be very subtle and even impossible to detect on plain x-ray studies.

Today, conservative treatment of scaphoid fractures is (again) a widely accepted treatment for undisplaced scaphoid fractures and, apparently, is not accelerated by PEMF. However, I still believe that CT scans are mandatory before conservative treatment is initiated to rule out significant rotation or displacement of the 2 fragments.

K. Megerle, MD

Diagnostic accuracy of imaging modalities for suspected scaphoid fractures: meta-analysis combined with latent class analysis
Yin Z-G, Zhang J-B, Kan S-L, et al (Tianjin Orthopaedic Hosp, China)
J Bone Joint Surg Br 94-B:1077-1085, 2012

Follow-up radiographs are usually used as the reference standard for the diagnosis of suspected scaphoid fractures. However, these are prone to errors in interpretation. We performed a meta-analysis of 30 clinical studies on the diagnosis of suspected scaphoid fractures, in which agreement data between any of follow-up radiographs, bone scintigraphy, magnetic resonance (MR) imaging, or CT could be obtained, and combined this with latent class analysis to infer the accuracy of these tests on the diagnosis of suspected scaphoid fractures in the absence of an established standard. The estimated sensitivity and specificity were respectively 91.1% and 99.8% for follow-up radiographs, 97.8% and 93.5% for bone scintigraphy,

97.7% and 99.8% for MRI, and 85.2% and 99.5% for CT. The results were generally robust in multiple sensitivity analyses. There was large between-study heterogeneity for the sensitivity of follow-up radiographs and CT, and imprecision about their sensitivity estimates.

If we acknowledge the lack of a reference standard for diagnosing suspected scaphoid fractures, MRI is the most accurate test; follow-up radiographs and CT may be less sensitive, and bone scintigraphy less specific.

▶ This is a very thorough study using advanced statistical analysis to evaluate previous studies through the use of meta-analysis and latent class analysis. Understanding this article requires a hefty amount of statistics background.

Latent class analysis uses a technique to devise a model to look at multiple variables. It has been defined as follows: It is a finite mixture model used to identify underlying (latent) subgroups within a population based on individuals' responses to multiple observed variables. Factor analysis is based on continuous latent variables, whereas latent class analysis is based on categorical latent variables. This technique is useful in the case of diagnostic modalities for scaphoid fractures because there is no defined standard diagnostic test against which to compare other testing modalities.

Two issues have made the diagnosis of scaphoid fractures difficult to study. The first, mentioned previously, is the lack of a defined standard. Is edema on a magnetic resonance imaging (MRI) a fracture? Is the loss of cortical continuity on one cut of a computed tomography (CT) a fracture? The second issue is the relatively low prevalence of true fractures among suspected fractures. This makes it very difficult to assess the accuracy of diagnostic tests.

This study attempts to overcome these difficulties through the use of latent class analysis. The basic conclusions of the article are that MRI remains the most sensitive and specific test available. Bone scan is also sensitive, but not very specific. CT and follow-up radiographs have specificity about equal to MRI, but not nearly the sensitivity.

I have relied on MRI to be the best test for patients with suspected scaphoid fractures. Patients that present with radial wrist pain and initially negative radiographs are typically placed in a thumb spica splint. If they have significant pain, a cast is placed instead, because it is more comforting. If their pain and tenderness persists for more than a week (which is when I am typically seeing them for the first time, their initial visit usually being in an emergency room or primary care physician's office), then I obtain an MRI. MRI is the most sensitive and specific imaging modality available. It can also point to other etiologies for their pain if fracture is ruled out. I typically use CT scans to evaluate radiograph-diagnosed scaphoid fractures for displacement, scaphoid nonunions for deformity and bone quality, and healing fractures for completeness of healing.

T. Hughes, MD

Interobserver Variability Among Radiologists for Diagnosis of Scaphoid Fractures by Computed Tomography

de Zwart AD, Beeres FJP, Kingma LM, et al (Landsteiner Inst, The Hague; Leiden Univ Med Centre, The Netherlands)
J Hand Surg 37A:2252-2256, 2012

Purpose.—To determine the interobserver variability among radiologists for computed tomography (CT) diagnosis of scaphoid fractures.

Methods.—Four specialized musculoskeletal radiologists evaluated the CT scans of 150 consecutive patients who were clinically suspected of having sustained a scaphoid fracture but whose scaphoid-specific radiographs were normal. The radiologists were asked to determine the presence or absence of a scaphoid fracture and to localize the fracture. Interobserver agreement was calculated using the kappa statistic.

Results.—The radiologists diagnosed between 11 (7%) and 22 (15%) scaphoid fractures; the kappa value was 0.51.

Conclusion.—Agreement on the presence of a scaphoid fracture and its location on a CT scan was moderate among the 4 radiologists. This finding raises the question as to whether scaphoid fractures could be under- or over-diagnosed in daily practice when CT is used to exclude or confirm a fracture. This should be kept in mind when interpreting clinical and radiological results in patients with suspected scaphoid fractures.

▶ All surgeons who see patients with hand and wrist injuries are familiar with the problem of the rule out scaphoid fracture. Up to 20% of scaphoid fractures may not be evident on plain radiographs. A number of studies have evaluated computed tomography (CT) as a superior diagnostic test in this situation.[1-6] There has been enthusiasm in practice and in the literature for the use of CT scans to avoid delays, unnecessary immobilization, and the additional cost of other imaging modalities, such as magnetic resonance imaging (MRI). This study evaluated 150 consecutive patients who had CT scans, and the scans were interpreted by 4 radiologists. In this study, there was disagreement as to the presence of a scaphoid fracture in half of the patients in which a fracture was seen on a CT scan. Although this study used one CT scan protocol and other studies reporting superior agreement have used thinner slice reformations, most surgeons lack control over the protocols used on a large percentage of their patients. The reader has to conclude that CT scans in practice may have higher false-positive and false-negative results than expected from reading the literature. There are clear drawbacks to all of the modalities proposed for this situation; at this time, there is no clear evidence-based algorithm that is definitively superior. Currently when I am faced with this scenario, I immobilize patients in a short arm cast and have them return for new scaphoid x-rays at 2 to 3 weeks. If the x-rays are negative, but the exam still shows tenderness at the scaphoid, I will obtain an MRI scan.

P. Blazar, MD

References

1. Ty JM, Lozano-Calderon S, Ring D. Computed tomography for triage of suspected scaphoid fractures. *Hand (N Y)*. 2008;3:155-158.
2. Adey L, Souer JS, Lozano-Calderon S, Palmer W, Lee SG, Ring D. Computed tomography of suspected scaphoid fractures. *J Hand Surg Am*. 2007;32:61-66.
3. Roolker W, Tiel-van Buul MM, Ritt MJ, Verbeeten B Jr, Griffioen FM, Broekhuizen AH. Experimental evaluation of scaphoid X-series, carpal box radiographs, planar tomography, computed tomography, and magnetic resonance imaging in the diagnosis of scaphoid fracture. *J Trauma*. 1997;42:247-253.
4. Memarsadeghi M, Breitenseher MJ, Schaefer-Prokop C, et al. Occult scaphoid fractures: comparison of multidetector CT and MR imaging—initial experience. *Radiology*. 2006;240:169-176.
5. Cruickshank J, Meakin A, Breadmore R, et al. Early computerized tomography accurately determines the presence or absence of scaphoid and other fractures. *Emerg Med Australas*. 2007;19:223-228. Erratum in: *Emerg Med Australas*. 2007 Aug;19(4):387.

Volar Fixed-Angle Plating of Distal Radius Fractures: Screws Versus Pegs—A Biomechanical Study in a Cadaveric Model

Mehling I, Klitscher D, Mehling AP, et al (Univ Med Ctr of the Johannes Gutenberg-Univ of Mainz, Germany; BG Unfallklinik, Frankfurt am Main, Germany)

J Orthop Trauma 26:395-401, 2012

Objectives.—The purpose of this biomechanical study was to determine whether a multidirectional fixed-angle plate with locking screws or with locking pegs in the distal fragment would optimize fixation of Orthopaedic Trauma Association (OTA) type A3 distal radius fractures.

Methods.—Eight pairs of fresh—frozen human distal radii were used. Extra-articular distal radius fractures were created and stabilized with a multidirectional volar fixed-angle plate. The radii were randomized into 2 matched-paired groups. The distal fragment in Group I was stabilized with 7 locking screws. The distal fragment in Group II was fixed with 7 locking pegs. The proximal fragment in both groups was fixed with 3 screws. The specimens were tested under torsion and axial compression during static and cyclic tests. Finally, load-to-failure tests were performed under torsion.

Results.—After 1000 cycles, 99% of the median torsional stiffness remained in the group using screws, whereas only 76% of the median stiffness under torsion remained in the group using pegs ($P = 0.018$). Under axial compression, median stiffness remained at 93% in the group using screws after 1000 cycles compared with a median of 0% in the group using pegs ($P = 0.018$).

Conclusions.—This biomechanical study showed a statistically significant difference between the locking screw and locking smooth peg configuration with regard to stiffness of the constructs after 1000 cycles. The use of locking screws as opposed to smooth locking pegs for OTA type A3 extra-articular distal radius fractures optimizes construct stability.

▶ The authors compare smooth peg and screw fixation in locked volar plating for Orthopaedic Trauma Association (OTA) type A3 fractures. They clearly show that screw fixation was superior to smooth peg fixation when the construct was exposed to torque and axial load. This was a well-executed and designed study, and the results are clear. The results have clinical importance for those who operatively fix these fractures. Screws can be more difficult to use in osteopenic or comminuted bone. Having said that, the hand surgeon treating distal radius fractures with volar fixed angled plating has to be cognizant of tendon issues and potential rupture of dorsal tendons if the screws are prominent dorsally or along the radial styloid. Careful plate placement has great importance now and in the future when using threaded screws instead of smooth pegs. Judicious use of locked threaded screws appears to allow for a more stable construct, but further clinical study is indicated to compare these cadaver studies with patient outcomes.

C. Carroll, MD

Predictors of fracture following suspected injury to the scaphoid
Duckworth AD, Buijze GA, Moran M, et al (Royal Infirmary of Edinburgh, UK)
J Bone Joint Surg Br 94-B:961-968, 2012

A prospective study was performed to develop a clinical prediction rule that incorporated demographic and clinical factors predictive of a fracture of the scaphoid. Of 260 consecutive patients with a clinically suspected or radiologically confirmed scaphoid fracture, 223 returned for evaluation two weeks after injury and formed the basis of our analysis. Patients were evaluated within 72 hours of injury and at approximately two and six weeks after injury using clinical assessment and standard radiographs. Demographic data and the results of seven specific tests in the clinical examination were recorded.

There were 116 (52%) men and their mean age was 33 years (13 to 95; SD 17.9). In 62 patients (28%) a scaphoid fracture was confirmed. A logistic regression model identified male gender ($p = 0.002$), sports injury ($p = 0.004$), anatomical snuff box pain on ulnar deviation of the wrist within 72 hours of injury ($p < 0.001$), and scaphoid tubercle tenderness at two weeks ($p < 0.001$) as independent predictors of fracture. All patients with no pain at the anatomical snuff box on ulnar deviation of the wrist within 72 hours of injury did not have a fracture (n = 72, 32%). With four independently significant factors positive, the risk of fracture was 91%.

Our study has demonstrated that clinical prediction rules have a considerable influence on the probability of a suspected scaphoid fracture. This will help improve the use of supplementary investigations where the diagnosis remains in doubt.

▶ The diagnosis of a scaphoid fracture can be difficult, but failure to make such a diagnosis can lead to stiffness, pain, loss of function secondary to nonunion, and collapse. This study looked at a prospective series of patients with wrist trauma and looked at 7 factors related to physical examination. They noted males with sports injuries were at greatest risk for a scaphoid fracture. Anatomic snuff box pain with the wrist pronated and scaphoid tubercle tenderness were key factors to consider when diagnosing an occult scaphoid fracture within the first week after injury. The presence of 4 clinical factors led to a greater than 90% predictive chance for the fracture to be identified. The article has well-considered statistical analyses and has great significance for all who treat wrist injuries. The observations ring true for any population. The strength of a clinical examination can be very helpful given the limited access to and cost for advanced studies. As more midlevel providers assess these injuries, these clinical guidelines will be useful to ensure proper evaluation and referral in a cost-sensitive world.

C. Carroll, MD

The Effect of the Dorsal Intercarpal Ligament on Lunate Extension After Distal Scaphoid Excision

Kamal RN, Chehata A, Rainbow MJ, et al (The Warren Alpert Med School of Brown Univ and Rhode Island Hosp, Providence; Western General Hosp, Victoria, Australia; Universitat de Barcelona, Spain; et al)
J Hand Surg 37A:2240-2245, 2012

Purpose.—After a distal scaphoid excision, most wrists develop a mild form of carpal instability—nondissociative with dorsal intercalated segment instability. Substantial dysfunctional malalignment is only occasionally seen. We hypothesized that distal scaphoid excision would lead to carpal instability—nondissociative with dorsal intercalated segment instability in cadavers and that the dorsal intercarpal (DIC) ligament plays a role in preventing such complications.

Methods.—We used 10 cadaver upper extremities in this experiment. A customized jig was used to load the wrist with 98 N. Motion of the capitate and lunate was monitored using the Fastrak motion tracking system. Five specimens had a distal scaphoid excision first, followed by excision of the DIC ligament, whereas the other 5 specimens first had excision of the DIC ligament and then had a distal scaphoid excision. Rotation of the lunate and capitate was calculated as a sum of the relative motions between each intervention and was compared with its original location before intervention (control) for statistical analysis.

Results.—Distal scaphoid excision and subsequent DIC ligament excision both led to significant lunate extension. DIC ligament excision alone resulted in lunate flexion that was not statistically significant. After DIC ligament excision, distal scaphoid excision led to significant lunate extension.

Capitate rotation was minimal in both groups, verifying that the overall wrist position did not change with loading.

Conclusions.—Distal scaphoid excision leads to significant lunate extension through an imbalance in the force couple between the scaphotrapezio-trapezoidal joint and the triquetrum-hamate joint. The DIC ligament may serve as a secondary stabilizer to the lunocapitate joint and prevent further lunate extension with the wrist in neutral position.

Clinical Relevance.—The development of a clinically symptomatic carpal instability—nondissociative with dorsal intercalated segment instability with lunocapitate subluxation after distal scaphoid excision may be due to an incompetent DIC ligament.

▶ This cadaveric study analyzed the relative roles of the distal scaphoid and dorsal intercarpal (DIC) ligament in wrist biomechanics. The authors demonstrated that excision of the distal scaphoid in a loaded wrist resulted in lunate extension and ensuing dorsal intercalated segmental instability (DISI) deformity. This was accentuated if the DIC ligament was also transected. Transection of the DIC alone, however, did not result in a discernable instability pattern. The study concluded that the DIC ligament may be an important secondary stabilizer following distal scaphoid excision.

The presented results have significant clinical implications: Distal scaphoid excision has been gaining in popularity both in the treatment of scaphotrapezio-trapezoidal arthritis and for distal scaphoid nonunions. It is currently unknown whether cases of symptomatic DISI after distal scaphoid excision are directly related to incompetence of the DIC. This study seems to indicate, however, that dorsal ligamentous structures should be spared when performing distal scaphoid excisions. Thus, surgeons should approach these procedures through a volar approach whenever possible.

T. D. Rozental, MD

Functional Outcome of Open Reduction of Chronic Perilunate Injuries

Massoud AHA, Naam NH (Al Azhar Univ, Cairo, Egypt; Southern Illinois Univ and Southern Illinois Hand Ctr, Effingham)
J Hand Surg 37A:1852-1860, 2012

Purpose.—Perilunate injuries are complex and occasionally go unrecognized acutely. Open reduction and internal fixation is a valid treatment option for these injuries. The purpose of this study was to evaluate the functional outcome of treating chronic perilunate injuries with open reduction and internal fixation.

Methods.—Between 1998 and 2007, we treated 24 patients for chronic perilunate injuries. We excluded 5 patients from this study because they underwent proximal row carpectomy or limited wrist arthrodesis. We treated the remaining 19 patients with open reduction and internal fixation. Mean time from injury to surgery was 29 weeks. All patients were men, with a mean age of 27 years. A total of 13 patients had fracture dislocations (group 1); of these, 11 were transscaphoid and 2 were transscaphoid transcapitate fracture dislocations. Six patients had perilunate dislocations (group 2).

Results.—Postoperative follow-up averaged 58 months. All carpal fractures healed at an average of 18 weeks. At final evaluation, the average pain scores during rest, daily activities, and manual work on a 20-point visual analog scale were 0, 2, and 3, respectively, with no significant difference between groups. The active extension and flexion of the wrist averaged 39% and 52% of the uninjured side, respectively. Grip strength averaged 87% of the uninvolved extremity. According to the Mayo wrist scoring system, 58% of all patients (69% of group 1 and 33% of group 2) achieved good to excellent results. A total of 18 patients returned to their original work activities; 14 patients (74%) were very satisfied. No patients required secondary procedures.

Conclusions.—Despite late presentation, patients with chronic perilunate injuries can be treated with open reduction internal fixation, with satisfactory results. Patients with lesser arc injuries have less successful outcome. Patients with irreducible dislocations or major articular damage may require wrist salvage procedures.

▶ These authors present a retrospective analysis of a relatively large number of patients treated for the somewhat rare presentation of a missed perilunate injury. This is certainly one of the largest case series reported in which patients were treated primarily and preferentially with open reduction and internal fixation (ORIF) if possible (as opposed to proximal row carpectomy [PRC] or other salvage procedures). Overall, it does help guide treatment decisions and prognosis estimation for a challenging problem. They confirm that even chronic perilunate injuries (up to 9 months after injury) are indeed surgically reducible, and that articular surfaces are usually still acceptable for ORIF (only 5 of 24 patients were irreducible or not amenable to ORIF because of chondral lesions).

The outcomes of the patients who underwent ORIF are generally comparable with the outcomes of patients who underwent a primary salvage procedure such as PRC (as sited in this article, and compared with other historical studies evaluating PRC performed for other pathologies).[1-3] This study clearly supports treatment of chronic perilunate dislocations with attempted ORIF instead of proceeding directly to a salvage procedure. The duration of follow-up was decent (average 5 years), but the need for future salvage surgeries in the longer term for this young and active patient population is yet to be determined. After ORIF, however, few bridges are burned, and several options for salvage in the future remain viable.

R. C. Chadderdon, MD

References

1. DiDonna ML, Kiefhaber TR, Stern PJ. Proximal row carpectomy: study with a minimum of ten years of follow-up. *J Bone Joint Surg Am.* 2004;86-A:2359-2365.
2. Tomaino MM, Delsignore J, Burton RI. Long-term results following proximal row carpectomy. *J Hand Surg Am.* 1994;19:694-703.
3. Cohen MS, Kozin SH. Degenerative arthritis of the wrist: proximal row carpectomy versus scaphoid excision and four-corner arthrodesis. *J Hand Surg Am.* 2001;26:94-104.

4 Dupuytren's Contracture

Percutaneous Needle Fasciotomy for Recurrent Dupuytren Disease
van Rijssen AL, Werker PMN (Isala Clinics, Zwolle, The Netherlands)
J Hand Surg 37A:1820-1823, 2012

Purpose.—Increasing options to treat Dupuytren disease include percutaneous needle fasciotomy (PNF), a minimally invasive technique that has proven to be effective for the treatment of primary disease. However, its effect on recurrent disease is not clear.

Methods.—We studied 30 patients with recurrent Dupuytren disease in 40 fingers, with a mean follow-up of 4.4 years. Primary outcome measures were total passive extension deficit reduction and interval to a second recurrence, defined as an increase of more than 30° compared with the result at the end of the previous treatment. We noted complications.

Results.—Total passive extension reduction was 76%. Percutaneous needle fasciotomy was especially effective for the metacarpophalangeal joint, with an average reduction of 93%, whereas the average reduction in the proximal interphalangeal joint was 57%. A total of 50% of patients did not develop a secondary recurrence during follow-up. The other 50% did, and we treated recurrence within an average of 1.4 years after PNF. By means of PNF, we postponed tertiary treatment an average of 2.9 years starting from the initial treatment for Dupuytren disease. We successfully treated all secondary recurrences by limited fasciectomy, according to patients' wishes. We noted no major adverse effects.

Conclusions.—Percutaneous needle fasciotomy can be applied effectively for recurrent disease; 50% of patients remain free of recurrence for a mean of 4.4 years. If a secondary recurrence occurs, it does so relatively early after treatment. Patients must therefore be willing to accept this uncertainty in the context of the advantages of PNF, such as fast recovery, low complication rate, and minimal invasiveness.

▶ This article analyzes the use of percutaneous needle fasciotomy for Dupuytren's contracture recurrence. The population of the study is a subset of patients from a prior randomized study (needle fasciotomy vs limited fasciectomy) the authors had completed. The current study consists of patients from that prior study who developed a recurrence within 5 years of the first procedure.

There were 30 patients who underwent needle fasciotomy for this recurrence. Nearly all of the patients had previously undergone needle fasciotomy, but a few had undergone limited fasciectomy. The needle fasciotomy was done according to accepted technique.

The study found that half of the patients who underwent this needle fasciotomy for recurrence had a second recurrence at an average of 4 years, and these patients later went on to a limited fasciectomy for their third procedure. All patients obtained improvements in range of motion whether the contracture was at the metacarpophalangeal joint, the proximal interphalangeal joint, or both. Not surprisingly, the metacarpophalangeal joints had more improvement in range of motion.

Those of us who perform needle aponeurotomy have a suspicion, which is that recurrence is common and repeat needle treatment is a reasonable option, and that is basically confirmed by this study.

J. B. Friedrich, MD, FACS

The consequences of different definitions for recurrence of Dupuytren's disease
Kan HJ, Verrijp FW, Huisstede BMA, et al (Erasmus Med Ctr, Rotterdam, The Netherlands)
J Plast Reconstr Aesthet Surg 66:95-103, 2013

Background.—Recurrence rates are important in the evaluation of the effectiveness of treatment for Dupuytren's disease (DD). In the literature, recurrence rates vary between 0% and 100%. The definition of recurrence of DD after treatment is inconsistently used. The aim of this study is to review all definitions of recurrence after treatment of DD and to evaluate the impact of using these definitions on a single cohort of patients treated for DD.

Methods.—A literature search was performed in PubMed and Embase to identify studies. Titles and abstracts were analysed to collect all articles that described recurrence rates or definitions of recurrence. Two independent reviewers selected relevant studies and extracted data. The different definitions of recurrence were applied on our data set of 66 patients.

Results.—Of the 113 articles reporting recurrent rates of DD, 56 (49%) presented a definition of recurrence. We could categorise the definitions into three groups. By applying the different definition on our data set of a randomised controlled trial, the recurrence rates ranged from 2% to 86%.

Conclusions.—In the literature, different definitions of recurrence of DD are used and many authors failed to define recurrence. This study shows that the wide range of reported recurrence rates may largely be contributed by inconsistency in recurrence definitions. As a result, it is difficult or even impossible to compare recurrence rates between different treatments reported in the literature. The study indicates that consensus on a recurrence definition is needed.

▶ The authors present a poignant finding associated with many articles that examine outcomes following treatment for Dupuytren's contracture. Much of how we define success following intervention is based on the incidence of recurrence. However, the authors shed light on not just the lack of definition of recurrence but also how inconsistent the definition of recurrence is seen in the literature. The study underscores the need for a universal definition of recurrence so treatment options can be appropriately compared. As newer studies are being published, reviewing outcomes of nonoperative interventions, such as collagenase injection and needle aponeurotomy, the need for a universal definition of recurrence will distill information from these treatments appropriately.

M. Rizzo, MD

The Use of Skeletal Extension Torque in Reversing Dupuytren Contractures of the Proximal Interphalangeal Joint

Agee JM, Goss BC (Hand Biomechanics Lab, Inc, Sacramento, CA)
J Hand Surg 37A:1467-1474, 2012

Dupuytren contracture of the proximal interphalangeal (PIP) joint can be reversed by an extension torque transmitted from an external device, the Digit Widget, by skeletal pins to the middle phalanx. This extension torque, generated by the same elastic bands dentists use to align teeth, gradually restores length to soft tissues palmar to the PIP joint's axis of rotation. Simultaneously, tissues dorsal to the joint's axis will shorten toward normal length as the PIP progressively straightens. Although the contractile nodules and bands of Dupuytren disease may be excised either before or after reversal of the joint's contracture, a 2-staged approach is preferred: (1) reverse the PIP flexion contracture, and (2) excise the diseased tissue from the straightened finger. We believe this 2-staged approach yields better results. In addition, it is technically easier to avoid injury to nerves and arteries while excising the nodules and bands, when one operates through palmar skin of more nearly normal length.

▶ Most experienced hand surgeons and therapists have abandoned the notion that external dynamic extension splinting will alter a chronic Dupuytren contracture of the proximal interphalangeal (PIP) joint. Patients cannot tolerate the skin pressure of these devices long enough for them to be effective. Perhaps serial casting might be effective but at the risk of PIP joint stiffness, that is, lost flexion, a poor trade. Almost 20 years ago, Messina[1] showed that an extension torque applied to the skeleton is tolerated and effective in straightening Dupuytren PIP joint contractures, but his device was very obtrusive. The clinical success prompted development of other devices such as the Pipster or the S-Quattro (Google these if you want to read more). The exceedingly clever John Agee, with the right brain of a bioengineer and the left brain of a hand surgeon, has developed a very elegant and adaptable device, the Digit Widget, which I now routinely use for severe recurrent PIP contractures. I agree with Agee that a 2-stage procedure is more likely to succeed, and I prefer to excise the poor proximal phalanx skin and place a large full thickness skin graft. We recently reviewed 16 recurrent PIP contractures, almost all of the fifth digit. There were no intra- or postoperative complications. Two years after surgery, the arc of PIP motion was 70% greater than preoperatively and only 1 finger showed any sign of recurrence. I no longer worry about the dreaded end-of-case white finger. This is a great addition to our surgical armamentarium.

V. R. Hentz, MD

Reference

1. Messina A, Messina J. The continuous elongation treatment by the TEC device for severe Dupuytren's contracture of the fingers. *Plast Reconstr Surg.* 1993;92(1):84-90.

Dupuytren Diathesis and Genetic Risk
Dolmans GH, de Bock GH, Werker PM (Univ Med Ctr Groningen and Univ of Groningen, the Netherlands)
J Hand Surg 37A:2106-2111, 2012

Purpose.—Dupuytren disease (DD) is a benign fibrosing disorder of the hand and fingers. Recently, we identified 9 single nucleotide polymorphisms (SNPs) associated with DD in a genome-wide association study. These SNPs can be used to calculate a genetic risk score for DD. The aim of this study was to test whether certain clinical characteristics (including the DD diathesis features) of patients with DD are associated with a high genetic risk score.

Methods.—Between 2007 and 2010, we prospectively invited all DD patients (1,120 in total) to participate. Clinical characteristics were noted using patient- and doctor-completed questionnaires, and blood was obtained for DNA analysis. We analyzed a total of 933 subjects with genetic and clinical data. The 9 previously identified DD SNPs were used to calculate a weighted genetic risk score. Patients were categorized into high and low genetic risk score groups, according to their weighted genetic risk score. Logistic regression was performed to study the association of clinical characteristics with a high genetic risk score.

Results.—In a univariate regression model, patients with an age of onset of DD younger than 50 years, a family history positive for DD, knuckle pads, and Ledderhose disease were statistically significantly associated with a high genetic risk score. In an additional analysis using high and low genetic risk groups that deviate further from the median, Ledderhose disease was no longer significantly associated with DD.

Conclusions.—Patients with DD who present with these diathesis features, and predominantly patients with knuckle pads, are more likely to carry more risk alleles for the discovered DD SNPs than patients without these diathesis features.

Clinical Relevance.—These markers may prove useful in predicting disease progression or recurrence.

▶ Predicting the course of Dupuytren's disease (DD) remains a challenge for the practicing hand surgeon. Previous work has identified several clinical character-istics associated with more aggressive disease or diathesis, including onset at a young age, ectopic disease, family history, and bilateral hand disease. This study was performed by a group that had previously identified genetic alleles associated with DD. They then developed a Dupuytren's genetic risk score using the presence of these genetic traits. The purpose of the study was to assess whether a high genetic risk score was associated with clinical signs of Dupuyt-ren's diathesis.

The study looked at 566 patients with DD and correlated their clinical findings with those of genetic testing. Their analysis confirmed that a higher value on the genetic risk score was associated with clinical traits known to be associated with more severe disease. The second analysis, which assessed the clinical traits asso-ciated with the group of patients with the highest genetic risk scores, was partic-ularly interesting. It found that the presence of knuckle pads had by far the highest odds of having a high genetic score. This study concluded that the more risk alleles a patient has, the more aggressive the clinical picture.

This is a strong study based on a large group of patients with DD. The major weakness is that each subject's clinical picture was a snapshot in time, and although the picture may seem aggressive, without longitudinal data, we cannot yet conclude that a higher genetic risk is associated with a more aggressive clinical course.

A hand surgery goal continues to be clarifying the genetic underpinnings of DD. If we understand the mechanisms, then interventions could be designed to prevent progression. This study is one more step toward a transition from reac-tionary to preventative treatment of DD.

C. Curtin, MD

Steroid Injection and Needle Aponeurotomy for Dupuytren Contracture: A Randomized, Controlled Study
McMillan C, Binhammer P (Sunnybrook Health Sciences Centre, Toronto, Ontario, Canada)
J Hand Surg 37A:1307-1312, 2012

Purpose.—To compare flexion deformity at 6 months in patients with Dupuytren contracture who had percutaneous needle aponeurotomy (PNA) combined with a series of triamcinolone acetonide (TA) injections to that of patients who had PNA alone.

Methods.—Forty-seven patients with Dupuytren disease who were candi-dates for PNA (at least 1 contracture of at least 20°) participated in the study. Patients were randomized either to receive TA injections immediately following and 6 weeks and 3 months after the procedure or to receive no injections. Injections were administered into cords. The number of injections and the amount of TA per injection was determined based on the number of digits involved and the cord size. All subjects returned for 3 follow-up visits after the procedure, and contractures were measured using a goniometer. Change in total active extension deficit (TAED) was analyzed using a repeated measures analysis of variance to assess for differences between groups, time points, and interaction between group and time point. Descriptive statistics were calculated for all variables of interest. Continuous measures were summarized using means and standard deviations.

Results.—There was no significant difference in TAED between groups before cord aponeurotomy. Correction at 6 months was 87% of preoperative TAED for the TA group versus 64% for the control group. This difference was statistically significant. The amount of TA administered did not correlate with TAED improvement.

Conclusions.—The study group who received TA in combination with PNA experienced a significantly greater degree of correction of flexion deformity at 6 months than those who had PNA alone.

▶ With the ever-growing interest in the role of nonoperative treatments for Dupuytren's disease, there has been an increasing trend in the use of collagenase and percutaneous needle aponeurotomy (PNA) in the management of this disorder.[1-3] Despite early promising results in the correction of contractures with PNA, longer-term follow-up studies have shown a recurrence rate ranging from 50% to 65%. Given the disease-modifying effects of corticosteroid injections, the authors have conducted a well-powered, prospective study comparing the efficacy of PNA alone with triamcinolone acetonide (TA) injections into the divided cord immediately, 6 weeks, and 3 months after PNA. Despite a lack of statistical significant differences, the total active extension deficit (TAED) of the TA-treated patients was greater than that of the PNA alone group. At 6 months posttreatment, correction of deformity was found to be significantly greater within the TA group, particularly at the proximal interphalangeal joint.

I commend the authors on their attempts to evaluate the benefit of adjuvant therapy to improving and maintaining corrections in TAED after PNA. Despite the promising results, there are a few methodologic concerns with the study. Patients were injected immediately, between points of release of the cord, at 6 weeks and at 3 months, in areas of palpable thickness along the treated cord after PNA. How were these time points decided? Additionally, given the lack of an objective tool to guide the accuracy of injection within the cord, such as ultrasound, it is difficult to determine the point of delivery of the corticosteroid injection. Indeed, the authors comment that "the TA suspension leaked out at the time of PNA through puncture sites" thereby limiting the drug's efficacy. Secondly, a range of steroid (8–48 mg) was administered per digit rather than a set amount, thereby making it very difficult to determine the therapeutic dose needed for maximum benefit. As highlighted by the authors, the correction seen in the steroid-treated patients may be a result of greater correction from PNA rather than from the TA. Other methodologic flaws include a lack of blinding by the treating physician, an absence of patient-reported outcomes, and no measure of patient compliance with postoperative splinting and therapy. Lastly, as pointed out by the authors, the length of follow-up of 6 months is limited, and long-term studies are needed to assess the efficacy of TA to maintain correction.

Not withstanding these limitations, I believe the authors should be congratulated on their attempts to try and assess the efficacy of an adjunctive treatment to PNA to improve and maintain contracture correction. With long-term follow-up studies needed to assess corticosteroid efficacy, an alternative therapeutic arm may be the injection of collagenase under ultrasound guidance into the cord after PNA.

S. Kakar, MD

References

1. Foucher G, Medina J, Navarro R. Percutaneous needle aponeurotomy: complications and results. *J Hand Surg Br.* 2003;28:427-431.
2. Van Rijssen AL, Werker PM. Percutaneous needle fasciotomy in Dupuytren's disease. *J Hand Surg Br.* 2006;31:498-501.
3. Ketchum LD, Donahue TK. The injection of nodules of Dupuytren's disease with triamcinolone acetonide. *J Hand Surg Am.* 2000;25:1157-1162.

Steroid Injection and Needle Aponeurotomy for Dupuytren Contracture: A Randomized, Controlled Study
McMillan C, Binhammer P (Sunnybrook Health Sciences Centre, Toronto, Canada)
J Hand Surg 37A:1307-1312, 2012

Purpose.—To compare flexion deformity at 6 months in patients with Dupuytren contracture who had percutaneous needle aponeurotomy (PNA) combined with a series of triamcinolone acetonide (TA) injections to that of patients who had PNA alone.

Methods.—Forty-seven patients with Dupuytren disease who were candidates for PNA (at least 1 contracture of at least 20°) participated in the study. Patients were randomized either to receive TA injections immediately following and 6 weeks and 3 months after the procedure or to receive no injections. Injections were administered into cords. The number of injections and the amount of TA per injection was determined based on the number of digits involved and the cord size. All subjects returned for 3 follow-up visits after the procedure, and contractures were measured using a goniometer. Change in total active extension deficit (TAED) was analyzed using a repeated measures analysis of variance to assess for differences between groups, time points, and interaction between group and time point. Descriptive statistics were calculated for all variables of interest. Continuous measures were summarized using means and standard deviations.

Results.—There was no significant difference in TAED between groups before cord aponeurotomy. Correction at 6 months was 87% of preoperative TAED for the TA group versus 64% for the control group. This difference was statistically significant. The amount of TA administered did not correlate with TAED improvement.

Conclusions.—The study group who received TA in combination with PNA experienced a significantly greater degree of correction of flexion deformity at 6 months than those who had PNA alone.

▶ Corticosteroid injection into Dupuytren nodules has been advocated by Ketchum and Donahue[1] as a way to diminish progression to the cord and contracture stage. Repeated injections seem to be necessary for durability. The authors studied whether the addition of corticosteroids at the time of needle aponeurotomy provides some benefit, at least for the short term. They concluded that this was the case, at least for proximal interphalangeal (PIP) joint contractures. Closer analysis of the data generates some concern regarding this conclusion. For example, the group that had the steroids started with 20° more extensor lag, although the average extensor lags at the metacarpophalangeal (MP) and PIP between the 2 groups were a little different. Thus, many more in the treatment group had both an MP and a PIP contracture, and I suspect many more in this group had a cord that bridged across both joints. This is the patient with a pretendinous cord and central cord who cannot extend the PIP joint when the MP joint is also extended but can sometimes fully passively extend the PIP joint when the MP joint is flexed. In this case, release of the cord in the palm results in extension of both joints. Perhaps the control group had more isolated PIP contractures or contractures associated with a lateral digital sheet cord or isolated abductor digiti minimi cord, for whom percutaneous needle aponeurotomy (PNA) is historically not as effective initially and certainly not as durable. In the current study, PNA was not as durable for PIP contractures in the controls, but were the authors treating equivalent groups? Perhaps not.

Note that there was really no difference between the 2 groups at the MP joint, in spite of statistical analysis. If the accepted error of a finger goniometer is about 5°, then there is no clinically relevant difference between the reported values. For the PIP joint, only at the 6-month interval was there a real difference. Also concerning is the author's use of active movement when essentially all others report passive extension deficits. Did the steroids help diminish the effects of the trauma of PNA? Tissues are injured and injuries healed by scar formation and scars have the tendency to contract.

V. R. Hentz, MD

Reference

1. Ketchum LD, Donahue TK. The injection of nodules of Dupuytren's disease with triamcinolone acetonide. *J Hand Surg Am.* 2000;25:1157-1162.

5 Compressive Neuropathies

Comparison of carpal tunnel release with three different techniques
Aslani HR, Alizadeh K, Eajazi A, et al (Shahid Beheshti Med Univ, Tehran, Iran)
Clin Neurol Neurosurg 114:965-968, 2012

Background.—Carpal tunnel syndrome is one of the most common compression neuropathies in the upper limbs and requires surgery if conservative treatment fails. This article compares the result of regular open incision, mid-palmar mini incision and endoscopic technique in carpal tunnel release.

Methods.—This is a clinical trial study on 105 patients (10 males, 95 females) within one year, who were surgical candidates. The surgery was done with regular open incision or with mid-palmar small incision. The clinical outcomes were evaluated one week, 4 weeks and 4 months post-surgery.

Results.—Relief and satisfaction were better in the first month in the endoscopic and mid-palmar mini incision group. All 3 techniques had similar outcomes after 4 months. In the 4-month follow-up, night pain relief, followed by parasthesia relief had the best improvement. Weakness was the symptom with the least improvement. Longer incision cases were associated with more delay to return to work.

Conclusion.—Carpal tunnel release with endoscopic and mini incision techniques have better early satisfaction rates compared to regular open incision, but no difference is seen between the two groups after four months.

▶ Most studies of different approaches to carpal tunnel release (CTR) compare the traditional open approach to endoscopic CTR (eCTR); fewer compare mini-open procedures to eCTR.[1] This article addresses this weakness while also comparing the open approach to both of these approaches.

A number of different approaches to CTR exist, but there has been no conclusive evidence that one is superior. Depending on their preference, surgeons use big open, mini open, 2 portal eCTR, 1 portal eCTR, 2 incision mini open, and 1 incision mini open. Available level 1 or 2 evidence is insufficient to state with certainty which technique should be used in which circumstances. Studies like this one should help address the question of which release, if any, is superior.

The study assessed a group of patients that had both clinical and electrodiagnostic confirmation of carpal tunnel syndrome. Patients were prospectively and randomly assigned to be released via open, mini open, or 2 portal eCTR; the results are summarized in the abstract. The study's major shortcoming was the absence of a validated scale for evaluating postoperative outcomes.

The results did not differ from the meta-analyses of various CTRs that have been published in that no one release was found to result in better outcomes than another. It did reinforce, however, that this lack of clarity on the question of superiority also applies to mini open releases.

The prospective nature of this study should be commended and other, larger, prospective multi-institutional studies should be encouraged. This study on its own is unlikely to change current practice patterns.

J. Frankenhoff, MD

Reference

1. Abrams R. Endoscopic versus open carpal tunnel release. *J Hand Surg Am.* 2009; 34:535-539.

Acute carpal tunnel syndrome in trauma

Jhattu H, Klaassen S, Ying C, et al (The Canberra Hosp, Australia)
Eur J Plast Surg 35:639-646, 2012

Carpal tunnel syndrome (CTS) is one of the commonest compression neuropathy. It carries significant employment and health care costs and causes much grief to patients. There are numerous causes for carpal tunnel syndrome; however, in this review, the authors concentrate on trauma as a primary etiology. CTS is essentially a compression of the median nerve within the carpal tunnel producing debilitating symptoms and signs. Early recognition of the clinical presentation of this syndrome is vital, since it is a surgical emergency and urgent release is indicated. The anatomy, etiology, pathogenesis, clinical features, investigations, and management with case presentation have been discussed in detail, referencing a diverse collection of textbooks and papers. A comprehensive literature review of 44 papers was performed, with compilation of current treatment guidelines and management. Picture illustrations of a case encountered by the authors are included for better understanding for clinicians and trainees. This article describes acute CTS in detail and provides information for correct and early diagnosis together with effective treatment. The risk factors and treatment options are discussed in detail with photographic illustrations, providing simple but comprehensive material for education of students and clinicians, therefore to improve outcome of patients with this potentially devastating condition.

▶ Although the title is "Acute carpal tunnel syndrome in trauma," the authors have provided a general overview of carpal tunnel syndrome (CTS). They discuss the anatomy of the carpal tunnel and symptoms of both idiopathic and acute CTS, including the role of electrodiagnostic and other imaging and pressure measurements for confirmation. They describe the etiology of acute CTS and provide a case example of acute CTS treated with decompression and fasciotomies of the hand. They close with a discussion of complications.

This article is a nice review of the topic and will be helpful for those involved in teaching medical students or residents not familiar with CTS, but it does not provide new information for the practicing hand surgeon.

W. C. Hammert, DDS, MD

The long-term post-operative electromyographic evaluation of patients who have undergone carpal tunnel decompression
Faour-Martín O, Martín-Ferrero MA, Almaraz-Gómez A, et al (Clinic Univ Hosp of Valladolid, Spain)
J Bone Joint Surg Br 94-B:941-946, 2012

We present the electromyographic (EMG) results ten years after open decompression of the median nerve at the wrist and compare them with the clinical and functional outcomes as judged by Levine's Questionnaire. This retrospective study evaluated 115 patients who had undergone carpal tunnel decompression at a mean of 10.47 years (9.24 to 11.36) previously. A positive EMG diagnosis was found in 77 patients (67%), including those who were asymptomatic at ten years.

It is necessary to include both clinical and functional results as well as electromyographic testing in the long-term evaluation of patients who have undergone carpal tunnel decompression particularly in those in whom revision surgery is being considered. In doubtful cases or when there are differing outcomes, self-administered scales such as Levine's Questionnaire should prevail over EMG results when deciding on the need for revision surgery.

▶ Carpal tunnel release is a reliable surgery, and recurrence of carpal tunnel syndrome after release is fairly rare. The authors attempt to characterize the electrophysiologic changes of the operated hand 10 years after release. Although the study overall is a good one, the most glaring problem is that the authors continually refer to the electrophysiologic testing used as electromyographic (EMG), even though it is actually nerve conduction studies that are used to assess impairments in the median nerve at the carpal tunnel. EMG and nerve conduction study are not interchangeable terms.

The authors identified 115 patients who had undergone carpal tunnel release 10 years prior to the study and who were willing to undergo repeat examination and electrophysiologic testing. This in and of itself is a laudable accomplishment. Interestingly, most patients had distinct improvements when compared with the preoperative nerve conduction studies, but the velocities remained below what the testers had considered normal. Specifically, 67% of all patients had what would be considered a positive diagnosis in the 10-year testing, and 57% of asymptomatic patients had a positive nerve conduction study. An even higher percentage (81%) of symptomatic patients had a positive nerve conduction study. Although the authors also used the Levine scale in evaluating these patients at 10 years, this did not seem to add much to the final data other than correlating positively with motor latency and inversely with sensory conduction velocity.

Although this study is unable to explain why there appear to be long-term changes in the nerve as seen on electrophysiologic testing following carpal tunnel release, those changes appear to persist and only partially resolve following surgery.

J. B. Friedrich, MD, FACS

Effect of Splinting and Exercise on Intraneural Edema of the Median Nerve in Carpal Tunnel Syndrome—An MRI Study to Reveal Therapeutic Mechanisms
Schmid AB, Elliott JM, Strudwick MW, et al (The Univ of Queensland, St Lucia (Brisbane), Australia; Northwestern Univ, Chicago, IL; et al)
J Orthop Res 30:1343-1350, 2012

Splinting and nerve and tendon gliding exercises are commonly used to treat carpal tunnel syndrome (CTS). It has been postulated that both modalities reduce intraneural edema. To test this hypothesis, 20 patients with mild to moderate CTS were randomly allocated to either night splinting or a home program of nerve and tendon gliding exercises. Magnetic resonance images of the wrist were taken at baseline, immediately after 10 min of splinting or exercise, and following 1 week of intervention. Primary outcome measures were signal intensity of the median nerve at the wrist as a measure of intraneural edema and palmar bowing of the carpal ligament. Secondary outcome measures were changes in symptom severity and function. Following 1 week of intervention, but not immediately after 10 min, signal intensity of the median nerve was reduced by ~11% at the radioulnar level for both interventions ($p = 0.03$). This was accompanied by a mild improvement in symptoms and function ($p < 0.004$). A similar reduction in signal intensity is not observed in patients who only receive advice to remain active. No changes in signal intensity were identified further distally ($p > 0.28$). Ligament bowing remained unchanged ($p > 0.08$). Intraneural edema reduction is a likely therapeutic mechanism of splinting and exercise.

▶ This report, comparing nerve gliding exercise and splinting by completing a study of mild-to-moderate patients with carpal tunnel syndrome after 1 week of either treatment, was well structured. Data collection to achieve a sample size was adequate, exploratory in nature, and based on current literature. In any study, a greater study sample would be better because of the dropout rate. The methodology, the results, and ensuing discussion were clearly stated. Discussion of how the reduction in intraneural edema is the therapeutic mechanism or benefit, most likely at 11%, which was also found 3 months postoperatively, was factual and obvious in the study results. Discussion on ligament bowing and elevated carpal tunnel pressure was well described and brought out interesting factors of causation, based on literature by Seradge et al.[1] This article is also useful because it warrants future studies with larger populations and the acknowledgment of the patient-specific function scale improvement clinical relevance.[2]

S. Kranz, OTR/L, CHT

References

1. Seradge H, Jia YC, Owens W. In vivo measurements of carpal tunnel pressure in the functioning hand. *J Hand Surg (Am).* 1995;20:855-859.
2. Stratford P, Gill C, Westaway M, et al. Assessing disability and change on individual patients: a report of a patient specific measure. *Physiother Can.* 1995;47:258-363.

Accuracy of Ultrasonography and Magnetic Resonance Imaging in Diagnosing Carpal Tunnel Syndrome Using Rest and Grasp Positions of the Hands
Horng Y-S, Chang H-C, Lin K-E, et al (Buddhist Tzu Chi General Hosp, Taipei Branch, Taiwan; Tzu Chi Univ, Hualien, Taiwan; Natl Taiwan Univ, Taipei; et al)
J Hand Surg 37A:1591-1598, 2012

Purpose.—To compare the accuracy of ultrasonography and magnetic resonance imaging (MRI) in diagnosing carpal tunnel syndrome (CTS) in both the rest and grasp positions. We postulated that the diagnostic accuracy could be improved by imaging hands in the grasp position rather than in the rest position.

Methods.—Fifty patients with CTS and 45 healthy volunteers received a package of questionnaires and had a physical examination and a nerve conduction study. Ultrasonography and MRI images were recorded in both the rest and grasp positions for each participant.

Results.—There were significant differences between the patients and the healthy volunteers regarding patient-reported outcomes, the results of physical examinations, the nerve conduction studies, and the ultrasonography and MRI imaging. The area under the receiver operating characteristic curve of ultrasonography was significantly improved by measuring the bowing of the flexor retinaculum in the grasp position than by measuring that in the rest position. The diagnostic accuracy of ultrasonography was similar to that of MRI when we used a combination of the measurements of the cross-sectional area of the median nerve in the rest position and the bowing of the flexor retinaculum in the grasp position.

Conclusions.—The accuracies of MRI and ultrasonography for diagnosing CTS were improved by measuring the bowing of the flexor retinaculum in the grasp position. Ultrasonography can be an adequate screening method for CTS if clinicians combine the cross-sectional area of the median nerve in the rest position and the bowing of the flexor retinaculum in the grasp position.

Type of Study/Level of Evidence.—Diagnostic I.

▶ The authors compare the accuracies of magnetic resonance imaging (MRI) and ultrasonography for the diagnosis of carpal tunnel syndrome (CTS) in resting and grasp positions of the hand. They conclude that by combining different measurement positions, ultrasonography can reach similar levels of diagnostic accuracy as MRI scans.

Although the methodology seems quite sound (except for the higher body mass index in the patient groups, which might be a confounding variable), I am still not convinced about the necessity for any imaging study for the diagnosis of CTS. The authors demonstrate that the diagnostic accuracy is best for severe cases of CTS, which were defined as greater impairment in the nerve conduction studies. Typically, imaging is unnecessary for these patients. The only possible indication for additional imaging would be for patients who complain of typical symptoms but have normal electrodiagnostic tests. However, for this group of patients, the diagnostic accuracy is rather poor for both imaging modalities. Because the overall risk of complications is rather low for the procedure, I would still consider offering open carpal tunnel release to patients with typical symptoms, even if the electrodiagnostic studies were normal.

K. Megerle, MD

Predicting the Outcome of Revision Carpal Tunnel Release
Beck JD, Brothers JG, Maloney PJ, et al (Geisinger Med Ctr, Danville, PA)
J Hand Surg 37A:282-287, 2012

Purpose.—To test the hypothesis that the result of steroid injection in the carpal tunnel in a patient with recurrent carpal tunnel symptoms would serve as a good predictor of the outcome of later carpal tunnel release (CTR).

Methods.—We conducted a retrospective review of all patients who underwent revision CTR for recurrent or persistent carpal tunnel syndrome over a 2-year period at our institution. A total of 28 wrists in 23 patients met inclusion criteria. We evaluated patients to determine whether preoperative factors or the result of injection predicted the outcome of revision CTR. We used a multivariate logistic regression analysis to predict surgical success when multiple preoperative findings were considered.

Results.—Of the 23 wrists that had relief from injection, 20 had symptom improvement with surgery. Although they did not reach statistical significance, the sensitivity and positive predictive value for injection alone predicted outcome of revision CTR in 87%. No patient characteristic or physical examination finding predicted successful revision CTR. Multivariate logistic regression analysis combining preoperative injection results with physical examination findings (numbness and/or motor weakness in median nerve distribution, positive Durkin test, and positive Phalen test) provided a sensitivity of 100% and a specificity of 80%.

Conclusions.—In a small group of patients with recurrent carpal tunnel syndrome, cortisone injection into the carpal tunnel was not, by itself, a statistically significant predictor of successful revision surgery. However, relief from injection as a diagnostic test for predicting successful revision CTR was found to have both a high sensitivity and a positive predictive value. Coupled with the components of the physical examination, injection provides a good screening test to establish surgical success with revision CTR.

Type of Study/Level of Evidence.—Therapeutic III.

▶ This article by Beck et al provides some data confirming what many hand surgeons have used in clinical practice; that is, that in equivocal cases of carpal tunnel syndrome or in recurrent cases of carpal tunnel syndrome, steroid injection can be an excellent diagnostic test for carpal tunnel syndrome. In my practice, patients with negative electromyogram studies or atypical symptoms are occasionally seen. In those patients, I would inject corticosteroid into the carpal canal and ask the patient to return 1 month thereafter. At 1-month follow-up, I would ask if their symptoms had improved. Those who had noticed improvement would be candidates for open carpal tunnel release. Invariably, if they are not released, the symptoms recur several months after the injection.

This article showed that in a small cohort of patients with recurrent carpal tunnel syndrome, relief after injection had high sensitivity and a positive predictive value for success in revision carpal tunnel release. There is an additional point in the article: The authors spend some time documenting the presence or absence of an intact flexor retinaculum at time of reoperation. However, this is difficult to assess because even patients with full release of the transverse carpal ligament will have scar tissue that can mimic this finding.

J. Chang, MD

Treatment of Carpal Tunnel Syndrome by Members of the American Society for Surgery of the Hand: A 25-Year Perspective
Leinberry CF, Rivlin M, Maltenfort M, et al (Thomas Jefferson Univ, Philadelphia, PA; Univ of Utah, Salt Lake City)
J Hand Surg 37A:1997-2003, 2012

Purpose.—In 1987, Duncan et al reported on a survey of the members of the American Society for the Surgery of the Hand (ASSH) about their practices in treating carpal tunnel syndrome (CTS). To better understand changes in the treatment of CTS over the past 25 years, we repeated the survey while incorporating present-day controversies.

Methods.—With the approval of the ASSH, an Internet-based survey was e-mailed to all members of the Society. This included 33 primary questions focusing on 4 areas of study: surgeon demographic information, nonoperative treatment, surgical technique, and postoperative care. A total of 1,463 surveys were delivered and 707 surveys were completed and returned, for a response rate of 48%. Responses were compared with the responses from Duncan et al. published 25 years ago.

Results.—In contrast to the practice patterns identified 25 years ago, this survey identified several changes in current clinical practices including the following statistically significant findings: Preoperatively, surgeons have increased the use of splints and corticosteroid injections, treat nonoperatively longer, and have narrowed their surgical indications. Regarding surgical technique, surgeons now are using tourniquets less, infiltrate the carpal tunnel with corticosteroids less, and place deep sutures less often. Furthermore, performing concomitant procedures along with release of the transverse carpal ligament has decreased. Orthotic use and duration postoperatively also decreased.

Conclusions.—Although significant differences are evident between management of CTS between 1987 and 2011, no consensus has emerged.

▶ The authors have carefully repeated a study done 25 years ago to look at trends related to care of carpal tunnel syndrome. Perusal is important to see where care has changed, and the findings reflect my own personal experience. As surgeons, we may be more conservative and have narrowed our indications in an attempt to minimize poor outcomes and poorly selected surgical candidates. Tourniquet use, deep stitches, and steroid use for injections have decreased as well. Concomitant procedures performed with the release of the transverse carpal ligament and splinting after surgery have also decreased. Cost may be a driving factor in the changes, but no clear consensus emerges. This article is interesting to consider but does not lead to any significant conclusions that would lead to a change in practice patterns concerning carpal tunnel syndrome in 2013. My own experience over the same period would mirror these findings as well, although I did not complete the survey for time management reasons as opposed to technology concerns.

C. Carroll, MD

Carpal Tunnel Syndrome and Radiographically Evident Basal Joint Arthritis of the Thumb in Elderly Koreans
Shin CH, Paik N-J, Lim J-Y, et al (Seoul Natl Univ Bundang Hosp, Seongnam, South Korea)
J Bone Joint Surg Am 94:e120.1-e120.6, 2012

Background.—Previous studies have suggested a high prevalence of carpal tunnel syndrome in patients seeking treatment for basal joint arthritis of the thumb. The purpose of this study was to compare the prevalence of carpal tunnel syndrome between individuals with and those without radiographic evidence of basal joint arthritis of the thumb in the general elderly Korean population, and to determine if there is a correlation between the severity of carpal tunnel syndrome shown by electrophysiological studies and the severity of basal joint arthritis as seen on radiographs.

Methods.—We evaluated hand radiographs and nerve conduction studies of 192 men and 176 women (more than sixty-five years of age) who participated in the Korean Longitudinal Study on Health and Aging. The basal joint of the thumb was assigned a grade for osteoarthritis of 0 to 4 on radiographs with use of the Kellgren and Lawrence criteria. The diagnosis of carpal tunnel syndrome was based on the combination of a positive response to survey questions and a positive nerve conduction study. Motor distal latency and motor conduction velocity were measured to assess the electrophysiological severity of carpal tunnel syndrome.

Results.—The prevalence of carpal tunnel syndrome was 16.7% in the group with basal joint arthritis and 10.9% in the group without basal joint arthritis, a difference that was not significant ($p = 0.249$). Neither motor distal latency nor motor conduction velocity was significantly correlated with the severity of the basal joint arthritis in the entire group of 368 study subjects ($p = 0.154$ and $p = 0.662$, respectively) or in those with carpal tunnel syndrome ($p = 0.603$ and $p = 0.998$, respectively).

Conclusions.—This study of Koreans who were more than sixty-five years of age showed that the prevalence of carpal tunnel syndrome is similar in patients with and those without radiographic findings of basal joint arthritis of the thumb. We found no correlation between the electrophysiological severity of carpal tunnel syndrome and the severity of basal joint arthritis.

▶ This study seeks to investigate the correlation of carpal tunnel syndrome (CTS) and basal joint arthritis of the thumb in the general population of elderly Koreans. Several investigators have suggested that the prevalence of CTS in patients with basal joint arthritis of the thumb is higher than that in the normal population. The results of the article, however, indicate that these 2 conditions are not associated. Furthermore, it was found that the severity of basal joint arthritis of the thumb had no correlation with CTS prevalence.

As the authors point out, the limitation of this study is that CTS was diagnosed on the dominant hand in a healthy population by electrodiagnosis only. Positive screening results for CTS were not diagnostically confirmed by clinical evaluation, which is considered to be the most appropriate diagnostic tool. The results may not apply to other ethnic groups, especially to caucasians, as the prevalence of basal joint arthritis of the thumb is different according to race.

Another limitation is that the investigation was carried out only on the dominant hand.

Despite the limitations, this study is the first investigation showing statistical evidence that there is no relationship between CTS and basal joint arthritis of the thumb in the Korean population.

M. S. S. Choi, MD

Recurrent or Persistent Cubital Tunnel Syndrome

Ehsan A, Hanel DP (Kaiser Permanente Los Angeles Med Ctr, CA; Univ of Washington, Seattle, WA)
J Hand Surg 37A:1910-1912, 2012

Background.—Patients complaining of numbness of the ring and small fingers, decreased dexterity, and perhaps weakness may be candidates for subcutaneous ulnar nerve transposition to address their cubital tunnel syndrome. However, problems may again trouble these patients and the question becomes, Are these recurrent or persistent symptoms? The diagnosis and management of cubital tunnel syndrome that appears to have recurred were evaluated according to the best available evidence.

Current Approaches.—Often cubital tunnel syndrome is only reported at an advanced stage, which indicates that symptoms have gone unnoticed for an extended period of time. Patients who are convinced that surgery will help them tend to report improvements that are not indicated by nerve physiology. They interpret the "return" of symptoms as recurrence or worsening of the problem. It is agreed that patients who have new or continued symptoms after undergoing ulnar nerve decompression at the elbow do not respond as well to surgery as the typical patient with cubital tunnel syndrome. Treatment approaches include nerve decompression and neurolysis, coverage with muscle flaps, and nerve wrapping using vein or synthetic agents. The indication for surgery is controversial, with various courses chosen.

Current Evidence.—The available studies tend to be small, few in number, and retrospective case series in design. No consensus has emerged concerning a reference standard for diagnosing persistent or recurrent symptoms. It can be hard to distinguish between patients' misperceptions and real changes in status. Lacking a control group, it is possible to misinterpret outcomes, whether objective or subjective. Placebo effect, self-limited disease course, and regression to the mean may explain the response reported. Telling patients that their numbness, weakness, or atrophy is permanent and being unable to explain the process precisely can contribute to patient dissatisfaction and the demand for further interventions that can prove useless.

Recommendations.—Currently it is advisable to counsel patients that revision surgery has unpredictable and sometimes unsatisfactory results compared to their initial surgery. Mood disorders can significantly influence the patient's perception of the outcome. If persistent ulnar nerve compression is likely, patients should be offered ulnar nerve external neurolysis beginning proximal and extending distal to the site of the index procedure along with submuscular transposition. If neuromas of the medial antebrachial cutaneous nerve (MABCN) are found, they are excised and the nerve branch is transposed into the muscle of the upper arm. Vein wrapping is reserved for patients with extensive scarring or those who have undergone more than two previous ulnar surgeries. Early postoperative mobilization is encouraged to permit neural gliding and diminish scar adhesions.

Conclusions.—Further research is needed to compare different revision techniques objectively using reliable outcome measures. Studies should be multicenter prospective cohort studies to obtain the most useful information. The influence of pathophysiology on outcome, especially mood factors, should be closely studied.

▶ The management of patients with recurrent or persistent cubital tunnel syndrome continues to be a vexing problem, both in terms of diagnosis and treatment. The authors present an evidence-based review of the management of recurrent ulnar neuropathy in a 38-year-old patient who had previously undergone a subcutaneous ulnar nerve transposition. They succinctly highlight the shortcomings within the literature, namely, the lack of objective diagnostic criteria and a paucity of prospective controlled trials comparing the milieu of revision surgeries.

From the limited retrospective case series, ulnar nerve neurolysis and submuscular transposition appears to be the procedure of choice, with a success rate of 75% to 78%. Patients tend to respond favorably with respect to a reduction in pain when compared with improvements in paresthesia and strength. Common findings at secondary surgery include a persistent or incompletely excised intermuscular septum, dense perineural fibrosis, and neuromas of the medial antebrachial cutaneous nerve.[1,2]

A discordant relationship exists between surgeons' and patients' expectations after revision cubital tunnel surgery. Within a cohort of 38 patients, 21% of patients were reported as being symptom free by their treating surgeon compared with only 3% of patients reporting complete resolution. As has been reported in the management of carpal tunnel syndrome,[3] this may be in part related to the role of mood disorders as a predictor of patient dissatisfaction and disability.[4-6]

S. Kakar, MD

References

1. Gabel GT, Amadio PC. Reoperation for failed decompression of the ulnar nerve in the region of the elbow. *J Bone Joint Surg Am.* 1990;72A:213-219.
2. Vogel RB, Nossaman BC, Rayan GM. Revision anterior submuscular transposition of the ulnar nerve for failed subcutaneous transposition. *Br J Plast Surg.* 2004;57:311-316.
3. Mackinnon SE, Novak CB. Operative findings in reoperation of patients with cubital tunnel syndrome. *Hand (N Y).* 2007;2:137-143.
4. Bartels RH, Grotenhuis JA. Anterior submuscular transposition of the ulnar nerve. For post-operative focal neuropathy at the elbow. *J Bone Joint Surg Br.* 2004;86: 998-1001.
5. Lozano Calderón SA, Paiva A, Ring D. Patient satisfaction after open carpal tunnel release correlates with depression. *J Hand Surg Am.* 2008;33:303-307.
6. Straub TA. Endoscopic carpal tunnel release: a prospective analysis of factors associated with unsatisfactory results. *Arthroscopy.* 1999;15:269-274.

Repair of Distal Biceps Ruptures

Baratz M, King GJW, Steinmann S (Drexel Univ, Pittsburgh, PA; Univ of Western Ontario, London, Ontario, Canada; Mayo Clinic, Rochester, MN)
J Hand Surg 37A:1462-1466, 2012

Background.—Distal biceps ruptures can cause permanent loss of 30% to 50% of supination strength if left unrepaired. However, the best treatment, surgical approach, timing of repair, fixation method, and postoperative management regimen for these injuries remain undetermined. The evidence currently available was reviewed.

Treatment Options.—Untreated rupture of the distal biceps can cause varying degrees of loss of supination strength and flexion strength. However, endurance and the eventual functional outcome appear not to be affected by nonsurgical treatment.

Surgical approaches include a single-incision anterior option and a two-incision, combined anteroposterior approach. Some laboratory data indicate the two-incision approach offers advantages over the single-incision approach, but these differences may not be meaningful to the patient. Generally it is recommended that repair be done within 2 weeks of injury to avoid perhaps doubling the incidence of complications. However, direct repair has been performed more than 31 days after injury with a return of supination strength ranging from 47% to 103% of preinjury levels.

Some evidence supports newer methods of fixation, but no clinical studies support this position. Postoperative management can extend for varying lengths of time, with immobilization generally imposed for 3 to 6 weeks, although some practitioners allow immediate motion. Most clinicians do not allow strengthening for 3 months after injury. Complications that occur with surgical repair include dysesthesias in the distribution of the lateral antebrachial cutaneous nerve, heterotopic bone formation, nerve injury, arterial injury, fracture of the radius, and repeat rupture. Only the dysesthesias are common.

Limitations.—The current evidence is generally based on relatively small, uncontrolled, retrospective case series. There are also challenges in determining forearm rotation and supination and flexion strength accurately. It is difficult to isolate the contribution of biceps contraction to supination strength and endurance. In addition, the median and average postrepair supination values can cover a wide range, although they are typically around 90%.

Conclusions and Recommendations.—The approach to biceps repair can be varied depending on surgeon preference. Fixation aids of many types can be used with satisfactory results. Delaying repair will likely increase complications but does not ultimately affect outcome. Direct repairs are not recommended when the flexion angle required exceeds 90°. Patients should be immobilized for 2 to 5 days, then begin self-assisted active flexion and extension exercises. In the first 4 weeks, self-assisted active forearm rotation is done with the elbow flexed 90°. Three months after surgery, the patient can begin strengthening exercises and resume full activity. Very muscular patients may be treated with indomethacin for 2 weeks as a prophylaxis against forming heterotopic ossification, but it is also acceptable to use indomethacin routinely or not at all.

▶ The authors present a case of an acute distal biceps tendon rupture and discuss the up-to-date evidence regarding treatment options to enable the surgeon to best counsel the patient. There is good evidence to suggest that without surgery, the patient will most likely experience weakness in flexion and supination strength in the arm. Classical teaching is that the patient will lose 30% flexion strength and 40% supination strength. More recent studies suggest that patients may also lose endurance with supination. The most common risks associated with surgery are heterotopic ossification, lateral antecubital neuritis, or posterior interosseous nerve palsy. Equivocal results have been shown with both a single-incision technique vs a 2-incision technique. A single-incision technique may have a higher risk of posterior interosseous nerve palsy. A 2-incision technique may have a higher risk of heterotopic ossification. Biomechanical studies have shown superiority of interference screw fixation. Bioresorbable anchors have been reported to cause osteolysis at the radial tuberosity. Fractures sustained using the traditional technique with transosseous tunnels have also been reported. The surgeon should choose the technique with which he or she has become most familiar. The results for surgical fixation are positive and reliable overall.

E. Cheung, MD

Diagnosing ulnar neuropathy at the elbow using magnetic resonance neurography

Keen NN, Chin CT, Engstrom JW, et al (Univ of California San Francisco)
Skeletal Radiol 41:401-407, 2012

Introduction.—Early diagnosis of ulnar neuropathy at the elbow is important. Magnetic resonance neurography (MRN) images peripheral nerves. We evaluated the usefulness of elbow MRN in diagnosing ulnar neuropathy at the elbow.

Methods.—The MR neurograms of 21 patients with ulnar neuropathy were reviewed retrospectively. MRN was performed prospectively on 10 normal volunteers. The MR neurograms included axial T1 and axial T2 fat-saturated and/or axial STIR sequences. The sensitivity and specificity of MRN in detecting ulnar neuropathy were determined.

Results.—The mean ulnar nerve size in the symptomatic and normal groups was 0.12 and 0.06 cm^2 ($P < 0.001$). The mean relative signal intensity in the symptomatic and normal groups was 2.7 and 1.4 ($P < 0.01$). When using a size of 0.08 cm^2, sensitivity was 95% and specificity was 80%.

Discussion.—Ulnar nerve size and signal intensity were greater in patients with ulnar neuropathy. MRN is a useful test in evaluating ulnar neuropathy at the elbow.

▶ The stated goals of this study were to "assess the sensitivity and specificity of magnetic resonance neurography (MRN) for ulnar neuropathy at the elbow, to develop initial standards for the use of MRN in evaluating ulnar neuropathy, and to demonstrate that changes in the appearance of the nerve on MRN can complement current diagnostic modalities in difficult cases." It did not accomplish any of these.

This is unfortunate, because an objective test to diagnose ulnar neuropathy other than an electromyogram (EMG)/nerve conduction study (NCS) would be welcomed. Most patients find the EMG/NCS test unpleasant, and the results are very much operator-dependent.

The study population comprised individuals whom neurologists referred to radiology with a presumptive diagnosis of ulnar neuropathy. The diagnosis was based on a purely clinical basis. Only 12 of the 21 patients had an EMG/NCS.

Of those 12, 3 had a normal study and 1 showed only a median neuropathy. Eight of the 21 patients had an EMG/NCS consistent with ulnar neuropathy.

Confounding matters further was that 5 patients had prior elbow surgery and yet another 5 had a history of trauma to the elbow. In addition, the magnetic resonance protocol was not consistent in all the patients. Some (8) had additional T1-weighted spin echo images after intravenous (IV) gadopentetate, and the others received no IV contrast.

The authors went on to say that since these studies were performed, better imaging techniques (newer fat-suppression techniques) have become available, which may change the accuracy of the results.

Based on this, I believe that this study does not provide a basis for any sort of statement about MRN standards. I do look forward to their future work because this modality is clearly in its infancy, and alternatives to the EMG/NCS are needed.

J. Frankenhoff, MD

Predictors of Surgical Outcomes Following Anterior Transposition of Ulnar Nerve for Cubital Tunnel Syndrome: A Systematic Review

Shi Q, MacDermid JC, Santaguida PL, et al (McMaster Univ, Hamilton, Ontario, Canada; St Joseph's Health Centre, London, Ontario, Canada)
J Hand Surg 36A:1996-2001.e6, 2011

Purpose.—Although cubital tunnel syndrome is the second most common nerve entrapment neuropathy, few studies explore potential predictor(s) of surgical outcomes. The purpose of this systematic review was to determine which factors affect the postoperative outcome for patients who undertake anterior transposition of the ulnar nerve.

Methods.—We included all studies reporting predictor(s) of clinical, electrophysiological study, or functional outcome after any anterior transposition of the ulnar nerve. We searched the Cochrane Central Register of Controlled Trials, MEDLINE, EMBASE, and CINAHL from 1980 to April 2011 and reference lists of articles. Two reviewers performed study selection, assessment of methodological quality, and data extraction independently of each other.

Results.—We assessed 26 studies including 2 randomized controlled trials, 10 cohort studies, and 14 case series. Overall, the methodological quality of the studies ranged from low to moderate. Six aspects of prognosis were sufficiently studied for a narrative evidence synthesis on age, duration of symptom, severity of operative status, preoperative electrodiagnostic testing results, type of surgery, and work compensation status. Evidence was conflicting across studies in terms of both the direction and intensity of the impact of these 6 potential predictors on surgical outcomes.

Conclusions.—Because of conflicting results, we were unable to conclude which predictor(s) affect surgical outcomes after anterior transposition of the ulnar nerve. Surgeons who are aware of only a limited number of prognostic studies and their limited scope of evidence may not appreciate the extent of the inconsistency about whether factors commonly viewed as prognostic actually have a noteworthy impact on outcomes achieved. Such factors may be identified in the future with higher-quality studies, because limitations in the current research undoubtedly contribute to the controversies observed.

▶ Cubital tunnel syndrome surgery is common, but the outcome is not uniformly good. Predictors of outcome would be helpful for decision making and patient education. However, this is hindered by a paucity of predictor information for surgical outcomes. This is partly due to the lack of well-conceived and well-executed clinical studies studying possible predictors. Another reason is that research in this area is complicated by different surgical techniques to treat the condition, differences in patient populations, and the numerous possible outcome measures.

This systematic review attempted to shed some light onto possible predictors by combining the results from various studies. However, no conclusive predictors were found: poor methodology, small sample sizes, and conflicting results were among the reasons cited. The authors suggest that one of the key contributions of this work is to highlight the inconsistency in the reported literature about possible predictors.

In light of this, surgeons should consider the key finding of this study when deciding on anterior transposition: There is a lack of clear evidence on which factors predict outcomes following this surgery for cubital tunnel syndrome. However, surgeons' own experience can add weight to their own decision making. An audit of their own practice, or their institution's experience, will help profile their own patients to enable better patient education and clinical decision making.

A. Chong, MD

Therapeutic Implications of the Radiographic "Drop Sign" Following Elbow Dislocation
Pipicelli JG, Chinchalkar SJ, Grewal R, et al (Western Univ, London, Ontario, Canada; St Joseph's Health Care, London, Ontario, Canada)
J Hand Ther 25:346-353, 2012

A radiographic drop sign following elbow trauma is an abnormality that is controversial with limited information describing optimal management. The consequences of this complex clinical situation includes limited motion, pain, and joint impingement, which may lead to joint stiffness and contracture formation. These authors describe the therapeutic implications of this radiographic finding and present a treatment approach in order to enhance patient outcomes (Figs 1 and 5, Table 1).

▶ A radiographic drop sign represents a measurable increase in the ulnohumeral joint space (Fig 1). It commonly occurs in the setting of elbow instability and can be indicative of persistent instability. Certainly, in the setting of elbow trauma,

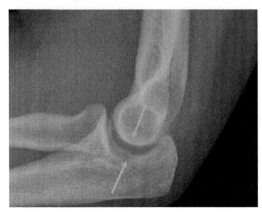

FIGURE 1.—A drop sign is a radiographically measurable increase in ulnohumeral joint distance evident on lateral radiograph. (Reprinted from Journal of Hand Therapy. Pipicelli JG, Chinchalkar SJ, Grewal R, et al. Therapeutic implications of the radiographic "drop Sign" following elbow dislocation. *J Hand Ther.* 2012;25:346-353, Copyright 2013, with permission from the American Society of Hand Therapists.)

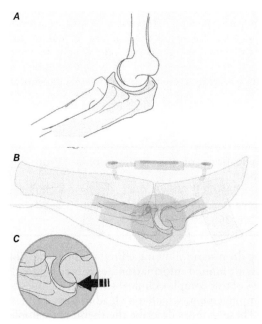

FIGURE 5.—A. Schematic of drop sign. B. Schematic of an elbow in approximately 30° of elbow extension with an unresolved drop sign. C. Schematic of static-progressive elbow extension orthosis with an unresolved drop sign. This form of splinting will likely cause posterior joint impingement, hinging, inflamation, and pain. (Reproduced With Permission of Techniques in Hand and Upper Extremity Surgery. 2011;15:198−208). (Reprinted from Journal of Hand Therapy. Pipicelli JG, Chinchalkar SJ, Grewal R, et al. Therapeutic implications of the radiographic "drop Sign" following elbow dislocation. *J Hand Ther.* 2012;25:346-353, Copyright 2012, with permission from the American Society of Hand Therapists.)

TABLE 1.—Overhead, Isometric, and Isotonic Exercise Regime

Weeks	Exercise Regime	Frequency
0–6	1. Overhead active elbow flexion and extension within established safe arc of motion. Elbow extension is advanced by 108 increments on a weekly basis. 2. Overhead active pronation and supination with the elbow positioned at 90°.	Exercises are performed every 1–2 h during the day for 10 to 20 repetitions.
	3. Isometric co-contraction of brachialis, biceps, and triceps.	Exercises are performed 4 to 6 times per day for 5 to 10 repetitions. Each repetition is held for 5-10 sec in duration.
2–6	Isotonic exercise of the wrist flexors and extensors	Exercises are performed 1 to 2 times per day for 15–30 repetitions using a 1–2 lb weight.
	Isotonic exercise of the digital flexors and extensors	Exercises are performed 1 to 2 times per day for 15–30 repetitions using a stress ball or thera-putty.
Radiographic drop sign reduced and joint stability confirmed by physician		
6–8	AROM and PROM permitted in all directions	Exercises are performed every 1–2 h during the day for 8–15 repititions.
8–12	Progressed to isotonic strengthening of the elbow flexors, extensors, forearm rotators, and shoulder. Mobilization splinting applied as necessary.	Exercises are performed 1 to 2 times per day for 15–30 repititions using lightweights or resistive bands.

injury, swelling, and edema in the muscles about the elbow, which act as dynamic stabilizers, can exacerbate the sag seen in the setting of ligament injury.

The authors suggest referral to therapy within 3 to 5 days after an elbow dislocation to initiate active mobilization of the elbow within the established safe arc of motion and according to the constraints dictated by the presence of associated ligamentous injuries.

In the setting of lateral collateral ligament injuries, the forearm is positioned in pronation, whereas in the setting of medial collateral ligament injuries, the forearm is supinated. If both sides are injured, then a neutral position is preferred.

Patients are given a resting splint set at 80° to 90° degrees of flexion. Specifics regarding the suggested treatment algorithm are noted in Table 1.

After this treatment, algorithm results in correction of the drop sign within 2 to 6 weeks in most cases. If it does not, then care should be taken to assure that hinging does not occur, particularly with application of static progressive joint splints (Fig 5).

J. E. Adams, MD

Acute carpal tunnel syndrome in trauma
Jhattu H, Klaassen S, Ying C, et al (The Canberra Hosp, Australia)
Eur J Plast Surg 35:639-646, 2012

Carpal tunnel syndrome (CTS) is one of the commonest compression neuropathy. It carries significant employment and health care costs and causes much grief to patients. There are numerous causes for carpal tunnel syndrome; however, in this review, the authors concentrate on trauma as a primary etiology. CTS is essentially a compression of the median nerve within the carpal tunnel producing debilitating symptoms and signs. Early recognition of the clinical presentation of this syndrome is vital, since it is a surgical emergency and urgent release is indicated. The anatomy, etiology, pathogenesis, clinical features, investigations, and management with case presentation have been discussed in detail, referencing a diverse collection of textbooks and papers. A comprehensive literature review of 44 papers was performed, with compilation of current treatment guidelines and management. Picture illustrations of a case encountered by the authors are included for better understanding for clinicians and trainees. This article describes acute CTS in detail and provides information for correct and early diagnosis together with effective treatment. The risk factors and treatment options are discussed in detail with photographic illustrations, providing simple but comprehensive material for education of students and clinicians, therefore to improve outcome of patients with this potentially devastating condition.

▶ This article provides an excellent review of the pathogenesis, etiology, and treatment for acute carpal tunnel syndrome. The authors performed a literature review of nearly 45 papers and used this information to provide treatment guidelines.

Common etiologies were primarily trauma based, including distal radius and scaphoid fractures, crush injuries, penetrating trauma (eg, stab or gunshot wounds), dislocations, and iatrogenic causes. The authors reviewed the anatomy associated with carpal tunnel syndrome and the clinical presentation.

Based on their literature review, the article clearly favors immediate surgical intervention as the treatment that affords the optimal outcome and recovery. Unfortunately, surgery associated with acute carpal tunnel inherits increased complexity and complication rates.

This article provides a concise overview of acute carpal tunnel syndrome and its treatment based on an extensive literature review.

M. Rizzo, MD

Predicting the Outcome of Revision Carpal Tunnel Release
Beck JD, Brothers JG, Maloney PJ, et al (Geisinger Med Ctr, Danville, PA)
J Hand Surg 37A:282-287, 2012

Purpose.—To test the hypothesis that the result of steroid injection in the carpal tunnel in a patient with recurrent carpal tunnel symptoms would serve as a good predictor of the outcome of later carpal tunnel release (CTR).

Methods.—We conducted a retrospective review of all patients who underwent revision CTR for recurrent or persistent carpal tunnel syndrome over a 2-year period at our institution. A total of 28 wrists in 23 patients met inclusion criteria. We evaluated patients to determine whether preoperative factors or the result of injection predicted the outcome of revision CTR. We used a multivariate logistic regression analysis to predict surgical success when multiple preoperative findings were considered.

Results.—Of the 23 wrists that had relief from injection, 20 had symptom improvement with surgery. Although they did not reach statistical significance, the sensitivity and positive predictive value for injection alone predicted outcome of revision CTR in 87%. No patient characteristic or physical examination finding predicted successful revision CTR. Multivariate logistic regression analysis combining preoperative injection results with physical examination findings (numbness and/or motor weakness in median nerve distribution, positive Durkin test, and positive Phalen test) provided a sensitivity of 100% and a specificity of 80%.

Conclusions.—In a small group of patients with recurrent carpal tunnel syndrome, cortisone injection into the carpal tunnel was not, by itself, a statistically significant predictor of successful revision surgery. However, relief from injection as a diagnostic test for predicting successful revision CTR was found to have both a high sensitivity and a positive predictive value. Coupled with the components of the physical examination, injection provides a good screening test to establish surgical success with revision CTR.

Type of Study/Level of Evidence.—Therapeutic III.

▶ This small series looked at the ability of response to steroid injection to predict the result after revision carpal tunnel release. The differences were not statistically significant (20 of 23 responders improved with second surgery vs 3 of 5 nonresponders), but the authors conclude that the procedure is worthwhile and note that the subset of patients with a response to injection, median sensory loss or thenar weakness, and positive Phalen or Durkan test all improved after the second surgery.

It is my opinion that injection is useful, but one must conclude that the case for routine use of injection to help select patients for reoperation after failed carpal tunnel release is, to use the Scottish legal term, "not proven" by this study.

P. C. Amadio, MD

Incidence of Carpal Tunnel Release: Trends and Implications Within the United States Ambulatory Care Setting
Fajardo M, Kim SH, Szabo RM (Univ of California, Davis, Sacramento)
J Hand Surg 37A:1599-1605, 2012

Purpose.—To investigate the changes, trends, and implications of carpal tunnel release (CTR) surgery within an ambulatory setting over the past decade in the United States.

Methods.—We undertook an analysis of ambulatory surgery center CTR cases using data from the National Survey of Ambulatory Surgery. The Centers for Disease Control and Prevention carried out this survey in 1996, and again in 2006. We searched the cases with the procedure codes indicative of CTR.

Results.—The number of CTR procedures increased by 38% (from 360,000 to 577,000) between 1996 and 2006. In 1996, 16% of all ambulatory CTRs were performed in freestanding ambulatory surgery centers (hospital-based centers were 84%), and the proportion increased to 49% in 2006. By 2006, greater than 99% of CTRs were performed in an ambulatory setting. There was a significant increase in women aged 50 to 59 years of age undergoing CTR.

Conclusions.—The minimal invasiveness of CTR combined with the advent of ambulatory care facilities has made CTR a predominantly outpatient procedure. In contrast to other reports, our study demonstrated a higher incidence of CTR within the United States in 2006 compared with 1996. Elderly women, in particular, with CTS were 3 times more likely to be treated surgically than other age groups. Further study is needed to better define factors influencing CTR indications.

Type of Study/Level of Evidence.—Prognostic II.

▶ This epidemiologic study by Szabo et al looked at demographic trends of carpal tunnel release (CTR) surgery in the United States using a national database in 1996 and 2006. These trends suggest a number of interesting findings, including a shift from the inpatient to outpatient setting, and an overall increase in CTR surgery, particularly in women 50 to 59 years of age. The authors also point out that CTR surgery performed in the outpatient setting is more efficient (30-minute average longer stay for the patient undergoing CTR at a hospital-based facility) as well as less costly (22% less). The authors also suggest that the future of CTR surgery may be office based and performed under straight local anesthesia, as it is typically performed in Canada. My own experience echoes these trends, with a shift in my practice away from the hospital to free-standing ambulatory surgery centers using local anesthesia with light sedation.

D. Zelouf, MD

Expected and Actual Improvement of Symptoms With Carpal Tunnel Release
Becker SJE, Makanji HS, Ring D (Massachusetts General Hosp, Boston)
J Hand Surg 37A:1324-1329, 2012

Purpose.—This study tested the null hypothesis that there is no difference between expected improvement and actual improvement of symptoms with carpal tunnel release (CTR). Secondary analyses addressed factors associated with both expected relief and actual relief of symptoms with carpal tunnel syndrome surgical release, predictors of arm-specific disability, and satisfaction with surgery.

Methods.—Sixty-six employed, English-speaking adult patients requesting limited-incision open CTR for electrodiagnostically confirmed carpal tunnel syndrome completed questionnaires before and after surgery. Before surgery, patients completed a survey regarding demographic data, expected improvement of symptoms with surgery, expected return to work after surgery, and validated questionnaires assessing arm-specific disability, job burnout, depressive symptoms, catastrophic thinking, and pain anxiety. An average of 6 ± 5 months (range, 40 d to 19 mo) after surgery, participants completed questionnaires regarding actual improvement of symptoms with surgery, actual return to work, satisfaction with surgery, and arm-specific disability.

Results.—Patients' actual and expected improvements with CTR were similar, with the exception of sleep disturbance, which was an average 0.3 points better than patients expected on a 5-point Likert scale. Lower postoperative disability was associated with men, less catastrophic thinking, and greater actual improvement of weakness with CTR. Fifty-three percent of the variation in satisfaction with treatment was associated with single status, more education, and relief of pain, sleep disturbance, and tingling.

Conclusions.—Actual relief of symptoms with CTR matched patients' expectations in an employed population. Satisfaction with treatment correlated with relief of symptoms.

▶ The authors found that expected and actual symptom improvement after carpal tunnel release is comparable. The point they make—in the end—is that preoperative expectations can significantly influence postoperative satisfaction. Not surprisingly, patient satisfaction was largely linked to actual relief of symptoms. An interesting finding is that relief of sleep disturbance significantly exceeded patient expectations. In addition, patients who expected to take fewer days off from work after surgery demonstrated higher expected improvements in sleep disturbance. Conversely, patients who experienced less actual improvement in their numbness postoperatively more frequently experienced changed work roles secondary to carpal tunnel syndrome before surgery. There is clearly a component of self-reliance and optimistic thinking that influences postoperative outcomes.

The strength of this study lies in its prospective cohort design. The study's weaknesses included limited power and the loss of 28% of enrolled patients, which may have skewed the final results. In addition, the questionnaire was administered at varying time frames with a range of 40 days to 19 months after surgery.

E. Shin, MD

Predictors of Surgical Outcomes Following Anterior Transposition of Ulnar Nerve for Cubital Tunnel Syndrome: A Systematic Review

Shi Q, MacDermid JC, Santaguida PL, et al (McMaster Univ, Hamilton, Ontario, Canada; St Joseph's Health Centre, London, Ontario, Canada)
J Hand Surg 36A:1996-2001.e6, 2011

Purpose.—Although cubital tunnel syndrome is the second most common nerve entrapment neuropathy, few studies explore potential predictor(s) of surgical outcomes. The purpose of this systematic review was to determine which factors affect the postoperative outcome for patients who undertake anterior transposition of the ulnar nerve.

Methods.—We included all studies reporting predictor(s) of clinical, electrophysiological study, or functional outcome after any anterior transposition of the ulnar nerve. We searched the Cochrane Central Register of Controlled Trials, MEDLINE, EMBASE, and CINAHL from 1980 to April 2011 and reference lists of articles. Two reviewers performed study selection, assessment of methodological quality, and data extraction independently of each other.

Results.—We assessed 26 studies including 2 randomized controlled trials, 10 cohort studies, and 14 case series. Overall, the methodological quality of the studies ranged from low to moderate. Six aspects of prognosis were sufficiently studied for a narrative evidence synthesis on age, duration of symptom, severity of operative status, preoperative electrodiagnostic testing results, type of surgery, and work compensation status. Evidence was conflicting across studies in terms of both the direction and intensity of the impact of these 6 potential predictors on surgical outcomes.

Conclusions.—Because of conflicting results, we were unable to conclude which predictor(s) affect surgical outcomes after anterior transposition of the ulnar nerve. Surgeons who are aware of only a limited number of prognostic studies and their limited scope of evidence may not appreciate the extent of the inconsistency about whether factors commonly viewed as prognostic actually have a noteworthy impact on outcomes achieved. Such factors may be identified in the future with higher-quality studies, because limitations in the current research undoubtedly contribute to the controversies observed.

▶ Shi et al set out to answer an important and perplexing question: How can I tell if this patient with ulnar nerve entrapment will get better with surgery? The authors performed a systematic review of the literature addressing prognostic factors for outcome after anterior transposition of the ulnar nerve. They specifically looked at whether patient age, duration of symptoms, severity of preoperative status, preoperative electrodiagnostic testing, type of surgery (submuscular or subcutaneous transposition), or workers compensation status correlated with postoperative outcome.

They encountered many of the usual problems seen with systematic reviews: variation in study design and quality, limited power from small numbers, and inconsistency of outcome measures. For example, only a few studies addressed type of surgery and workers compensation status. Some outcomes were based on patients' recall of their symptoms prior to surgery. With each of the 6 prognostic factors examined, some studies supported a correlation, and some refuted any correlation, leaving the authors to report no consistent relationship between these 6 prognostic factors and results after anterior transposition of the ulnar nerve.

Use of a standard outcome measure for ulnar nerve entrapment and better study design may result in identification of prognostic factors in the future, but for now we remain in the dark.

C. M. Ward, MD

The outcome of carpal tunnel decompression in patients with diabetes mellitus

Jenkins PJ, Duckworth AD, Watts AC, et al (Queen Margaret Hosp, Dunfermline, UK)
J Bone Joint Surg Br 94-B:811-814, 2012

Diabetes mellitus is recognised as a risk factor for carpal tunnel syndrome. The response to treatment is unclear, and may be poorer than in non-diabetic patients. Previous randomised studies of interventions for carpal tunnel syndrome have specifically excluded diabetic patients. The aim of this study was to investigate the epidemiology of carpal tunnel syndrome in diabetic patients, and compare the outcome of carpal tunnel decompression with non-diabetic patients. The primary endpoint was improvement in the QuickDASH score. The prevalence of diabetes mellitus was 11.3% (176 of 1564). Diabetic patients were more likely to have severe neurophysiological findings at presentation. Patients with diabetes had poorer QuickDASH scores at one year post-operatively ($p = 0.028$), although the mean difference was lower than the minimal clinically important difference for this score. After controlling for underlying differences in age and gender, there was no difference between groups in the magnitude of improvement after decompression ($p = 0.481$). Patients with diabetes mellitus can therefore be expected to enjoy a similar improvement in function.

▶ This article aims to investigate the epidemiology of carpal tunnel syndrome (CTS) in diabetic patients and their outcome after surgical treatment. Of the patients who received carpal tunnel release (CTR) in a single hand center in a Scotland, 11.3% had diabetes mellitus (DM). The mean age of diabetic patients was significantly higher than that of normoglycemic patients (58.4 vs 54.7 years).

Although there were poorer QuickDASH scores in the patients with DM treated with CTR at 1 year postoperative follow-up, this difference was lower than a clin-ically important difference. There was no difference of health-related life quality after CTR between diabetic and nondiabetic patients.

So far, there has been little information about the outcome of carpal tunnel surgery in diabetic patients, as many prospective studies excluded this patient group.

The evidence provided in this study of 1564 CTS patients is useful for hand surgeons in preoperative counseling of patients with diabetes, as it suggests that these patients do similarly well to normoglycemic patients.

M. S. S. Choi, MD

Accuracy of Ultrasonography and Magnetic Resonance Imaging in Diagnosing Carpal Tunnel Syndrome Using Rest and Grasp Positions of the Hands

Horng Y-S, Chang H-C, Lin K-E, et al (Buddhist Tzu Chi General Hosp, Taipei Branch, Taiwan; Tzu Chi Univ, Hualien, Taiwan; Natl Taiwan Univ, Taipei; et al)
J Hand Surg 37A:1591-1598, 2012

Purpose.—To compare the accuracy of ultrasonography and magnetic resonance imaging (MRI) in diagnosing carpal tunnel syndrome (CTS) in both the rest and grasp positions. We postulated that the diagnostic accuracy could be improved by imaging hands in the grasp position rather than in the rest position.

Methods.—Fifty patients with CTS and 45 healthy volunteers received a package of questionnaires and had a physical examination and a nerve conduction study. Ultrasonography and MRI images were recorded in both the rest and grasp positions for each participant.

Results.—There were significant differences between the patients and the healthy volunteers regarding patient-reported outcomes, the results of physical examinations, the nerve conduction studies, and the ultrasonography and MRI imaging. The area under the receiver operating characteristic curve of ultrasonography was significantly improved by measuring the bowing of the flexor retinaculum in the grasp position than by measuring that in the rest position. The diagnostic accuracy of ultrasonography was similar to that of MRI when we used a combination of the measurements of the cross-sectional area of the median nerve in the rest position and the bowing of the flexor retinaculum in the grasp position.

Conclusions.—The accuracies of MRI and ultrasonography for diagnosing CTS were improved by measuring the bowing of the flexor retinaculum in the grasp position. Ultrasonography can be an adequate screening method for CTS if clinicians combine the cross-sectional area of the median nerve in the rest position and the bowing of the flexor retinaculum in the grasp position.

Type of Study/Level of Evidence.—Diagnostic I.

▶ Even though carpal tunnel syndrome (CTS) is a clinical diagnosis, supportive diagnostic tests are commonly employed.[1] The current gold standard for confirming CTS is electrodiagnostic testing (nerve conduction study [NCS]/ electromyogram [EMG]). Other possible tests, such as magnetic resonance neurography (MRN) and ultrasonography (US), are on the horizon and may ultimately prove to be more objective, sensitive, and specific than electrodiagnostics.

Objective, reproducible tests prior to a surgical release would be helpful. This feeling is shared by the American Academy of Orthopaedic Surgeons and drives the current recommendation to obtain a NCS/EMG in suspected cases of CTS prior to surgical release.[2] Because of the lack of good data, they recommend against the use of newer diagnostic tools: "The physician should not routinely evaluate patients suspected of having carpal tunnel syndrome with new technology, such as magnetic resonance imaging, computed tomography, and pressure-specified sensorimotor devices in the wrist and hand."

Studies like this one have the potential to change that recommendation. Previous studies[3-6] have assessed the accuracy, sensitivity, and specificity of MRN and US. They have not yet shown them to be better than electrodiagnostics, especially with respect to specificity.

This study examined whether studying the nerve with the hand in the grasp position increases the diagnostic accuracy of CTS using both MRN and US. It showed that the accuracy of US began to approach that of MRN when a combination of the cross-sectional area measurements in rest and grasp positions was used.

This is encouraging because US is certainly less expensive and better tolerated by patients. Unfortunately, the accuracy of both MRN and US was better in electrodiagnostically severe cases. This obviously limits the usefulness of these modalities as current screening tools. Further investigations like this may ultimately determine imagings' final positioning in the diagnostic armamentarium.

J. Frankenhoff, MD

References

1. Jablecki CK, Andary MT, Floeter MK, et al. Practice parameter: Electrodiagnostic studies in carpal tunnel syndrome. Report of the American Association of Electrodiagnostic Medicine, American Academy of Neurology, and the American Academy of Physical Medicine and Rehabilitation. *Neurology.* 2002;58:1589-1592.
2. American Academy of Orthopaedic Surgeons. AAOC-website. http://www.aaos.org/Research/guidelines/guide.asp. Accessed September, 2008.
3. Wiesler, Chloros GD, Cartwright MS, Smith BP, Rushing J, Walker FO. The use of diagnostic ultrasound in carpal tunnel syndrome. *J Hand Surg Am.* 2006;31: 726 732.
4. Khachi, Skirgaudes M, Lee WP, Wollstein R. The clinical applications of peripheral nerve imaging in the upper extremity. *J Hand Surg Am.* 2007;32:1600-1604.
5. Deniz, Oksüz E, Sarikaya B, et al. Comparison of the diagnostic utility of electromyography, ultrasonography, computed tomography, and magnetic resonance imaging in idiopathic carpal tunnel syndrome determined by clinical findings. *Neurosurgery.* 2012;70:610-616.
6. Kwon BC, Jung KI, Baek GH. Comparison of sonography and electrodiagnostic testing in the diagnosis of carpal tunnel syndrome. *J Hand Surg Am.* 2008;33: 65-71.

6 Nerve

Clinical outcomes following brachialis to anterior interosseous nerve transfers: Report of 4 cases
Ray WZ, Yarbrough CK, Yee A, et al (Washington Univ School of Medicine, St Louis, MO)
J Neurosurg 117:604-609, 2012

The surgical management of lower brachial plexus injuries remains a challenging problem. Although nerve transfers have improved clinical outcomes following brachial plexus injuries, the majority of work has focused on upper trunk injuries. Complete lower plexus injuries often lack suitable donors for either nerve or tendon transfers. The authors describe their experience with isolated lower trunk injuries utilizing the nerve to the brachialis to reinnervate the anterior interosseous nerve.

▶ Isolated lower plexus injuries are extremely uncommon in comparison to upper plexus and complete plexus injuries, reflecting the relative paucity of literature and surgical techniques available in regard to their treatments. As opposed to upper plexus lesions, there is a shortage of appropriate donors for nerve and tendon transfers to restore hand function. The authors propose a novel nerve transfer for reinnervation of the anterior interosseous nerve, with the assumption that the brachialis is an expendable donor (which the authors appropriately justify). Although this is a small case series of 4 patients, their reported results suggest significant improvement in hand function. There is little time spent on surgical technique, but the schematic drawing and well-labeled intraoperative pictures are excellent.

Based on the authors' description, however, it seems only 3 of the 4 patients truly had isolated lower plexus injuries. Case 2 is presented as the patient having "regained some weak motor response in his... biceps and radial wrist extension" prior to undergoing nerve transfer. This implies that the musculocutaneous nerve (and, thus, nerve to the brachialis) was perhaps regenerating, and it is generally contraindicated to use this type of nerve as a donor. This also directly contradicts their later advice in the discussion section: "the brachialis represents a strong motor donor when elbow flexion is normal, but we believe it should only be used when elbow flexion is normal." Other than this discrepancy, this is another innovative and thoughtful approach to the treatment of a complex problem. For surgeons who treat brachial plexus patients, this technique should be considered for restoration of partial hand function in the isolated lower plexus patient.

R. C. Chadderdon, MD

Ultrasound in Pediatric Peripheral Nerve Injuries: Can This Affect Our Surgical Decision Making? A Preliminary Report

Lee J, Bidwell T, Metcalfe R (Middlemore Hosp, Otahuhu, New Zealand; Starship Hosp, Grafton, Auckland, New Zealand)
J Pediatr Orthop 33:152-158, 2013

Background.—The treatment of closed fractures with associated peripheral nerve palsy is controversial. Traditionally, the nerve palsy is managed with watchful waiting and subsequent neurophysiological studies if no improvement is seen within 4 months. This may not be necessary if nerve integrity can be imaged acutely with ultrasound scan. We present a case series of pediatric patients with closed upper limb injuries and associated peripheral nerve palsy who underwent ultrasound scanning to assess nerve integrity.

Methods.—A retrospective review of patients attending Starship Children's Hospital between May 2008 and April 2010 with closed upper limb injuries and associated peripheral nerve palsy was undertaken. Those patients up to and including the age of 14 years (skeletally immature) with complete clinical records available were included.

Results.—Complete clinical records were available for 24 patients who fit the inclusion criteria for the period of May 2008 to April 2010. Fifteen patients were managed expectantly and showed signs of spontaneous nerve recovery at a mean of 4 weeks. One patient proceeded to theater for early exploration where an intact but kinked nerve was found. Eight patients underwent ultrasound examination of their nerves; on the basis of the ultrasound findings, 3 proceeded to theater for nerve repair or neurolysis and 5 were managed expectantly with first signs of nerve recovery seen at a mean of 12 weeks for the surgical group, and 13.2 weeks for the nonsurgical group.

Conclusions.—Ultrasound examination of peripheral nerves provides pathomorphologic information that can aid our clinical decision-making process and identify those patients who would benefit from early surgical intervention. In our case series, ultrasound findings correlated with intraoperative findings and clinical recovery.

Level of Evidence.—Level III evidence retrospective comparative study.

▶ Peripheral nerve injuries associated with closed fractures have a high rate of spontaneous recovery. Because of this, many surgeons watch these expectantly, and, as this article supports, will be rewarded with a good outcome. The problem is that some patients do need surgical intervention—these patients are often referred late and explored late. The ability to identify which patients will fail expectant observation would be extremely useful. Though there will be patients who have intact nerves but will still fail observation, the ability to visualize the nerves, either through magnetic resonance imaging (MRI) or ultrasound (US), will identify at least some of the patients that will benefit from early exploration. This study supports this concept. Weaknesses of the article include an extremely small sample size of 8 patients. Although the abstract suggests that 24 patients were in the study, 16 of those never underwent US and should have been excluded! Because US is a useful modality in adults, it stands to reason that it will be useful in pediatric patients that, in general, should have less adipose tissue and smaller limbs than their adult counterparts. Additionally, the ability to lie still while an MRI is being performed is often lacking in the pediatric population, adding to the appeal of US as the modality of choice for nerve visualization.

J. Isaacs, MD

Effectiveness of Fibrin Adhesive in Facial Nerve Anastomosis in Dogs Compared With Standard Microsuturing Technique
Attar BM, Zalzali H, Razavi M, et al (Isfahan Univ of Med Sciences, Iran)
J Oral Maxillofac Surg 70:2427-2432, 2012

Purpose.—Epineural suturing is the most common technique used for peripheral nerve anastomosis. In addition to the foreign body reaction to the suture material, the surgical duration and difficulty of suturing in confined anatomic locations are major problems. We evaluated the effectiveness of fibrin glue as an acceptable alternative for nerve anastomosis in dogs.

Methods.—Eight adult female dogs weighing 18 to 24 kg were used in the present study. The facial nerve was transected bilaterally. On the right side, the facial nerve was subjected to epineural suturing; and on the left side, the nerve was anastomosed using fibrin adhesive. After 16 weeks, the nerve conduction velocity and proportion of the nerve fibers that crossed the anastomosis site were evaluated and compared for the epineural suture (right side) and fibrin glue (left side). The data were analyzed using the paired t test and univariate analysis of variance.

Results.—The mean postoperative nerve conduction velocity was 29.87 ± 7.65 m/s and 26.75 ± 3.97 m/s on the right and left side, respectively. No statistically significant difference was found in the postoperative nerve conduction velocity between the 2 techniques ($P = .444$). The proportion of nerve fibers that crossed the anastomotic site was 71.25% ± 7.59% and 72.25% ± 8.31% on the right and left side, respectively. The histologic evaluation showed no statistically significant difference in the proportion of the nerve fibers that crossed the anastomotic site between the 2 techniques ($P = .598$).

Conclusions.—The results suggest that the efficacies of epineural suturing and fibrin gluing in peripheral nerve anastomosis are similar.

▶ Ok. Fibrin glue works to hold nerve ends together. We can stop killing lab animals to prove this point over and over again. The main concern with using fibrin glue as a coaptation aid is that the nerve ends can pull apart. This has been shown in rat hind limbs.[1] Additionally, we showed in the lab that fibrin glue resisted gapping but did not add significant holding strength to nerve repairs over a couple of 8-0 sutures.[2] This study looking at dog fascial nerves is perhaps an easier test of the efficacy of fibrin glue than studies already done. Specifically because there is little tension on this repair—unlike a moving rat hind limb–the dogs most likely did not stress these repairs very much.

It should be pointed out that use of fibrin glue for nerve repairs is not approved by the US Food and Drug Administration. Additionally, the authors of this study held the nerve ends together for 60 seconds as the fibrin glue initially set up. Three minutes is the more commonly recommended initial set-up period.

J. Isaacs, MD

References

1. Maragh H, Meyer BS, Davenport D, Gould JD, Terzis JK. Morphofunctional evaluation of fibrin glue versus microsuture nerve repairs. *J Reconstr Microsurg.* 1990; 6:331-337.
2. Isaacs JE, McDaniel CO, Owen JR, Wayne JS. Comparative analysis of biomechanical performance of available "nerve glues". *J Hand Surg Am.* 2008;33:893-899.

A new nerve coaptation technique using a biodegradable honeycomb-patterned film
Okui N, Yamamoto M, Fukuhira Y, et al (Nagoya Univ, Japan)
Microsurgery 32:466-474, 2012

We developed a biodegradable poly-lactide (PLA) film with a honeycomb-patterned porous structure (honeycomb film). This study investigated the use of this film in neurorrhaphy. Three types of PLA film were tested following bilateral sciatic nerve transection and neurorrhaphy in 35 rats: 7- and 10-µm thick honeycomb films, and cast film with no porous structures. Initially, following two-stitch neurorrhaphy, 40 limbs (20 rats) underwent wrapping in 7- or 10-µm honeycomb film, cast film, no wrapping, or extra two-stitch neurorrhaphy (8 limbs each). Breaking strength was tested 2 days postoperatively. Another 30 limbs (15 rats) then underwent wrapping in 7- or 10-µm honeycomb film, cast film, no wrapping, or sham operation (six limbs each). Histological and functional analyses were performed 6 weeks postoperatively. Breaking strength was significantly higher for the 10-µm honeycomb film than for no wrapping ($P = 0.013$), although no significant difference was observed between the 7-µm honeycomb and no wrapping ($P = 0.085$). Breaking strength for the cast film was almost equal to that for no wrapping ($P = 0.994$). Extra two-stitch (four-stitch) neurorrhaphy was significantly stronger than all groups, except the 10-µm honeycomb group. No significant difference was observed between the 10-µm honeycomb and the four-stitch ($P = 0.497$). No negative effects on functional recovery were identified. No adhesions or inflammation were observed between the film and surrounding tissues in the honeycomb groups. Honeycomb film may offer a suitable reinforcing material for adhesion-free neurorrhaphy.

▶ Developing the perfect alternative techniques for neurorrhaphy is a common aspiration of nerve surgeons and nerve researchers. The imperfections of suture techniques notwithstanding, the market potential of an effective tool for nerve coaptation is obvious. Still, no one has managed to find a way to replace sutures. Fibrin glue and nerve connectors (small conduits sutured into place) are probably the most successful alternatives, but fibrin glue doesn't provide reliable holding strength and nerve connectors still require the use of stitches. Okui et al offer a new and promising approach to this problem. Their invention is basically a thin, pliable, absorbable sheet specifically manufactured to generate substantial surface tension. This surface tension seems to hold the nerve well enough that the sheeting seemed to fail prior to the sheet-nerve surface interface. It is surprising, therefore, that the film was not able to adequately hold the coapted nerves well enough on its own. I think that this is an important contribution to nerve surgery, and I believe we will be seeing more of this type of surgical tool, but, in its present form, this will not replace the need for sutures.

J. Isaacs, MD

Use of Bioabsorbable Nerve Conduits as an Adjunct to Brachial Plexus Neurorrhaphy

Wolfe SW, Strauss HL, Garg R, et al (Hosp for Special Surgery, NY; Weill Med College of Cornell Univ, NY)

J Hand Surg 37A:1980-1985, 2012

Purpose.—The use of bioabsorbable conduits in digital nerve repair has demonstrated increased efficacy compared to direct repair (for gaps ≤ 4mm) and nerve grafting (for gaps ≥8 mm) for sensory recovery in a level 1 human trial. Although nonhuman primate studies on mixed motor-sensory nerves have documented comparable efficacy of the bioabsorbable nerve conduits when compared to nerve repair or grafting, there is minimal human clinical data on motor recovery following bioabsorbable nerve conduit repair. This study investigates the outcomes of bioabsorbable nerve conduits in pure motor nerve reconstruction for adult traumatic brachial plexus injuries.

Methods.—Over a 3-year period, 21 adult patients had 1 or more nerve-to-nerve transfers for traumatic brachial plexus palsy performed using the operative microscope. Ten nerve transfers were performed by advancing the nerve ends into a semi-permeable type I collagen conduit stabilized with 8-0 nylon sutures (conduit-assisted neurorrhaphy). Twenty-eight concurrent nerve transfers were performed using standard end-to-end neurorrhaphy and 8-0 or 9-0 nylon sutures. Clinical evaluation using the Medical Research Council grading system (MRC) was performed at 1 and 2 years postoperatively. Postoperative electromyographic studies were performed in 28 of 38 transfers at final follow-up.

Results.—Thirty transfers (17 patients) were available for 2-year follow-up evaluation. All 10 transfers performed with nerve conduits demonstrated clinical recovery and electromyographic reinnervation at 2 years. Eighteen of 20 transfers performed without conduits demonstrated clinical recovery.

Conclusions.—Although no statistical difference in functional recovery was seen in nerve transfers performed with collagen nerve conduits or by traditional neurorrhaphy, this pilot series demonstrated clinical and electromyographic recovery in 10 of 10 motor nerve repairs performed using conduits. These findings warrant continued investigation into the efficacy of conduit-assisted repair for motor nerves, especially in regards to operative time, precision of repair, and speed of nerve recovery.

Type of Study/Level of Evidence.—Therapeutic IV.

▶ Suture repair of peripheral nerves and elements of the brachial plexus is technically challenging, time consuming, and, at least theoretically, generates scar tissue at the coaptation site that could hinder axonal regeneration. The use of conduits as nerve connectors is a relatively recent concept. Advantages include a protected microenvironment between approximated nerve stumps in which a concentrated neurogenic milieu can be collected—scar tissue is blocked from invading and axons blocked from escaping. Even though sutures are still used, fewer are used for nerve repairs, and they are placed away from the nerve ends. Perhaps most importantly, the opposing fascicles should all be facing each other in contrast to epineurial suture repairs in which many fascicles are pooched to the side. Despite these extensive theoretical benefits of nerve connectors, or conduit-assisted neurorrhaphy, there are few studies offering clinical support for their usage. This study, although not extensive, is a welcomed contribution. I wish the authors had opted to include intercostal nerve transfers because this is an area when the nerve connector is especially useful. Trying to suture these tiny nerve strands to a distal stump can be quite technically challenging. Using fibrin glue to secure 2 or 3 strands together and introducing these en bloc into the nerve connector is a useful technique.

Additionally, the number of sutures used for each neurorrhaphy would be interesting comparative information. This study will affect surgical practice although additional investigation would be appropriate before widespread adoption of this technique occurs.

J. Isaacs, MD

The Effects of Denervation, Reinnervation, and Muscle Imbalance on Functional Muscle Length and Elbow Flexion Contracture Following Neonatal Brachial Plexus Injury
Weekley H, Nikolaou S, Hu L, et al (Cincinnati Children's Hosp Med Ctr, OH)
J Orthop Res 30:1335-1342, 2012

The pathophysiology of paradoxical elbow flexion contractures following neonatal brachial plexus injury (NBPI) is incompletely understood. The current study tests the hypothesis that this contracture occurs by denervation-induced impairment of elbow flexor muscle growth. Unilateral forelimb paralysis was created in mice in four neonatal (5-day-old) BPI groups (C5-6 excision, C5-6 neurotomy, C5-6 neurotomy/repair, and C5-T1 global excision), one non-neonatal BPI group (28-day-old C5-6 excision), and two neonatal muscle imbalance groups (triceps tenotomy ± C5-6 excision). Four weeks post-operatively, motor function, elbow range of motion, and biceps/brachialis functional lengths were assessed. Musculocutaneous nerve (MCN) denervation and reinnervation were assessed immunohistochemically. Elbow flexion motor recovery and elbow flexion contractures varied inversely among the neonatal BPI groups. Contracture severity correlated with biceps/brachialis shortening and MCN denervation (relative axon loss), with no contractures occurring in mice with MCN reinnervation (presence of growth cones). No contractures or biceps/brachialis shortening occurred following non-neonatal BPI, regardless of denervation or reinnervation. Neonatal triceps tenotomy did not cause contractures or biceps/brachialis shortening, nor did it worsen those following neonatal C5-6 excision. Denervation-induced functional shortening of elbow flexor muscles leads to variable elbow flexion contractures depending on the degree, permanence, and timing of denervation, independent of muscle imbalance.

▶ The pediatric musculoskeletal system is dynamic. On one side of the spectrum, macrodactyly and hemihypertrophy have been associated with lipofibromatous hamartomas of the nerves serving the area of overgrowth. On the other side, denervation may be the cause of muscle undergrowth. We know that the affected arm in children with brachial plexus birth palsies or other conditions that lead to loss of lower motor neuron function will be smaller than the unaffected arm. This study lends further evidence to the theory that muscle denervation leads to less robust longitudinal muscle growth, which, in turn, leads to joint contractures. A similar study by the same group looking at the denervation of muscles about the shoulder showed that stunted muscle growth in the rotator cuff from denervation led to the types of joint contractures and deformities seen in children with brachial plexus birth palsies. Muscle imbalance in the shoulder has been blamed for glenohumeral dysplasia and internal rotation contractures because the external rotators are usually more affected than the internal rotators. Applying the same logic to the elbow would predict elbow extension contractures, which are rarely seen in this population. The theory of muscle denervation directly leading to stunted muscle growth is appealing because it explains both the contractures seen at the elbow and the shoulder.

D. A. Zlotolow, MD

Comparison of Initial Nonoperative and Operative Management of Radial Nerve Palsy Associated With Acute Humeral Shaft Fractures

Liu G-Y, Zhang C-Y, Wu H-W (Third Xiangya Hosp of Central South Univ, Changsha, China; Hunan Cancer Hosp, Changsha, China)
Orthopedics 35:702-708, 2012

The optimal treatment approach for the initial management of radial nerve palsy associated with humeral shaft fractures has yet to be conclusively determined. The authors performed a systematic review of the literature to identify studies that compared the outcomes after initial nonoperative and operative management for radial nerve palsy associated with acute humeral shaft fractures. A meta-analysis of the data from these studies was also performed to determine whether recovery from radial nerve palsy was more favorable in one approach compared with the other. The primary outcome was recovery from radial nerve palsy and the secondary outcome was complaints after treatment. Nine articles (1 prospective observational and 8 retrospective) were included in the meta-analyses. Operative management showed no improved recovery from radial nerve palsy compared with nonoperative management. Nonoperative management was associated with a decreased risk of complaints relative to operative management. Recovery from radial nerve palsy associated with acute humeral shaft fractures is not influenced by the initial management approach.

▶ Recovery from radial nerve palsy may be affected by several factors, including mechanism of injury, extent of nerve injury, and the location of the humeral fracture. The findings from the current systematic review and subsequent meta-analysis suggest that recovery from radial nerve palsy associated with acute humeral shaft fractures is not significantly influenced by the initial management approach (nonoperative or operative). Instances of radial nerve palsy associated with humeral shaft fracture should be considered on a case-by-case basis. Initial nonoperative management should be favored, unless there is great bony displacement or angulation or open fracture. The patient can be counseled that the nerve palsy will most likely recover. A radial nerve exploration is indicated if the nerve is not showing signs of recovery after a few months. However, nerve exploration may be technically more difficult in the face of nonunion, malunion, and the presence of scar tissue, which develops over time. Unfortunately, an insufficient number of patients in this study did not allow the authors to perform meaningful subgroup analyses to determine whether the outcome of initial management is affected by these factors. The results of the current meta-analyses are limited by the available evidence. For example, the quality of the studies that are currently available is relatively low. Only a small number of studies were identified, and none were randomized controlled trials. The specific operative management approaches varied between studies (plate, nail, or undefined operative method).

E. Cheung, MD

Axonal regeneration and motor neuron survival after microsurgical nerve reconstruction

Fox IK, Brenner MJ, Johnson PJ, et al (Washington Univ School of Medicine, Saint Louis, MO; Southern Illinois Univ School of Medicine, Springfield, IL)
Microsurgery 32:552-562, 2012

Rodent models are used extensively for studying nerve regeneration, but little is known about how sprouting and pruning influence peripheral nerve fiber counts and motor neuron pools. The purpose of this study was to identify fluctuations in nerve regeneration and neuronal survival over time. One hundred and forty-four Lewis rats were randomized to end-to-end repair or nerve grafting (1.5 cm graft) after sciatic nerve transection. Quantitative histomorphometry and retrograde labeling of motor neurons were performed at 1, 3, 6, 9, 12, and 24 months and supplemented by electron microscopy. Fiber counts and motor neuron counts increased between 1 and 3 months, followed by plateau. End-to-end repair resulted in persistently higher fiber counts compared to the grafting for all time points ($P < 0.05$). Percent neural tissue and myelin width increased with time while fibrin debris dissipated. In conclusion, these data detail the natural history of regeneration and demonstrate that overall fiber counts may remain stable despite pruning.

▶ This is a large-scale experimental study on nerve regeneration performed on the sciatic nerve in Lewis rats. The authors aimed at identifying the regenerative procedures that take place after nerve repair and nerve grafting and their appearance related to time. Unlike most previous studies, this work is based on a long observation period (24 months).

A total of 144 experimental animals were divided in 2 groups. One received sciatic nerve transection and primary suture. In the other group, a 5-mm piece of sciatic nerve was resected. This gap was reconstructed with isogenic 15-mm sciatic nerve grafts from 36 donor rats.

The sciatic nerves were harvested after 1, 3, 6, 9, 12, and 24 months. Nerve regeneration was assessed by quantitative histomorphometry. The survival of motor neurons in the ventral horn of the spinal cord was investigated with fluorescence microscopy after retrograde labeling with fast blue.

The overall finding is that nerve regeneration was significantly slower and less complete after grafting as compared with the cut-and-repair group. The counts for myelinated fibers reached normal values after 1 month in the repaired sciatic nerves distal to the neurorrhaphy, whereas no myelinated fibers had crossed the second suture line in the grafted group. Both groups reached a plateau of regeneration after 3 months. Most of the clearance for fiber debris occurred during the first 9 months in both groups. Regeneration of motor neurons in the ventral horn was observed at 1 month. After 3 months, the number of recovered motor neuron bodies was higher in the repair group compared with the grafted group; however, this was not statistically significant. Signs of nerve maturity, such as myelination and percent of neural tissue within a nerve, increased over a 12-month period.

The findings of this article could have a direct influence on the clinical practice of peripheral nerve surgery. Tension-free nerve suture is a well-established dogma, which led reconstructive surgeons to decide in favor of nerve grafting, whenever there was doubt about the degree of tension. Considering the poor results of recovery after grafting, there may be a shift back toward primary repair in borderline cases.

Based on this large-scale, long-term experiment, the article sheds light on the natural course of nerve regeneration after primary repair and nerve grafting. The observations made in this study are significant, as knowledge of the regenerative sequence allows further studies to be designed more efficiently, especially in terms of their duration.

M. S. S. Choi, MD

Factors Affecting Outcome of Triceps Motor Branch Transfer for Isolated Axillary Nerve Injury

Lee J-Y, Kircher MF, Spinner RJ, et al (Catholic Univ of Korea, Seoul; Mayo Clinic, Rochester, MN)

J Hand Surg 37A:2350-2356, 2012

Purpose.—Triceps motor branch transfer has been used in upper brachial plexus injury and is potentially effective for isolated axillary nerve injury in lieu of sural nerve grafting. We evaluated the functional outcome of this procedure and determined factors that influenced the outcome.

Methods.—A retrospective chart review was performed of 21 patients (mean age, 38 y; range, 16—79 y) who underwent triceps motor branch transfer for the treatment of isolated axillary nerve injury. Deltoid muscle strength was evaluated using the modified British Medical Research Council grading at the last follow-up (mean, 21 mo; range, 12—41 mo). The following variables were analyzed to determine whether they affected the outcome of the nerve transfer: the age and sex of the patient, delay from injury to surgery, body mass index (BMI), severity of trauma, and presence of rotator cuff lesions. The Spearman correlation coefficient and multiple linear regression were performed for statistical analysis.

Results.—The average Medical Research Council grade of deltoid muscle strength was 3.5 ± 1.1. Deltoid muscle strength correlated with the age of the patient, delay from injury to surgery, and BMI of the patient. Five patients failed to achieve more than M3 grade. Among them, 4 patients were older than 50 years and 1 was treated 14 months after injury. In the multiple linear regression model, the delay from injury to surgery, age of the patient, and BMI of the patient were the important factors, in that order, that affected the outcome of this procedure.

Conclusions.—Isolated axillary nerve injury can be treated successfully with triceps motor branch transfer. However, outstanding outcomes are not universal, with one fourth failing to achieve M3 strength. The outcome of this procedure is affected by the delay from injury to surgery and the age and BMI of the patient.

▶ Isolated paralysis of the deltoid after glenohumeral dislocation is all too often merely observed. Because many spontaneously recover, there is the tendency on the part of physicians to think that such injuries will all resolve, and the result is frequently referral only after 1 year or longer. Similarly, because there are reports of good outcomes of both grafting and nerve transfer in patients more than 12 months after injury, there is the tendency to try something because the outcomes of muscle transfers to restore shoulder abduction are generally poor. The current study provides useful information for decision making. The patient with an intact rotator cuff and a normal supraspinatus usually has full shoulder abduction but lacks endurance in maintaining the arm overhead. If the functional demands are limited, the injury more than 9 months old, and the arm heavy, perhaps this patient should just live with his or her deficit. One criticism is with the illustration, which portrays the motor branch to the long head of the triceps as essentially equivalent to that of the anterior part of the axillary nerve. In fact, there is frequently a sizable mismatch. A second criticism, as the authors note, is that recovery can be a long time coming. More than a year is needed to really assess results, and this is even more critical when the interval between injury and surgery is long. I have had patients with a disappointing result at 1 year postoperatively, although with good evidence of deltoid activation, who return at 3 years much stronger.

V. R. Hentz, MD

Acute Transfer of Superficial Radial Nerve to the Medial Nerve: Case Report
Rodriguez-Lorenzo A, Söfteland MB, Audolfsson T (Uppsala Univ Hosp, Sweden)
Ann Plast Surg 69:547-549, 2012

Distal nerve transfers have proven to be an important addition to the armamentarium for reconstruction of peripheral nerve injuries. As new nerve transfer procedures are developed, the indications for their uses continue to broaden. We report a case of a 77-year-old male who had a 9-cm-long gap of the median nerve after experiencing an avulsion injury to his right forearm. This was successfully treated by transferring superficial radial nerve to the median nerve at the carpal tunnel level, thus restoring thumb, index, and first web sensation. Our report emphasizes that nerve transfers in the emergency setting may be the treatment of first choice in cases where conventional nerve grafting is known to result in poorer outcomes such as in long nerve gaps or in the elderly patient population.

▶ Nerve transfers are an increasingly popular and logical approach to complex upper extremity peripheral nerve injuries. Initially reported by Oberlin for reinnervation of the biceps using ulnar nerve fascicles, nerve transfers use an expendable distal, donor nerve (or redundant fascicles) to innervate a target, more proximally injured peripheral nerve. This technique has rapidly been gaining popularity because of its high success rate, and the indications and techniques are also rapidly evolving. This case report highlights a less well-described technique for the restoration of median nerve sensation following irreparable median nerve injury with a particular focus on the role of patient age.

This challenging case involves a 77-year-old man with a 9-cm segmental loss of the median nerve in the proximal forearm distal to the anterior interosseous nerve takeoff. Traditional approaches for sensory restoration, such as autograft (sural nerve cable grafts), allograft, and nerve conduits, would be expected to yield lower outcomes in this case given the size of the nerve gap and the patient's age. The authors chose to perform a nerve transfer of the superficial radial nerve to the median nerve acutely with a concomitant carpal tunnel release and opponensplasty. At 9 months, the patient achieved 7-mm 2-point discrimination but without proper locognosia. Although the patient did not have any initial donor site morbidity, a late superficial burn in the radial sensory distribution did occur but healed uneventfully.

The technique of radial sensory nerve-to-median nerve transfer for the restoration of median nerve sensation has been successfully reported.[1-3] This case has relevance to clinical practice in 2 ways: First, it adds to the body of literature supporting the use of a radial sensory nerve-to-median nerve transfer to reliably restore protective median nerve sensation. Second, and perhaps more importantly, it demonstrates the ability of even elderly patients to achieve satisfactory sensory restoration after nerve transfer, especially in the acute setting.

Other nerve transfer options in this case would have included lateral antebrachial cutaneous nerve transfer, more distal selective transfer of the radial sensory nerve branches into the index radial digital and thumb digital nerves, or a fourth web to first web digital nerve transfer. Our literature presently does not support one technique over another, but like the authors' report, I have found the technique of radial sensory nerve-to-median nerve successful for restoring protective sensation to the hand. More reliable, however, has been fourth web to first web digital nerve transfer. These techniques all offer a shorter time to reinnervation compared with long proximal nerve grafting techniques.

One additional technique option if the transfer is made slightly more distally is to internally neurolyse the median nerve motor branch out of the donor nerve to avoid unwanted axonal regeneration into the motor branch if an opponensplasty is being performed simultaneously, and a carpal tunnel release is being performed. Lastly, although it may not have influenced the results of this case, sensory reeducation programs have been shown to improve cortical adaptation for localization of touch and should be considered in these cases.

G. Gaston, MD

References

1. Harris RI. The treatment of irreparable nerve injuries. *Can Med Assoc J.* 1921;11: 833-841.
2. Turnbull F. Radial-median anastomosis. *J Neurosurg.* 1948;5:562-566.
3. Hara Tsuyama N, Furusawa S. An attempt to regain sensations in the median nerve by transferring the superficial radial nerve to the median nerve. *Operation.* 1973;27: 551-558.

The Effect of Collagen Nerve Conduits Filled with Collagen-Glycosaminoglycan Matrix on Peripheral Motor Nerve Regeneration in a Rat Model

Lee J-Y, Giusti G, Friedrich PF, et al (The Catholic Univ of Korea, Suwon, South Korea; Mayo Clinic, Rochester, MN; et al)
J Bone Joint Surg Am 94:2084-2091, 2012

Background.—Bioabsorbable unfilled synthetic nerve conduits have been used in the reconstruction of small segmental nerve defects with variable results, especially in motor nerves. We hypothesized that providing a synthetic mimic of the Schwann cell basal lamina in the form of a collagen-glycosaminoglycan (GAG) matrix would improve the bridging of the nerve gap and functional motor recovery.

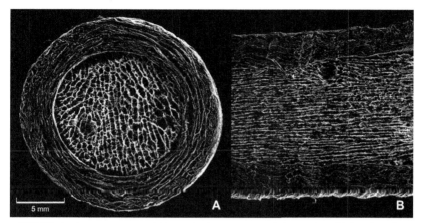

FIGURE 1.—Transverse (A) and longitudinal (B) sections of the conduit filled with collagen-glycosaminoglycan (GAG) matrix viewed by scanning electron microscopy (SEM). The pore channels in the collagen-GAG matrix are axially aligned to mimic the Schwann cell basal lamina as a mechanism to effectively support bridging across a critical-sized nerve defect. The bar is 0.5 mm long. (Reprinted from Lee J-Y, Giusti G, Friedrich PF, et al. The effect of collagen nerve conduits filled with collagen-glycosaminoglycan matrix on peripheral motor nerve regeneration in a rat model. *J Bone Joint Surg Am.* 2012;94:2084-2091, with permission from the Journal of Bone and Joint Surgery, Incorporated. Http://jbjs.org/.)

Methods.—A unilateral 10-mm sciatic nerve defect was created in eighty-eight male Lewis rats. Animals were randomly divided into four experimental groups: repair with reversed autograft, reconstruction with collagen nerve conduit (1.5-mm NeuraGen, Integra LifeSciences), reconstruction with collagen nerve conduit filled with collagen matrix, and reconstruction with collagen nerve conduit filled with collagen-GAG (chondroitin-6-sulfate) matrix. Nerve regeneration was evaluated at twelve weeks on the basis of the compound muscle action potential, maximum isometric tetanic force, and wet muscle weight of the tibialis anterior muscle, the ankle contracture angle, and nerve histomorphometry.

Results.—The use of autograft resulted in significantly better motor recovery compared with the other experimental methods. Conduit filled with collagen-GAG matrix demonstrated superior results compared with empty conduit or conduit filled with collagen matrix with respect to all experimental parameters. Axon counts in the conduit filled with collagen-GAG matrix were not significantly different from those in the reversed autograft at twelve weeks after repair.

Conclusions.—The addition of the synthetic collagen basal-lamina matrix with chondroitin-6-sulfate into the lumen of an entubulation repair significantly improved bridging of the nerve gap and functional motor recovery in a rat model.

Clinical Relevance.—Use of a nerve conduit filled with collagen-GAG matrix to bridge a motor or mixed nerve defect may result in superior functional motor recovery compared with commercially available empty collagen conduit. However, nerve autograft remains the gold standard for reconstruction of a segmental motor nerve defect (Fig 1).

▶ Hollow tube conduits are now regularly used for peripheral nerve repair, although their utility is tempered by length limitations. A fibrin clot must form within the tube and between nerve stumps to act as a scaffold that Schwann cells (and subsequently axons) can use to bridge the gap. The problem is that this fibrin clot becomes unstable with progressively longer gaps: no clot, no regeneration. The idea of introducing a matrix to stabilize the fibrin clot or to act in its place is not new. In this article, the authors have chosen a collagen-glycosaminoglycan (GAG) matrix with axially aligned channels to mimic the Schwann cell basal lamina present in nerve autograft (Fig 1). Although the concept worked better than a hollow tube, it did not prove to be equal to nerve autograft in the rodent model used in this study. Based on this study, the collagen-GAG matrix has potential, but by itself it does not seem to be the secret formula that will propel conduit nerve repairs above autograft.

J. Isaacs, MD

Functional Outcome Following Nerve Repair in the Upper Extremity Using Processed Nerve Allograft

Cho MS, Rinker BD, Weber RV, et al (San Antonio Military Med Ctr, Fort Sam, Houston, TX; Univ of Kentucky, Lexington; Inst for Nerve, Hand, and Reconstructive Surgery, Rutherford, NJ; et al)

J Hand Surg 37A:2340-2349, 2012

Purpose.—Reconstruction of peripheral nerve discontinuities with processed nerve allograft has become increasingly relevant. The RANGER Study registry was initiated in 2007 to study the use of processed nerve allografts in contemporary clinical practice. We undertook this study to analyze outcomes for upper extremity nerve repairs contained in the registry database.

Methods.—We identified an upper extremity–specific population within the RANGER Study registry database consisting of 71 nerves repaired with processed nerve allograft. This group was composed of 56 subjects with a mean age of 40 ± 17 years (range, 18–86 y). We analyzed data to determine the safety and efficacy of processed nerve allograft. Quantitative data were available on 51 subjects with 35 sensory, 13 mixed, and 3 motor nerves. The mean gap length was 23 ± 12 mm (range, 5–50 mm). We performed an analysis to evaluate response-to-treatment and to examine sensory and motor recovery according to the international standards for motor and sensory nerve recovery.

Results.—There were no reported implant complications, tissue rejections, or adverse experiences related to the use of the processed nerve allografts. Overall recovery, S3 or M4 and above, was achieved in 86% of the procedures. Subgroup analysis demonstrated meaningful levels of recovery in sensory, mixed, and motor nerve repairs with graft lengths between 5 and

TABLE 4.—Summary of Results of Most Repaired Nerves in the Upper Extremity Reporting Quantitative Data

Factor	n	Age (y)	Preoperative Interval (d)	Follow-Up (d)	Gap (mm)	Complex[a]	Lacerations	Neuromas	Meaningful Recovery[b]
Digital nerves	35	46 ± 14 (23–68)	190 ± 349 (0–1,460)	306 ± 184 (40–717)	19 ± 9 (5–40)	5	24	6	31 of 35 (89%)
Median nerve	8	28.2 ± 7 (20–38)	369 ± 278 (14–725)	230.5 ± 111 (131–442)	33 ± 13 (10–50)	2	4	2	6 of 8 (75%)
Ulnar nerve	3	42 ± 24 (25–70)	27 ± 38 (3–71)	323 ± 54 (270–378)	27 ± 6 (20–30)	2	1	0	2 of 3 (67%)

[a]Complex mechanisms include amputations, avulsions, and blast injuries.
[b]Meaningful recovery is defined as S3-S4 or M3-M5 on the MRCC scale.

TABLE 5.—Comparison With Historical Reference Literature

Study	n	Gap (mm)	Nerve Injury	Repair Technique	Positive Outcomes[a]
Kallio[21]	77	<50	Digital	Autograft	60%
Frykman and Gramyk[22]	141	<50	Digital	Autograft	88%
Kim et al[23]	15		Median	Autograft	67%
Kim et al[24]	7		Ulnar	Autograft	57%
Frykman and Gramyk[22]			Median	Autograft	80%
Frykman and Gramyk[22]			Ulnar	Autograft	60%
Vastamäki et al[33]	14	≤35	Ulnar	Autograft	57%
Lohmeyer et al[5]	12	5–18	Digital	NeuraGen[b] type 1 bovine collagen tube	75%
Wangensteen and Kalliainen[4]	64	3–25	Digital and mixed	NeuraGen[b] type 1 bovine collagen tube	43%
Chirac et al[27]	16	2–25	Digital	Neurolac[c] copolyester poly(DL-lactide-ε-caprolactone) tube	44%
Chirac et al[27]	12	2–25	Median and ulnar	Neurolac[c] copolyester poly(DL-lactide-ε-caprolactone) tube	8%

Editor's Note: Please refer to original journal article for full references.
[a]As reported, based on individual study parameters for acceptable recovery: M3-M5 and S3-S4 by MRCC.
[b]Integra LifeSciences, Plainsboro, NJ.
[c]Polyganics; Groningen, Netherlands.

50 mm. The study also found meaningful levels of recovery in 89% of digital nerve repairs, 75% of median nerve repairs, and 67% of ulnar nerve repairs.

Conclusions.—Our data suggest that processed nerve allografts offer a safe and effective method of reconstructing peripheral nerve gaps from 5 to 50 mm in length. These outcomes compare favorably with those reported in the literature for nerve autograft, and exceed those reported for tube conduits (Tables 4 and 5).

▶ This is a report focusing on upper extremity nerve reconstruction but using reprocessed (and already reported) data from a multicenter registry study on decellularized nerve allograft reconstruction. The manuscript is meant to emphasize that results obtained with this repair tool are comparable with other positive outcomes published on upper extremity nerve reconstruction (using autograft and nerve conduits; Table 5)[1]. Additionally, the report highlights that decellularized nerve allograft can be used successfully in the reconstruction of median and ulna nerves (Table 4). Important points worth emphasizing include no adverse reactions, and this off the shelf option in many cases can be as effective as more morbid options such as nerve autograft. Weaknesses of the article include its retrospective nature and a lack of consistent outcome assessment tools (assessments based on individual institutions' standards of care). As more and more data are reported on this novel nerve repair tool, surgeons will be more comfortable choosing it for overcoming nerve gaps all over the body. This study suggests (as other studies have) that this is very promising technology.[2]

J. Isaacs, MD

References

1. Whitlock EL, Tuffaha SH, Luciano JP, et al. Processed allografts and type I collagen conduits for repair of peripheral nerve gaps. *Muscle Nerve.* 2009;39:787-799.
2. Johnson PJ, Newton P, Hunter DA, Mackinnon SE. Nerve endoneurial microstructure facilitates uniform distribution of regenerative fibers: a post hoc comparison of midgraft nerve fiber densities. *J Reconstr Microsurg.* 2011;27:83-90.

Supercharged End-to-Side Anterior Interosseous to Ulnar Motor Nerve Transfer for Intrinsic Musculature Reinnervation
Barbour J, Yee A, Kahn LC, et al (Washington Univ School of Medicine, St Louis, MO)
J Hand Surg 37A:2150-2159, 2012

Functional motor recovery after peripheral nerve injury is predominantly determined by the time to motor end plate reinnervation and the absolute number of regenerated motor axons that reach target. Experimental models have shown that axonal regeneration occurs across a supercharged end-to-side (SETS) nerve coaptation. In patients with a recovering proximal ulnar nerve injury, a SETS nerve transfer conceptually is useful to protect and preserve distal motor end plates until the native axons fully regenerate. In addition, for nerve injuries in which incomplete regeneration is anticipated, a SETS nerve transfer may be useful to augment the regenerating nerve with additional axons and to more quickly reinnervate target muscle. We describe our technique for a SETS nerve transfer of the terminal anterior interosseous nerve (AIN) to the pronator quadratus muscle (PQ) end-to-side to the deep motor fascicle of the ulnar nerve in the distal forearm. In addition, we describe our postoperative therapy regimen for these transfers and an evaluation tool for monitoring progressive muscle reinnervation. Although the AIN—to—ulnar motor group SETS nerve transfer was specifically designed for ulnar nerve injuries, we believe that the SETS procedure might have broad clinical utility for second- and third-degree axonotmetic nerve injuries, to augment partial recovery and/or "babysit" motor end plates until the native parent axons regenerate to target. We would consider all donor nerves currently utilized in end-to-end nerve transfers for neurotmetic injuries as candidates for this SETS technique.

▶ The appeal of the supercharged end-to-side nerve procedure is obvious: to augment and increase the numbers of regenerating axons without sacrificing any native regenerated or regenerating axons (such as would occur with a redo repair or a distal nerve transfer). A functional proximal stump is fed into the side of an intact but compromised nerve (hence, supercharging it). Indeed, the initial animal model investigation in 2005 demonstrated that axons would grow from a proximal nerve stump into the side of a distal nerve and provide meaningful motor innervation of the downstream muscle.[1] However, despite subsequent supportive follow-up rodent studies,[2,3] the technique was slow to translate to clinical settings. Conceptualization of the dispersion process of the axons to muscle fibers throughout the muscle belly was not clear. McCallister et al had demonstrated that axons could travel in the epineural space in rabbit nerves,[4] so it is possible that the axons could use this space as a conduit to reach denervated muscle (though this is not clear, and some percentage of axons certainly may find appropriate conventional pathways). Once reaching the muscle, however, do the axons then continue to follow neural connective tissues or do they randomly disseminate to nearby muscle fibers as might be seen with direct muscle neurotization (implantation)? Additionally, it is concerning that 2 separate nerve signals trying to fire the same muscle could result in asynchronous contractions or nerve signals could interfere with each other.[2] Ueda and Harii demonstrated that a neurotization procedure with a separate donor nerve did not improve subsequent muscle recovery following regeneration of native axons[5]—a situation (in a rodent model) analogous to using the distal anterior interosseus nerve as a donor to compete with regenerating ulna nerve axons. Stated differently, there should be concerns that we do not understand the mechanism by which this process works and that the supercharged end-to-side nerve repair is a surgery likely to work in rats, but not necessarily in people.

Technique guides typically imply that a described procedure is an accepted and standard surgery that should be routinely offered to patients based on the clinical scenarios outlined in the article.

The supercharged end-to-side nerve repair is a fascinating and compelling idea, but it certainly has not been proven to a level satisfactory for widespread clinical utilization. Much more basic science and controlled clinical studies should be completed and assessed in a peer review fashion before this procedure can be considered anything more than experimental.

J. Isaacs, MD

References

1. Isaacs J, Allen D, Chen LE, Nunley J 2nd. Reverse end-to-side neurotization. *J Reconstr Microsurg*. 2005;21:43-48. discussion 49—50.
2. Isaacs JE, Cheatham S, Gagnon EB, Razavi A, McDowell CL. Reverse end-to-side neurotization in a regenerating nerve. *J Reconstr Microsurg*. 2008;24:489-496.
3. Fujiwara T, Matsuda K, Kubo T, et al. Axonal supercharging technique using reverse end-to-side neurorrhaphy in peripheral nerve repair: an experimental study in the rat model. *J Neurosurg*. 2007;107:821-829.
4. McCallister WV, McCallister EL, Trumble SA, Trumble TE. Overcoming peripheral nerve gap defects using an intact nerve bridge in a rabbit model. *J Reconstr Microsurg*. 2005;21:197-206.
5. Ueda K, Harii K. Prevention of denervation atrophy by nerve implantation. *J Reconstr Microsurg*. 2004;20:545-553.

Peripheral Nerve Injuries in Sports-Related Surgery: Presentation, Evaluation, and Management: AAOS Exhibit Selection

Maak TG, Osei D, Delos D, et al (Hosp for Special Surgery, NY)
J Bone Joint Surg Am 94:e121.1-e121.10, 2012

Peripheral nerve injuries during sports-related operative interventions are rare complications, but the associated morbidity can be substantial. Early diagnosis, efficient and effective evaluation, and appropriate management are crucial to maximizing the prognosis, and a clear and structured algorithm is therefore required. We describe the surgical conditions and interventions that are commonly associated with intraoperative peripheral nerve

TABLE 1.—Surgical Anatomy: Important Landmarks and Relationships

Surgical anatomy: upper extremity
  Shoulder arthroscopy (axillary, musculocutaneous, subscapular nerves)

Posterior portal	Located 3-4 cm superior to axillary nerve in quadrangular space[31]
Anterior portal	Musculocutaneous, axillary, and subscapular nerves lie inferior and lateral to coracoid process at level of anterior portal. Brachial plexus lies medial to coracoid process at level of anterior portal[31]
Lateral portal	Axillary nerve enters deep surface of deltoid approximately 5 cm distal to lateral aspect of acromion. Smaller branches may enter deltoid 1 cm distal to lateral aspect of acromion

  Elbow arthroscopy (musculocutaneous, radial, medial antebrachial cutaneous, median, ulnar nerves)

Midlateral portal	Lies 7 mm from posterior antebrachial cutaneous nerve[32]
Posterolateral portal	Lies 20 mm from medial antebrachial cutaneous nerve (MABCN) and 25 mm from ulnar nerve[33]
Anteromedial portal	Lies 1 mm from MABCN, 4 mm from median nerve. Flexion of elbow and distention of joint with saline solution increases distance of portal from median nerve to 14 mm[33]
Anterolateral portal	Lies 3 mm posterior to radial nerve, 7-11 mm with joint distention. Lies 2 mm anterior to posterior antebrachial cutaneous nerve

  Direct biceps repair (median, posterior interosseous nerves)
    Distal biceps insertion on radial tuberosity lies 12 mm from medial nerve, 18 mm from posterior interosseous nerve (PIN)[34]
    Lateral antebrachial cutaneous nerve injury is the most common (up to 40% in some series); median nerve injury is the most serious
    Steinmann pin fixation of the biceps should be performed directly posterior rather than at oblique 45° angle. At 0°, distance to PIN is 14 mm. At 45°, distance decreases to 8 mm
Surgical anatomy: lower extremity
  Periarticular knee surgery (peroneal, saphenous nerves)
    Peroneal nerve passes just beneath biceps tendon, crossing obliquely across fibula.[35] Anatomic variability can lead to iatrogenic injury; 20% of patients will have separate deep and superficial peroneal nerve at level of lateral joint line; 19% of patients will have continuation of common peroneal nerve below level of fibular neck[36]
    Saphenous nerve lies beneath sartorius muscle and passes distally between sartorius and gracilis tendons.[35]
    Sends off an anterior infrapatellar branch to the knee.
    Distal sartorial branch crosses inferolaterally at level of pes anserinus (lies in surgical field during anterior cruciate ligament surgery)
  Ankle arthroscopy (superficial peroneal nerve)
    Superficial peroneal nerve lies lateral to peroneus tertius tendon in 11.8% and at its lateral edge in 27.5%[30]

Editor's Note: Please refer to original journal article for full references.

TABLE 4.—Pertinent Motor and Sensory Innervation: Function and Signs Suggestive of Injury

Nerve-specific examination: upper extremity
  Axillary nerve

Muscles innervated	Middle and anterior deltoid (anterior division of axillary nerve), posterior deltoid, and teres minor (posterior division of axillary nerve)
Function	Shoulder abduction to 90°, transverse extension, and external rotation
Sensory contributions	Sensation over lateral aspect of proximal aspect of humerus
Injury findings	Weakness in shoulder forward flexion, numbness in lateral aspect of shoulder

  Radial nerve

Muscles innervated	Triceps brachii, brachioradialis, posterior compartment of forearm
Function	Elbow extension; forearm supination; wrist, finger, and thumb extension
Sensory contributions	Posterior brachial cutaneous nerve: sensation over posterior aspect of arm. Posterior antebrachial cutaneous nerve: sensation over middle 1/3 of posterior aspect of arm. Superficial branch of radial nerve: sensation to dorsoradial aspect of wrist and hand. Lateral branch: sensation to dorsoradial aspect of thumb. Medial branch: sensation to dorsum of index finger, middle finger, and radial aspect of ring finger
Injury findings	Elbow, wrist, and digit extensor weakness; dorsal arm, forearm, and hand numbness (1st thenar web space)

  Musculocutaneous nerve

Muscles innervated	Coracobrachialis, biceps brachii, brachialis
Function	Coracobrachialis: flexion and adduction of shoulder joint with arm flexed and laterally rotated at the shoulder joint, elbow flexed, and forearm supinated. Biceps brachii: forearm supination and resisted elbow flexion with forearm supinated. Brachialis: elbow flexion with neutral forearm rotation
Sensory contributions	Lateral antebrachial cutaneous nerve: provides sensation to volar lateral aspect of forearm
Injury findings	Weakness in elbow flexion and forearm supination; radial forearm numbness

  Ulnar nerve

Muscles innervated	Pronator teres, flexor carpi radialis, flexor digitorum superficialis, palmaris longus, flexor pollicis longus*, flexor digitorum profundus to index and middle fingers*, pronator quadratus*, abductor pollicis brevis, flexor pollicis brevis (superficial head), opponens pollicis, lumbricals to index and middle fingers (* = supplied by anterior interosseous branch)
Function	Wrist flexion and ulnar deviation, finger flexion, metacarpophalangeal joint flexion, proximal interphalangeal joint extension, finger abduction and adduction, thumb adduction and flexion
Sensory contributions	Dorsal branch of the ulnar nerve: sensation over dorsal ulnar aspect of hand. Common and proper digital nerves: sensation to small finger and ulnar aspect of ring finger
Injury findings	Interosseous and hypothenar wasting (Wartenberg sign, Froment sign), claw hand (with high ulnar nerve injury), decreased sensation to small finger and ulnar aspect of ring finger

  Median nerve

Muscles innervated	Triceps brachii, brachioradialis, posterior compartment of forearm
Function	Elbow extension; forearm supination; wrist, finger, and thumb extension
Sensory contributions	Palmar cutaneous branch: sensation to thenar area of hand. Common and proper digital nerves: sensation to volar aspect of thumb, index finger, middle finger, and radial aspect of ring finger
Injury findings	Loss of thumb interphalangeal joint flexion, index and long finger distal interphalangeal joint flexion, forearm pronation, and thumb opposition. Thenar atrophy; decreased sensation to thumb, index finger, long finger, and radial half of ring finger

(Continued)

Table 4.—(*Continued*)

Nerve-specific examination: lower extremity	
Sciatic nerve	
Muscles innervated	Semimembranosus, semitendinosus, biceps femoris
Function	Knee flexion
Sensory contributions	None in the thigh; provides sensation to the leg and foot via its distal branches
Injury findings	Weakness in knee flexion
Common peroneal nerve	
Muscles innervated	Peroneus longus, peroneus brevis, peroneous tertius, tibialis anterior, extensor hallucis longus, extensor digitorum longus
Function	Ankle dorsiflexion and eversion, toe extension
Sensory contributions	Lateral sural cutaneous nerve: sensation to posterior and lateral aspects of leg
	Medial dorsal cutaneous nerve: sensation to dorsum of foot, medial side of hallux, and 2nd-3rd toe web space
	Intermediate dorsal cutaneous nerve: sensation to dorsolateral aspect of foot and to 3rd-4th and 4th-5th toe web spaces
	Medial terminal branch of deep peroneal nerve: sensation to 1st web space
Injury findings	Foot drop and eversion weakness, dorsal foot numbness
Lateral femoral cutaneous nerve	
Muscles innervated	None
Sensory contributions	Sensation to anterolateral aspect of proximal aspect of thigh
Injury findings	Lateral thigh numbness
Saphenous nerve	
Muscles innervated	None
Sensory contributions	Sensation to medial aspect of thigh, leg, and foot
Injury findings	Medial thigh, leg, and foot numbness

injuries. In addition, we review the common postoperative presentations of patients with these injuries as well as the anatomic structures that are directly injured or associated with these injuries during the operation. Some examples of peripheral nerve injuries incurred during sports-related surgery include ulnar nerve injury during ulnar collateral ligament reconstruction of the elbow and elbow arthroscopy, median nerve injury during ulnar collateral ligament reconstruction of the elbow, axillary nerve injury during Bankart repair and the Bristow transfer, and peroneal nerve injury during posterolateral corner reconstruction of the knee and arthroscopic lateral meniscal repair. We also detail the clinical and radiographic evaluation of these patients, including the utility and timing of radiographs, magnetic resonance imaging (MRI), ultrasonography, electromyography (EMG), and nonoperative or operative management. The diagnosis, evaluation, and management of peripheral nerve injuries incurred during sports-related surgical interventions are critical to minimizing patient morbidity and maximizing postoperative function. Although these injuries occur during a variety of procedures, common themes exist regarding evaluation techniques and treatment algorithms. Nonoperative treatment includes physical therapy and medical management. Operative treatments include neurolysis, transposition, neurorrhaphy, nerve transfer, and tendon transfer. This article provides orthopaedic surgeons with a simplified, literature-based algorithm for evaluation and management of peripheral nerve injuries associated with sports-related operative procedures (Tables 1 and 4).

▶ This article tackles the difficult issue of iatrogenic nerve injuries associated with sports-related surgical procedures. It provides a basic overview of types of nerve injury as well as a diagnosis and treatment algorithm. The most useful information in this article is contained within 2 tables. Table 1 provides information on relevant nerve anatomy as it relates to common incision and portal placement. This list of common surgical exposures and the nerves at risk is a useful surgical resource. Table 4 provides information on sensory and motor functions of specific nerves that are most commonly injured with sports-related surgical procedures. This table is a quick guide to the exam of a patient with suspected nerve injury. Overall, the text in this article presents basic information for those who need a refresher, and the tables are excellent resources. The 1 weakness is that the treatment algorithm does not adequately stress the time-sensitive nature of major nerve injuries. The motor endplates begin to have irreversible changes at 12 months of denervation and, overall, earlier reinnervation results in better outcomes. Thus, early intervention should be considered as soon as there is indication of a severe nerve injury; this is especially true for more proximal injuries.

C. Curtin, MD

Fascicular Selection for Nerve Transfers: The Role of the Nerve Stimulator When Restoring Elbow Flexion in Brachial Plexus Injuries
Bhandari PS, Deb P (Armed Forces Med College and Command Hosp, Pune, India)
J Hand Surg 36A:2002-2009, 2011

Purpose.—Restoration of elbow flexion is an important goal in brachial plexus injuries. Double nerve transfers using fascicles from ulnar and median nerves have consistently produced good results without causing functional compromise to the donor nerve. According to conventional practice, these double nerve transfers are dependent on the careful isolation of ulnar and median nerve fascicles, which are responsible for wrist flexion, using a handheld nerve stimulator. Here we suggest that fascicular selection by nerve stimulation might not be a necessity when executing double nerve transfers for restoration of elbow flexion in brachial plexus injuries.

Methods.—This is a retrospective case control study in 26 patients with C5, C6 brachial plexus injuries that were managed with double nerve transfers between March 2005 and January 2008. Our technique consisted of transferring 2 fascicles, one each from the ulnar and the median nerve, directly onto the biceps and brachialis motor branches. Contrary to the standard practice, the ulnar or median nerve fascicles were selected without using a handheld nerve stimulator. Results were compared to 21 cases (control group) in which a nerve stimulator was used for fascicular selection. The denervation period ranged from 3 to 9 months.

Results.—Twenty-four patients of the study group experienced full restoration of elbow flexion, and 2 had an antigravity flexion of 120° and 110°. The EMG revealed the first sign of reinnervation of biceps and brachialis muscle at 9 ± 2 weeks and 11 ± 2 weeks, as compared to 9 ± 2 weeks and 12 ± 4 weeks in the control group. After surgery, the appearance of initial evidence of elbow flexion, the range and mean of elbow flexion strength, and the difference between preoperative and postoperative grip and pinch strengths were comparable in both groups. At 24 to 28 months follow-up, 19 patients of the study group had M4 power and 7 had M3, compared to 18 and 3 cases, respectively, in the control group. The *P* values for Medical Research Council grade, strength of elbow flexion, and range of elbow flexion between the 2 groups did not reveal any significant statistical difference.

Conclusions.—Double nerve transfer is a reliable technique for restoring elbow flexion in brachial plexus injuries. There is no advantage of using a nerve stimulator in selecting fascicles before performing the nerve transfer.

▶ It is well accepted that the restoration of elbow flexion is the primary reconstructive priority in treating patients who have brachial plexus injuries. Although a multitude of donor nerves have been used successfully for the restoration of elbow flexion (intercostal, thoracodorsal, medial pectoral, and spinal accessory), the Oberlin transfer has gained widespread popularity recently. Originally, Oberlin described using a single motor fascicle from the ulnar nerve into the biceps brachii motor branch.[1] This has since been modified to include a double fascicular nerve transfer adding a fascicle from the median nerve into the brachialis motor branch. Conventionally, the donor fascicles are selected by isolating motor fascicles responsible for wrist flexion using a nerve stimulator. This well-designed, retrospective, case-control study challenges the traditional thinking that fascicular selection using nerve stimulation is necessary.

The authors compared the results of 26 patients who underwent double fascicular nerve transfer without selective fascicular nerve stimulation with those of 21 controls. The transfer was performed with traditional selective fascicular stimulation. The methodology of the study was very sound with stringent outcome measurements, including weekly physical examinations and electromyography (EMG) to assess time to recovery. The 2 groups were very well matched in terms of patient demographics, time from injury to surgery, and type of injury. Conventional wisdom would have concerns for increased donor site morbidity (higher risk of loss of hand intrinsic strength or sensation) and diminished outcomes (assuming the chosen fascicle had fewer donor axons or was predominantly sensory).

The authors found no difference in the time to electrophysiologic evidence of reinnervation, time to initial clinical sign of recovery, ultimate elbow flexion strength, grip strength, pinch strength, and donor nerve morbidity. In the group without selective fascicular stimulation, donor nerve fascicles were chosen from the anterolateral aspect of the median and ulnar nerves. Initial EMG signs of recovery of the biceps appeared in both groups at a mean of 9 weeks, and initial flicker of active muscle contracture was seen clinically in both groups at a mean of

14 weeks. Antigravity elbow flexion was achieved in all patients in both groups at a mean of 9 months after surgery. At 2-year follow-up, 19 of 26 study patients had M4 strength (7 had M3) and 18 of 21 control patients had M4 strength (3 had M3).

This study adds more evidence that selective fascicular nerve stimulation may not improve outcomes in restoring elbow flexion after double fascicular nerve transfer when compared with simply using the most anterolateral fascicle of each nerve. Similar findings were reported by Bertelli and Ghizoni[2] in a recent report of Oberlin procedures. I applaud the authors for a very well-designed study, and, in an era of cost containment, time can be saved, and the cost of a nerve stimulator may be able to be avoided in some cases.

I would strongly caution, however, against generalizing these results to other nerve transfers. It is well accepted that proximally there is much more crossing over of nerve fibers and that progressively moving distal, fascicular orientation is greater. Applying this same concept more distally could risk higher donor nerve deficits and diminished results. Also, many surgeons, myself included, will utilize 2 donor fascicles from the median or ulnar nerve for double nerve transfers. Nonselective harvesting of 2 fascicles could risk higher rates of donor nerve morbidity. The precise location of the fascicles controlling wrist flexion in the median and ulnar nerves has been the source of much debate. This study was harvested from the anterolateral aspect of the nerve, and the results cannot be generalized to the situation of harvesting from a different intraneural location. Lastly, the additional time required for selective fascicular stimulation is frequently very small, and often the nerve stimulator is already being used during the case for the brachial plexus, so there is very little downside to selective stimulation in most cases.

G. Gaston, MD

References

1. Oberlin C, Béal D, Leechavengvongs S, Salon A, Dauge MC, Sarcy JJ. Nerve transfer to biceps muscle using a part of ulnar nerve for C5–C6 avulsion of the brachial plexus: anatomical study and report of four cases. *J Hand Surg Am.* 1994;19: 232-237.
2. Bertelli JA, Ghizoni MF. Nerve root grafting and distal nerve transfers for C5-C6 brachial plexus injuries. *J Hand Surg Am.* 2010;35:769-775.

Axonal regeneration and motor neuron survival after microsurgical nerve reconstruction

Fox IK, Brenner MJ, Johnson PJ, et al (Washington Univ School of Medicine, Saint Louis, MO; Southern Illinois Univ School of Medicine, Springfield)
Microsurgery 32:552-562, 2012

Rodent models are used extensively for studying nerve regeneration, but little is known about how sprouting and pruning influence peripheral nerve fiber counts and motor neuron pools. The purpose of this study was to identify fluctuations in nerve regeneration and neuronal survival over time. One hundred and forty-four Lewis rats were randomized to end-to-end repair or nerve grafting (1.5 cm graft) after sciatic nerve transection. Quantitative histomorphometry and retrograde labeling of motor neurons were performed at 1, 3, 6, 9, 12, and 24 months and supplemented by electron microscopy. Fiber counts and motor neuron counts increased between 1 and 3 months, followed by plateau. End-to-end repair resulted in persistently higher fiber counts compared to the grafting for all time points ($P < 0.05$). Percent neural tissue and myelin width increased with time while fibrin debris dissipated. In conclusion, these data detail the natural history of regeneration and demonstrate that overall fiber counts may remain stable despite pruning.

▶ Much of the basic science data upon which we have gained our understanding of the pathophysiology of peripheral nerve repair and regeneration have come from rodent models. Most studies have chosen arbitrary endpoints of time to analyze data. These studies naturally assume that these chosen time points allow meaningful comparison of the data when looking at multiple subgroups. This well-designed study allows direct comparison over time of nerve regeneration and neuronal survival between end-to-end repair vs nerve grafting in a rodent model.

Twelve rats per group (total 180) were analyzed at 1, 3, 6, 9, 12, and 24 months looking specifically at quantitative histomorphology of nerve regeneration as well as cell body labeling in the ventral horn to assess neuron survival. Histomorphometric data included nerve fiber density, number of myelinated fibers, myelin width, percentage of neural tissue present, and amount of fibrin debris.

By 3 months, the number of regenerating nerve fibers reached a plateau in both groups, but the nerve fibers became more mature with each additional month, increasing in myelination and neural tissue while decreasing in fibrin debris in both groups. This plateau was also seen in motor neuron cells in the anterior horn cells at 3 months. The mean fiber count in the repair group far exceeded the grafting group (13 850 vs 9102) at 3 months.

Interestingly, the pattern of nerve reinnervation was similar between the 2 groups, but at all time points there were greater nerve fiber counts in the repair vs grafting group. Nerve fiber density was not significantly different between the 2 groups. Percentage of neural tissue (indicating maturity of the regenerated nerves) continued to progress over the entire 24 months in both groups. For the repair group, percentage of neural tissue was 18% at 1 month, 37% at 3 months, and 52% at 24 months vs the grafting group, which was 0% at 1 month, 26% at 3 months, and 46% at 24 months. Myelinated fiber width (another indicator of nerve maturity) also increased over all time points between the 2 groups but at a more rapid rate in the repair group. Fiber debris cleared over the first 9 months in both groups but was a larger percentage of the nerve in the graft group (21% vs 5%). One not too surprising finding was that sections from the midportion of the isograft had very similar histomorphology to the primary repair graft at all time points.

The clinical relevance of this basic science study is that the bulk of the gain in mean fiber counts is seen in the first few months after repair or grafting, but then maturation of the peripheral nerve is seen for up to 24 months, at least in a rodent model. Despite similar time points for achieving mean fiber counts, the mean fiber counts were significantly higher in the repair group (nearly 50% higher than the grafting group).

G. Gaston, MD

Effects of Sensory Reeducation Programs on Functional Hand Sensibility after Median and Ulnar Repair: A Systematic Review
Miller LK, Chester R, Jerosch-Herold C (Univ of East Anglia, Queens Building, Norwich, UK; Norfolk and Norwich Univ Hosp, UK)
J Hand Ther 25:297-307, 2012

Introduction.—This is the first systematic review looking at the effectiveness of sensory re-education programmes on functional sensibility which focuses purely on clinical trials of adult patients with median and ulnar nerve injuries.

Methods.—A literature search of AMED, CINAHL, Embase and OVID Medline (from inception to July 2011) was undertaken. Studies were selected if they met the following inclusion criteria: controlled trials (with or without randomization) of sensory re-education, including early and late phase, in adults with median and/or ulnar nerve repair. Two independent assessors rated study quality and risk of bias using the 24 point Mac-Dermid Evaluation Tool.

Results.—A total of seven articles met the inclusion criteria representing five separate studies Study quality ranged from 13 to 33 out of 48 points on the Evaluation Tool. Due to heterogeneity of the interventions and outcomes assessed it was not possible to pool the results from all studies. There is limited evidence to support the use of early and late SR programmes.

Conclusion.—Further trials are needed to evaluate the effect of early and late sensory re-education which are adequately powered, include validated and relevant outcomes and which are reported according to CONSORT (Consolidated Standards of Reporting Trials) guidelines.

Level of Evidence.—2b.

▶ The authors initiated this study in an attempt to combine data from many studies and perform a meta-analysis. Though they note that a meta-analysis on sensory reeducation following nerve repair was published in 2007, the authors felt that there had been significant advances in the sensory reeducation philosophy and an updated analysis was in order. Among the new concepts worth mentioning, the most interesting may be the idea of starting the reeducation at the time of repair by using alternate sensory input (for example, audible signals to indicate that the fingertips are touching different surfaces). Unfortunately, the only thing the authors were really able to conclude was that the several studies identified in the past several years are of relatively poor quality—reeducation protocols are different in every study, several studies use completely subjective assessments, there is frequently poor blinding of the investigators, and the assessment and treatment tools are heterogenous. No meta-analysis was possible based on these inconsistencies. Supportive data for sensory reeducation are, for the most part, still lacking.

J. Isaacs, MD

Effects of Sensory Reeducation Programs on Functional Hand Sensibility after Median and Ulnar Repair: A Systematic Review

Miller LK, Chester R, Jerosch-Herold C (Univ of East Anglia, Norwich, UK)
J Hand Ther 25:297-307, 2012

Introduction.—This is the first systematic review looking at the effectiveness of sensory re-education programmes on functional sensibility which focuses purely on clinical trials of adult patients with median and ulnar nerve injuries.

Methods.—A literature search of AMED, CINAHL, Embase and OVID Medline (from inception to July 2011) was undertaken. Studies were selected if they met the following inclusion criteria: controlled trials (with or without randomization) of sensory re-education, including early and late phase, in adults with median and/or ulnar nerve repair. Two independent assessors rated study quality and risk of bias using the 24 point Mac-Dermid Evaluation Tool.

Results.—A total of seven articles met the inclusion criteria representing five separate studies Study quality ranged from 13 to 33 out of 48 points on the Evaluation Tool. Due to heterogeneity of the interventions and outcomes assessed it was not possible to pool the results from all studies. There is limited evidence to support the use of early and late SR programmes.

Conclusion.—Further trials are needed to evaluate the effect of early and late sensory re-education which are adequately powered, include validated and relevant outcomes and which are reported according to CONSORT (Consolidated Standards of Reporting Trials) guidelines.

Level of Evidence.—2b.

▶ This article dealt a systematic review of sensory rehabilitation programs using limited literature inclusion criteria. It was helpful to narrow the scope of the inclusion criteria, so the reader could quantify results on control trials for median and ulnar nerve repair, hence, sensory rehabilitation. It also did recognize the limitation of excluding non-English publications. It is impressive this was tabulated by 2 investigators. This article did an excellent job in reporting many of the comparisons of late vs early sensory rehabilitation and using scoring instruments (Preferred Reporting Items for Systematic Reviews and Meta-Analysis). It is a very difficult review topic of the interventions, as early- and late-stage controls are not the same in the outcomes or even these specific phases of recovery, frequency, or duration. Criteria are still variable on what is early or late sensory rehabilitation. This article cited specific steps needed to develop a validated impairment-based measure, including outcome functional activity. This article summarized well the limitation of available studies of sensory rehabilitation, whether late or early, in the discussion.

S. Kranz, OTR/L, CHT

Catastrophic complication of an interscalene catheter for continuous peripheral nerve block analgesia
Yanovski B, Gaitini L, Volodarski D, et al (Bnai Zion Med Ctr, Haifa, Israel; et al)
Anaesthesia 67:1166-1169, 2012

We report a catastrophic postoperative complication of a prolonged inter-scalene block performed under general anaesthesia. The course of the anaes-thetic was uneventful and the patient remained stable during his stay in the recovery area with the operative extremity paralysed and insensate. No further local anaesthetic was administered until later that day when the patient received 10 ml bupivacaine 0.25% through the catheter. Upon completion of the top-up dose, no change in the patient's status was noticed. The patient was next assessed 6.5 h later when he was found dead in his bed. A postmortem CT scan revealed the catheter to be sited intrathecally, presumably the result of dural sleeve penetration.

▶ The authors of this case report have described a complication resulting from regional anesthesia at their institution, which resulted in the death of a patient. This serves to remind us that procedures commonly done do have risks, and care should always be undertaken to provide the safest treatment possible.

The authors placed a catheter for regional anesthetic infusion after the admin-istration of general anesthesia. The catheter was felt to be in an appropriate posi-tion, but it was not tested. After surgery, the patient had good pain control, so the catheter was still not used. Later that evening, a bolus of anesthetic was given through the catheter without any change in the patient's examination or pain, but nothing else was done, and when the patient was reassessed approximately 6 hours later, he was found dead. This was apparently done before routine use of ultrasound scan, which could have prevented this complication, as the incorrect placement should have been determined. Ultrasound scan now seems to be routinely used in many institutions. This catastrophic event has changed protocol at the author's institution. An additional protocol that should help anyone involved with regional anesthesia or catheters for postoperative pain control would be monitoring after the initial bolus injection to make certain the catheter is in the appropriate position, and the desired effect occurs after the bolus.

W. C. Hammert, DDS, MD

Regional Anesthesia Improves Outcome After Distal Radius Fracture Fixation Over General Anesthesia

Egol KA, Soojian MG, Walsh M, et al (NYU Hosp for Joint Diseases; Norwalk Hosp, CT; SUNY Downstate Med School, Brooklyn, NY; et al)
J Orthop Trauma 26:545-549, 2012

Objective.—To compare the efficacy of anesthetic type on clinical outcomes after operative treatment of distal radius fractures.

Design.—Retrospective review of prospectively collected data.

Setting.—Academic medical center.

Patients.—One hundred eighty-seven patients with a distal radius fracture (OTA type 23) were identified within a registry of 600 patients.

Intervention.—Patients with operative distal radius fractures underwent open reduction and internal fixation with a volarly applied plate and screws under regional or general anesthesia.

Main Outcome Measurements.—Clinical, radiographic, and patient-based functional outcomes were recorded at routine postoperative intervals. Complications were recorded.

Results.—One hundred eighty-seven patients met inclusion criteria and had a minimum of 1-year follow-up. There were no differences between the groups with regard to patient demographics or fracture types treated. At both 3 and 6 months post surgery, pain was diminished among those patients who received a regional block. Wrist and finger range of motion for patients who received regional versus general anesthesia was improved at all follow-up points. Patients who received regional anesthesia also had higher functional scores as measured by the Disabilities of the Arm, Shoulder and Hand at 3 months ($P = 0.04$) and 6 months ($P = 0.02$).

Conclusion.—Patients who are candidates should be offered regional anesthesia when undergoing repair of a displaced distal radius fracture.

Level of Evidence.—Therapeutic Level III. See Instructions for Authors for a complete description of levels of evidence.

▶ In their article, Egol et al presented an interesting set of patients and examined their database of patients for differences in outcomes related to anesthesia choice at the time of surgery. One of the great strengths of the study is the existence of this database, which they've clearly taken a good deal of time and effort to develop. They have reported here a 5-year period of 600 distal radius fractures enrolled in the database. Their subset of patients is culled from this database. The authors are to be commended for keeping a significant amount of data about their patients and the patient outcomes in order to improve clinical outcomes. Additionally, they have set up their study with a clear null hypothesis and purpose. They have explained their indications for surgery, inclusion criteria, and exclusion criteria. They have a significant set of postoperative follow-up points, 5 in total, reaching out to a year postoperatively. Additionally, they used 2 validated outcome studies to judge the functional outcome of their patients.

Their null hypothesis was that the anesthetic type would have no effect on clinical- and patient-reported functional outcomes and that their purpose was to examine both the clinical and functional results after distal radius fracture surgery in 2 similar cohorts who differed only in the type of anesthesia they received at the time of surgery. Their methods do show several important weaknesses. First, they rightly stated this is a retrospective review; they do indicate that they collected the data prospectively, but a true prospective study would require that the purpose and hypothesis were established before the data were collected, so the data could be correctly structured for the question at hand. They haven't included whether or not any local or regional block was used at the time of surgery by the surgeon, which is very common with the use of general anesthesia, or whether all anesthesia types other than general anesthesia were omitted. Additionally, they state that the attending surgeons who decided on the type of treatment varied and that 3 were fellowship-trained orthopedic traumatologists, and 1 was a fellowship-trained orthopedic hand surgeon. They did feel that all 4 surgeons were similarly experienced in the treatment of distal radius fractures without breaking down exactly what this means. This allows for significant introduction of variation in surgeon technique, which could explain the differences seen.

It is also important to note that the patients were not randomized. This is a critical issue when dealing with multifactorial outcome results such as results of distal radius fracture fixation. Significant bias as to the patient type based on lack of randomization could have been easily introduced despite the fact that the 2 cohorts were similar when reviewed retrospectively. For example, the patients who received blocks tended to be smaller and female, which may have contributed significantly to their final outcome. No mention of workers' compensation status or legal status that would introduce significant secondary gains in the patient population was presented. And their statistical evaluation did not include a power study—this would have helped, particularly with a retrospective design. Also importantly, there is no mention of how the follow-up examinations were conducted. Was this done by a hand therapist? Was this done by a physician? Was the evaluator blinded to the type of anesthesia used and the physician? This is another source of important bias in the study.

Looking at their results, the authors do admit at one point that they recognized that the improvements seen are statistically significant but may not be clinically significant. Nevertheless, they go on to imply that their null hypothesis was correctly rejected.

They do have an interesting discussion of possible reasons for improvement. One possible explanation would be concomitant blockade of the sympathetic nervous system at the time of surgery, which is an interesting potential benefit of regional blockade for surgery. Interestingly, they had no reports of reflex sympathetic dystrophy in either group of patients, making this less likely to be a clinically significant phenomenon. A more interesting potential result is that the paralysis provided by muscular blockade in the patients who received a block may lead to less soft-tissue disruption at the time of surgery. This is an interesting possibility and bears further investigation as a potential for less iatrogenic tissue damage, particularly in elderly patients with less robust tissues.

Overall, I think that this article correctly notes that the improvements seen, although statistically significant, may not be clinically significant; however, that point is lost in the title that implies that there is both clinical and statistical significance in the difference between outcomes using regional anesthesia vs general anesthesia. I think on the whole, given the weaknesses of the study, their conclusions are poorly supported by statistical significance in the face of a faulty designed study with multiple areas for significant biased introduction. Given these weaknesses and that previous studies they quote showed no difference, further investigation into the outcomes of distal radius fracture treatment based on anesthetic choice are needed to support the idea that there is a superior outcome based on the anesthetic choice.

With no complications secondary to anesthesia and no complications secondary to surgery in either group, the differences the authors have shown would seem to be more likely a result of error despite statistical significance. Considering the number of places where significant bias is present in study design, treatment of the patient, and final evaluation of the patient, as outlined above, it is more likely than not that the null hypothesis has been wrongly rejected. Given the differences in anesthetic choice (block vs general anesthesia), a significant change that was the result of a change in the diagnosis of Reflex Sympathetic Dystrophy in these patients would be interesting.

D. Mastella, MD

Effects of Sensory Reeducation Programs on Functional Hand Sensibility after Median and Ulnar Repair: A Systematic Review

Miller LK, Chester R, Jerosch-Herold C (Univ of East Anglia, Norwich, UK)
J Hand Ther 25:297-307, 2012

Introduction.—This is the first systematic review looking at the effectiveness of sensory re-education programmes on functional sensibility which focuses purely on clinical trials of adult patients with median and ulnar nerve injuries.

Methods.—A literature search of AMED, CINAHL, Embase and OVID Medline (from inception to July 2011) was undertaken. Studies were selected if they met the following inclusion criteria: controlled trials (with or without randomization) of sensory re-education, including early and late phase, in adults with median and/or ulnar nerve repair. Two independent assessors rated study quality and risk of bias using the 24 point MacDermid Evaluation Tool.

Results.—A total of seven articles met the inclusion criteria representing five separate studies Study quality ranged from 13 to 33 out of 48 points on the Evaluation Tool. Due to heterogeneity of the interventions and outcomes assessed it was not possible to pool the results from all studies. There is limited evidence to support the use of early and late SR programmes.

Conclusion.—Further trials are needed to evaluate the effect of early and late sensory re-education which are adequately powered, include validated and relevant outcomes and which are reported according to CONSORT (Consolidated Standards of Reporting Trials) guidelines. *Level of Evidence.*—2b.

▶ The authors present an excellent review of the history and process of sensory reeducation (SR). Since SR has been widely used clinically since the 1970s when the first studies were published and then a systematic review was done in 2007 that indicated limited evidence for the effectiveness of SR, the authors appropriately decided it was time to review the evidence again. All published controlled trials to date that studied median or ulnar nerve lesions were reviewed with strict inclusion criteria. Of the 94 articles screened, a total of 7 studies met the criteria set forth and were included in this review.

As stated by the authors, "the quantity and quality of evidence remains limited." I appreciate their thorough review of published trials, noting the limitations of trials that were not randomized or blinded, small sample sizes, and use of SR interventions that were not described in detail. However, 2 studies did demonstrate that temporary forearm anesthesia combined with intensive SR improved tactile gnosis although the effects did not last beyond 6 weeks.

As a clinician who is asked to use evidence-based practice when formulating treatment plans, it is imperative that more research be done to validate SR, both phase I and phase II interventions. Because this review provides only limited evidence that SR improves functional sensibility after nerve repair, I look forward to further research.

S. J. Clark, OTR/L, CHT

The long-term post-operative electromyographic evaluation of patients who have undergone carpal tunnel decompression
Faour-Martín O, Martín-Ferrero MA, Almaraz-Gómez A, et al (Clinic Univ Hosp of Valladolid, Spain)
J Bone Joint Surg Br 94-B:941-945, 2012

We present the electromyographic (EMG) results ten years after open decompression of the median nerve at the wrist and compare them with the clinical and functional outcomes as judged by Levine's Questionnaire. This retrospective study evaluated 115 patients who had undergone carpal tunnel decompression at a mean of 10.47 years (9.24 to 11.36) previously. A positive EMG diagnosis was found in 77 patients (67%), including those who were asymptomatic at ten years.

It is necessary to include both clinical and functional results as well as electromyographic testing in the long-term evaluation of patients who have undergone carpal tunnel decompression particularly in those in whom revision surgery is being considered. In doubtful cases or when there are differing outcomes, self-administered scales such as Levine's Questionnaire should prevail over EMG results when deciding on the need for revision surgery.

▶ Carpal tunnel release (CTR) is one of the most common surgeries performed. The clinical results are generally good, but there is potential for recurrence. There is little published information on the long-term electrophysiologic results of patients after CTR. In particular, it is not known if late electrophysiologic findings correlate with the recurrence or resolution of carpal tunnel symptoms. This work sheds some light onto this issue.

In this study, 75.7% of eligible patients participated, so it provides a good representation of their population. There are a few key findings in the study:

1. Long-term electrophysiologic parameters show sustained improvement after CTR. However, sensory conduction velocity does not normalize, even in asymptomatic individuals.
2. There is significant correlation between the Levine's Questionnaire clinical scale and electrophysiologic findings.
3. There is a high incidence of electrophysiologic evidence of carpal tunnel syndrome in the long term even in the absence of symptoms.

These findings need to be considered when evaluating a patient after CTR. As the authors suggest, Levine's Questionnaire can be an important adjunct to clinical and electrophysiologic tests in the assessment of possible recurrent carpal tunnel syndrome after release.

A. Chong, MD

Comparison of muscle force after immediate and delayed reinnervation using nerve-muscle-endplate band grafting
Sobotka S, Mu L (Hackensack Univ Med Ctr, NJ)
J Surg Res 179:E117-E126, 2013

Background.—Because of poor functional outcomes of currently used reinnervation methods, we developed novel treatment strategy for the restoration of paralyzed muscles—the nerve-muscle-endplate band grafting (NMEG) technique. The graft was obtained from the sternohyoid muscle (donor) and implanted into the ipsilateral paralyzed sternomastoid (SM) muscle (recipient).

Methods.—Rats were subjected to immediate or delayed (1 or 3 mo) reinnervation of the experimentally paralyzed SM muscles using the NMEG technique or the conventionally used nerve end-to-end anastomosis. The SM muscle at the opposite side served as a normal control.

Results.—NMEG produced better recovery of muscle force as compared with end-to-end anastomosis. A larger force produced by NMEG was most evident for small stimulation currents.

Conclusions.—The NMEG technique holds great potential for successful muscle reinnervation. We hypothesize that even better muscle reinnervation and functional recovery could be achieved with further improvement of the environment that favors axon-end plate connections and accelerates axonal growth and sprouting (Fig 1).

▶ This is an interesting and thought-provoking study, although ultimately the conclusions offered will have minimal or no clinical impact. Essentially, the authors perform a neurotization procedure in which the donor nerve is transferred with a blood vessel and a chunk of muscle. In other words, a partial innervated muscle transfer is implanted within the denervated muscle. The authors suggest that harvesting the endplate band with the donor nerve in essence transfers endplates into the denervated muscle and improves final results. Their study supports this assertion.

Here are the problems with this conclusion:

1. The transferred muscle measures 6 × 6 × 3 mm—this is quite small except that the muscle being manipulated is the sternomastoid of a rat! The authors do not discuss how much muscle is being replaced, but how big can the rat sternocleidomastoid muscle be?

2. Comparison group is an end-to-end nerve repair of the motor branch to the sternomastoid of a rat. This is so small that a technically perfect repair would be quite difficult.

3. Essentially, in the 1-month and 3-month denervation groups, a chunk of denervated muscle is excised and replaced with innervated muscle.

4. In human skeletal muscles, the endplates are spread throughout the muscle.

5. Although the authors report statistical difference, the mean differences in contractile strength are 61% vs 70% of the control muscle, hardly a large difference in outcomes.

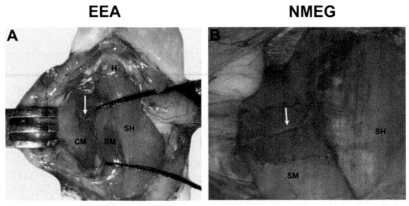

EEA　　　　　**NMEG**

FIGURE 1.—Photographs illustrating the reinnervation of a denervated SM muscle with the EEA procedure (A) and with the NMEG technique (B). Note that the SM nerve enters in the middle third of the muscle (A). An arrow in A indicates the anastomosed site of the transected SM nerve after the EEA procedure. A completed NMEG transplantation is shown in B. The transplanted NMEG with a visible nerve branch (arrow) was harvested from ipsilateral SH muscle. CM = cleidomastoid muscle; H = hyoid bone. (Reprinted from The Journal of Surgical Research. Sobotka S, Mu L. Comparison of muscle force after immediate and delayed reinnervation using nerve-muscle-endplate band grafting. *J Surg Res.* 2013;179:E117-E126, Copyright 2013, with permission from Elsevier.)

6. The authors focus a lot on low amplitude stimulation—the nerve-muscle-endplate band grafting—treated rats contract at a lower amplitude. The significance of this is merely conjecture and does not imply superiority of one technique over another.

7. The authors compare the results of their technique with clinical results as evidence that their technique offers substantial improvements over currently used techniques! Obviously, any repair will perform better in a rat than the best repair in a human.

8. Finally, there are almost no clinical scenarios in which a piece of muscle with an intact neurovascular pedicle can be transferred to a denervated muscle close enough that this leash will reach. In other words, this is a laboratory nerve repair that will not be usable in a human clinical situation.

This is an interesting idea that ultimately will not translate to humans.

J. Isaacs, MD

Functional Outcome Following Nerve Repair in the Upper Extremity Using Processed Nerve Allograft
Cho MS, Rinker BD, Weber RV, et al (Antonio Military Med Ctr, Fort Sam, Houston, TX; Univ of Kentucky, Lexington; Inst for Nerve, Hand, and Reconstructive Surgery, Rutherford, NJ; et al)
J Hand Surg 37A:2340-2349, 2012

Purpose.—Reconstruction of peripheral nerve discontinuities with processed nerve allograft has become increasingly relevant. The RANGER Study registry was initiated in 2007 to study the use of processed nerve allografts in contemporary clinical practice. We undertook this study to analyze outcomes for upper extremity nerve repairs contained in the registry database.

Methods.—We identified an upper extremity-specific population within the RANGER Study registry database consisting of 71 nerves repaired with processed nerve allograft. This group was composed of 56 subjects with a mean age of 40 ± 17 years (range, 18–86 y). We analyzed data to determine the safety and efficacy of processed nerve allograft. Quantitative data were available on 51 subjects with 35 sensory, 13 mixed, and 3 motor nerves. The mean gap length was 23 ± 12 mm (range, 5–50 mm). We performed an analysis to evaluate response-to-treatment and to examine sensory and motor recovery according to the international standards for motor and sensory nerve recovery.

Results.—There were no reported implant complications, tissue rejections, or adverse experiences related to the use of the processed nerve allografts. Overall recovery, S3 or M4 and above, was achieved in 86% of the procedures. Subgroup analysis demonstrated meaningful levels of recovery in sensory, mixed, and motor nerve repairs with graft lengths between 5 and

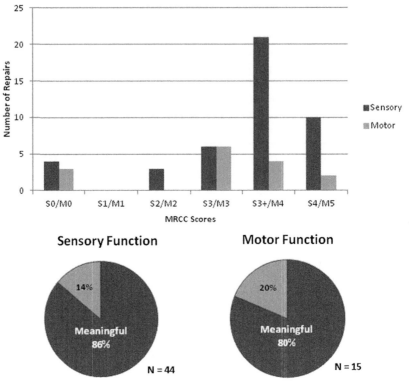

FIGURE 2.—Functional sensory and motor outcomes groups expressed by MRCC scores for the outcomes population reporting quantitative measures. Pie charts represent the percentage of subjects reporting meaningful recovery in each group. Bar charts represent the distribution of all MRCC scores for each group. We observed no significant difference ($P > .05$) between groups with $P = .68$. (Reprinted from The Journal of Hand Surgery. Cho MS, Rinker BD, Weber RV, et al. Functional outcome following nerve repair in the upper extremity using processed nerve allograft. *J Hand Surg.* 2012;37A:2340-2349, Copyright 2012, with permission from the American Society for Surgery of the Hand.)

50 mm. The study also found meaningful levels of recovery in 89% of digital nerve repairs, 75% of median nerve repairs, and 67% of ulnar nerve repairs.

Conclusions.—Our data suggest that processed nerve allografts offer a safe and effective method of reconstructing peripheral nerve gaps from 5 to 50 mm in length. These outcomes compare favorably with those reported in the literature for nerve autograft, and exceed those reported for tube conduits (Fig 2).

▶ The gold standard for reconstructing a peripheral nerve injury with a significant gap has been with autograft. The recent introduction of nerve allograft presents the opportunity to provide a tension-free repair without requiring a donor site. This study's goal was to provide functional outcomes for patients reconstructed with nerve allografts.

This is a retrospective review of 56 patients who had upper extremity nerves reconstructed with allograft for nerve gaps up to 5 cm. The authors looked at the percentage of patients who achieved meaningful recovery (greater or equal to S3/M3 on the Mackinnon modification of the Medical Research Council Classification scale). They found that 86% of those with sensory nerves and 80% with motor nerves achieved meaningful recovery, and there were no reports of implant complications (Fig 2).

This study provides data suggesting that nerve allografts are a useful tool for the surgeon faced with a nerve gap. The results for the motor nerves are particularly interesting and provide evidence that the role of nerve allograft may extend beyond noncritical sensory nerves. The study has some weaknesses. It is a retrospective chart review presenting a very heterogeneous group of patients. It is also important to consider that this study deals with nerve gaps less than 5 cm.

Off-the-shelf nerve allografts have become a helpful addition to my nerve repair tool kit. They are easy to work with in both preparation and handling in the operating room. They also save operating time and eliminate donor site morbidity. This study provides early evidence of efficacy and safety for these products. It also suggests that there may be expanding indications for nerve allografts.

C. Curtin, MD

Effects of Sensory Reeducation Programs on Functional Hand Sensibility after Median and Ulnar Repair: A Systematic Review
Miller LK, Chester R, Jerosch-Herold C (Univ of East Anglia, Norwich, UK)
J Hand Ther 25:297-307, 2012

Introduction.—This is the first systematic review looking at the effectiveness of sensory re-education programmes on functional sensibility which focuses purely on clinical trials of adult patients with median and ulnar nerve injuries.

Methods.—A literature search of AMED, CINAHL, Embase and OVID Medline (from inception to July 2011) was undertaken. Studies were selected if they met the following inclusion criteria: controlled trials (with or without randomization) of sensory re-education, including early and late phase, in adults with median and/or ulnar nerve repair. Two independent assessors rated study quality and risk of bias using the 24 point MacDermid Evaluation Tool.

Results.—A total of seven articles met the inclusion criteria representing five separate studies Study quality ranged from 13 to 33 out of 48 points on the Evaluation Tool. Due to heterogeneity of the interventions and outcomes assessed it was not possible to pool the results from all studies. There is limited evidence to support the use of early and late SR programmes.

Conclusion.—Further trials are needed to evaluate the effect of early and late sensory re-education which are adequately powered, include validated and relevant outcomes and which are reported according to CONSORT (Consolidated Standards of Reporting Trials) guidelines.

Level of Evidence.—2b.

▶ The aim of this systematic review was to provide an updated synthesis of clinical trials of adult patients with median (MN) and ulnar nerve (UN) injuries, excluding digital nerve injuries, with stricter criteria. Their search terms were *sensory relearning, sensory reeducation, hand,* and *upper limb.* Their inclusion criteria included controlled clinical trials with or without randomization, specific sensory relearning or sensory reeducation (SR) programs, adults with complete MN and/or UN lacerations with a sample size of greater than 10 people, and only English-language studies. To verify the quality of each study, MacDermid's Structured Effectiveness for Quality Evaluation of Study a 24-item, 48-point scale, was used.[1] It is generally accepted that studies with a score 1 to 20 are of low quality, scores of 21 to 34 are of moderate quality, and scores of 35 to 44 are of high quality. The included studies' scores ranged from 13 to 33.

SR is classified in 2 phases: early or phase I and late or phase II SR. Phase I begins within the first 24 hours postoperatively into the third and fourth month. Wynn-Parry and Salter defined the first published SR program, what is now considered *classic SR* or *late phase,*[2] which is defined as phase II in this article. Classic SR starts when re-innervation is confirmed by Tinel's in fingertips, or a Semmes Weinstein Monofilament Test (SWMT) notes sensation with the 4.31-sized monofilament, which is the loss of protective sensation level. Historically, this was when classic SR was initiated.[2]

The authors identified 94 studies, and 7 met inclusion criteria. They found there were 3 overarching comparative groups: phase II vs no intervention; phase I vs phase II, and phase II vs topical anesthesia. No meta-analysis was completed, as some studies did not completely outline their interventions for reproducibility, and complete information of some controlled groups' interventions was lacking.

The review found SR to be significantly effective in 3 major areas: (1) improved static and moving 2-point discrimination greater than control groups up to 2 years, (2) object recognition was significantly better in the experimental SR group at 2 years compared with the control group, and (3) significantly improved sensibility measured with SWMT up to 2 years after repair compared with the control groups. The authors concluded there is limited evidence to support phase I and II SR to improve MN and UN lesions at the wrist. The need for quality studies of well-defined intervention protocols of SR is emphasized by the authors.

V. H. O'Brien, OTD, OTR/L, CHT

References

1. MacDermid JC. The quality of clinical practice guidelines in hand therapy. *J Hand Ther.* 2004;17:200-209.
2. Parry CB, Salter M. Sensory re-education after median nerve lesions. *Hand.* 1976; 8:250-257.

7 Brachial Plexus

Outcome after transfer of intercostal nerves to the nerve of triceps long head in 25 adult patients with total brachial plexus root avulsion injury
Gao K, Lao J, Zhao X, et al (HuaShan Hosp, Shanghai, China)
J Neurosurg 118:606-610, 2013

Object.—The intercostal nerves (ICNs) have been used to repair the triceps branch in some organizations in the world, but the reported results differ significantly. The effect of this procedure requires evaluation. Thus, this study aimed to evaluate the outcome of ICN transfer to the nerve of the long head of the triceps muscle and to determine the factors affecting the outcome of this procedure.

Methods.—A retrospective review was conducted in 25 patients with global root avulsion brachial plexus injuries who underwent ICN transfer. The nerves of the long head of the triceps were the recipient nerves in all patients. The ICNs were used in 2 different ways: 2 ICNs were used as donor nerves in 18 patients, and 3 ICNs were used in 7 patients. The mean follow-up period was 5.6 years.

Results.—The effective rate of motor recovery in the 25 patients was 56% for the function of the long head of the triceps. There was no significant difference in functional recovery between the patients with 2 or 3 ICN transfers. The outcome of this procedure was not altered if combined with phrenic nerve transfer to the biceps branch. Patients in whom surgery was delayed 6 months or less achieved better results.

Conclusions.—The transfer of ICNs to the nerve of long head of the triceps is an effective procedure for treating global brachial plexus avulsion injuries, even if combined with phrenic nerve transfer to the biceps branch. Two ICNs appear to be sufficient for donation. The earlier the surgery is performed, the better the results achieved.

▶ Few American centers can match the volume of brachial plexus reconstruction seen in centers such as the Huashan Hospital in Shanghai. In 4 years, the senior author performed 95 intercostal (IC) to radial nerve branch to the long head of the triceps. This, in itself, is remarkable. It is, therefore, not only noteworthy, but also slightly disappointing that they only reported the outcomes on 25 patients! Their exclusion criteria (for the study, not for the surgery itself) are long and arbitrary and is a significant weakness of the study. Humerus fractures, rib fractures, and diabetes all affect brachial plexus patients, and we need to know if surgeries such as the one reported on in this study can help these patients, too! However, even with the study group optimized (by excluding less ideal patients), M3 or better is achieved slightly less than 60% of the time. As with many similar reports, the authors do not even include how many patients achieved M4 or M5 strength (which is really the desirable goal of all patients). Still, this article does support that IC nerves are an option for a group of patients in which the list of options is painfully short! Important secondary points that are worth emphasizing from this study: Two intercostals seem to be effective (instead of 3), and harvesting several intercostals (the senior author simultaneously transferred to the axillary nerve and thoracodorsal nerves) as well as the phrenic nerve did not seem to result in complications. The patients were able to fire both muscle groups (those innervated by the phrenic and those innervated by the ICs) independently. It should be noted that M3 in Asian populations is not the same in American patients, and respiratory effects not seen in Asian populations may still be a problem in American patients—both a result of the differences between American and Asian body habitus!

J. Isaacs, MD

Diagnostic accuracy of MRI in adults with suspect brachial plexus lesions: A multicentre retrospective study with surgical findings and clinical follow-up as reference standard
Tagliafico A, Succio G, Serafini G, et al (Univ of Genoa, Italy; Santa Corona Hosp, Pietra Ligure, Savona, Italy; et al)
Eur J Radiol 81:2666-2672, 2012

Objective.—To evaluate brachial plexus MRI accuracy with surgical findings and clinical follow-up as reference standard in a large multicentre study.

Materials and Methods.—The research was approved by the Institutional Review Boards, and all patients provided their written informed consent. A multicentre retrospective trial that included three centres was performed between March 2006 and April 2011. A total of 157 patients (men/women: 81/76; age range, 18—84 years) were evaluated: surgical findings and clinical follow-up of at least 12 months were used as the reference standard. MR imaging was performed with different equipment at 1.5T and 3.0T. The patient group was divided in five subgroups: mass lesion, traumatic injury, entrapment syndromes, post-treatment evaluation, and other.

Sensitivity, specificity with 95% confidence intervals (CIs), positive predictive value (PPV), pre-test-probability (the prevalence), negative predictive value (NPV), pre- and post-test odds (OR), likelihood ratio for positive results (LH+), likelihood ratio for negative results (LH−), accuracy and post-test probability (post-P) were reported on a per-patient basis.

Results.—The overall sensitivity and specificity with 95% CIs were: 0.810/0.914; (0.697−0.904). Overall PPV, pre-test probability, NPV, LH+, LH−, and accuracy: 0.823, 0.331, 0.905, 9.432, 0.210, 0.878.

Conclusions.—The overall diagnostic accuracy of brachial plexus MRI calculated on a per-patient base is relatively high. The specificity of brachial plexus MRI in patients suspected of having a space-occupying mass is very high. The sensitivity is also high, but there are false-positive interpretations as well.

▶ This large, multicenter study retrospectively examined magnetic resonance imaging (MRI) accuracy in brachial plexus lesions and confirms what we already know—MRI of the brachial plexus is useful in identifying mass lesions, scar tissue, and brachial plexitis. Traumatic lesions were frequently identified though specific localization, and prognosis was not expounded on. In other words, the MRIs in this study did not say that if 3 nerves are damaged they need to be fixed, rather, the MRI was able to identify that the plexus had suffered trauma.

It is worth mentioning that false positives were more common than false negatives, and poor quality MRIs were excluded from the study. This is useful information since the clinician can more comfortably use the MRI to rule out certain pathologies. The exclusion of poor quality MRIs makes sense (since clinically we could not use a poor quality MRI to guide decisions), but this certainly skews the results in favor of MRI as a testing modality.

In general, this is a good study that supports MRI usage.

J. Isaacs, MD

Grafting the C5 Root to the Musculocutaneous Nerve Partially Restores Hand Sensation in Complete Palsies of the Brachial Plexus

Bertelli JA, Ghizoni MF (Univ of the Southern of Santa Catarina (Unisul), Brazil)

Neurosurgery 71:259-263, 2012

Background.—In complete brachial plexus palsy, we have hypothesized that grafting to the musculocutaneous nerve should restore some hand sensation because the musculocutaneous nerve can drive hand sensation directly or via communication with the radial and median nerves.

Objective.—To investigate sensory recovery in the hand and forearm after C5 root grafting to the musculocutaneous nerve in patients with a total brachial plexus injury.

Methods.—Eleven patients who had recovered elbow flexion after musculocutaneous nerve grafting from a preserved C5 root and who had been followed for a minimum of 3 years were screened for sensory recovery in the hand and forearm. Six matched patients who had not undergone surgery served as controls. Methods of assessment included testing for pain sensation using Adson forceps, cutaneous pressure threshold measurements using Semmes-Weinstein monofilaments, and the static 2-point discrimination test. Deep sensation was evaluated by squeezing the first web space, and thermal sensation was assessed using warm and cold water.

Results.—All grafted patients recovered sensation in a variable territory extending from just over the thenar eminence to the entire lateral forearm and hand. Seven patients were capable of perceiving 2-0 monofilament pressure on the thenar eminence, palm, and dorsoradial aspect of the hand. All could differentiate warm and cold water. None recovered 2-point discrimination. None of the patients in the control group recovered any kind of sensation in the affected limb.

Conclusion.—Grafting the musculocutaneous nerve can restore nociceptive sensation on the radial side of the hand.

▶ This is an interesting study in which the authors note that patients with intact C5 roots and C6-T1 avulsions who underwent successful grafting of C5 to musculocutaneous nerve recovered pain and temperature sensation on the radial aspect of forearm and hand. Although they compared this with a group of non-grafted plexus avulsion injuries, a likely explanation is that the motive behind the study was a direct observation of this sensory recovery in some of their patients. They identified a subset of these patients and, indeed, the sensory recovery had occurred in all of them. Much of the article seems dedicated to answering criticisms of their study.

Certainly any sensation in the hand is better than nothing (and seems to help with pain perception as well), but it is hard to understand why grafting was not performed to the lateral cord, which would provide axons to the musculocutaneous and the sensory component of the median nerve, because this would be expected to further improve sensory recovery and in a more useful distribution than the radial side of the forearm. The authors describe that other nerves were graft from the C5 stump, but they do not describe the benefits of this exercise.

However, one important take-home message would be that the lateral antebrachial cutaneous nerve may not be the best option for grafting material, and it may facilitate some recovery of sensation if left in situ when grafting to the musculocutaneous nerve is planned.

J. Isaacs, MD

Upper Brachial Plexus Injuries: Grafts vs Ulnar Fascicle Transfer to Restore Biceps Muscle Function
Socolovsky M, Martins RS, Di Masi G, et al (Univ of Buenos Aires School of Medicine, Argentina; Univ of São Paulo Med School, Brazil)
Neurosurgery 71:ons227-ons232, 2012

Background.—Nerve transfers or graft repairs in upper brachial plexus palsies are 2 available options for elbow flexion recovery.

Objective.—To assess outcomes of biceps muscle strength when treated either by grafts or nerve transfer.

Methods.—A standard supraclavicular approach was performed in all patients. When roots were available, grafts were used directed to proximal targets. Otherwise, a distal ulnar nerve fascicle was transferred to the biceps branch. Elbow flexion strength was measured with a dynamometer, and an index comparing the healthy arm and the operated-on side was developed. Statistical analysis to compare both techniques was performed.

Results.—Thirty-five patients (34 men) were included in this series. Mean age was 28.7 years (standard deviation, 8.7). Twenty-two patients (62.8%) presented with a C5-C6 injury, whereas 13 patients (37.2%) had a C5-C6-C7 lesion. Seventeen patients received reconstruction with grafts, and 18 patients were treated with a nerve transfer from the ulnar nerve to the biceps. The trauma to surgery interval (mean, 7.6 months in both groups), strength in the healthy arm, and follow-up duration were not statistically different. On the British Medical Research Council muscle strength scale, 8 of 17 (47%) patients with a graft achieved ≥M3 biceps flexion postoperatively, vs 16 of 18 (88%) post nerve transfers ($P = .024$). This difference persisted when a muscle strength index assessing improvement relative to the healthy limb was used ($P = .031$).

Conclusion —The results obtained from ulnar nerve fascicle transfer to the biceps branch were superior to those achieved through reconstruction with grafts.

▶ Data in the medical literature seem to be continually growing in support of nerve transfers in place of long reconstructive nerve grafts. One of the most studied and successful transfers is the partial ulna to motor branch of biceps transfer. The authors of this study present their results of upper plexus injuries treated with this transfer vs those treated with long-graft reconstruction. Similar to other reports, the nerve transfer was clearly superior, even though patients undergoing this procedure had root avulsions, which theoretically implies more trauma and a worse prognosis when compared with the upper trunk rupture injuries that were grafted. The patient subgroups were otherwise quite evenly matched. One confounding factor not really discussed is that grafting across ruptured nerves has the potential for repairing within the zone of injury—a problem not associated with distal nerve transfers. Otherwise, the benefits of short regeneration lengths, high motor axon ratios, and a direct shot into the biceps are all well known and appreciated advantages of this technique. This article, although well done, does not offer anything new but confirms what is rapidly evolving to conventional wisdom among brachial plexus surgeons.

J. Isaacs, MD

Axillary nerve neurotization with the anterior deltopectoral approach in brachial plexus injuries
Jerome JTJ, Rajmohan B (Apollo Speciality Hosps, Madurai, Tamil Nadu, India)
Microsurgery 32:445-451, 2012

Combined neurotization of both axillary and suprascapular nerves in shoulder reanimation has been widely accepted in brachial plexus injuries, and the functional outcome is much superior to single nerve transfer. This study describes the surgical anatomy for axillary nerve relative to the available donor nerves and emphasize the salient technical aspects of anterior deltopectoral approach in brachial plexus injuries. Fifteen patients with brachial plexus injury who had axillary nerve neurotizations were evaluated. Five patients had complete avulsion, 9 patients had C5, six patients had brachial plexus injury pattern, and one patient had combined axillary and suprascapular nerve injury. The long head of triceps branch was the donor in C5,6 injuries; nerve to brachialis in combined nerve injury and intercostals for C5-T1 avulsion injuries. All these donors were identified through the anterior approach, and the nerve transfer was done. The recovery of deltoid was found excellent (M5) in C5,6 brachial plexus injuries with an average of 134.4° abduction at follow up of average 34.6 months. The shoulder recovery was good with 130° abduction in a case of combined axillary and suprascapular nerve injury. The deltoid recovery was good (M3) in C5-T1 avulsion injuries patients with an average of 64° shoulder abduction at follow up of 35 months. We believe that anterior approach is simple and easy for all axillary nerve transfers in brachial plexus injuries.

▶ In this small, 15-patient series, the authors describe their results and technique of axillary nerve neurotization through a deltopectoral approach. Numerous authors have prioritized shoulder abduction as second only to elbow flexion in importance for functional restoration after brachial plexus injuries. Nerve transfers in the management of brachial plexus injuries have gained widespread acceptance, and some studies report superior results to traditional nerve grafting. Donor nerves previously reported for transfer into the axillary nerve include a branch of the radial nerve, spinal accessory nerve, intercostal nerves, thoracodorsal nerve, and the medial pectoral nerve. The traditional approaches include the posterior approach (popularized by Leechavengvongs) and the axillary approach. The authors describe their experience using the deltopectoral approach.

In this series, all 15 patients had relatively low-energy injuries (all bike crashes) with a young median age of 26 years. Patients with 5 root avulsions were managed with intercostal to musculocutaneous and axillary nerve transfers (5 patients). Patients with isolated upper trunk injuries were managed with radial (long head triceps branch) to axillary nerve transfers and double fascicular nerve transfers for elbow flexion (9 patients). All of these transfers were done through a deltopectoral approach taking down the pectoralis minor tendon. The exposure allowed visualization of the radial, axillary, medial pectoral, and thoracodorsal nerves as well as the 3 cords. M5 (excellent) shoulder abduction was obtained in all upper trunk injuries (long head triceps branch transfer) and M3 (good) shoulder abduction in the pan plexus cohort (intercostal transfer).

In addition to the excellent results reported, there are several conceptual advantages of this approach. First, when used in combination with a plexus exploration and Oberlin or double fascicular transfer, it obviates the need to rotate the patient into the lateral decubitus position to perform the radial to axillary transfer for deltoid restoration. Second, the infraclavicular exposure, including nerve transfers for shoulder and elbow, can be done through 1 utilitarian approach. Finally, this approach allows neurotization into the entire axillary nerve because it is very proximal, thus innervating the posterior deltoid and teres minor that is often left out with a posterior approach (though can be addressed from a posterior approach as well).

The final appeal of this approach is the ability to visualize and consider multiple transfers (radial, thoracodorsal, and medial pectoral as well as median and ulnar nerve fascicles) through 1 approach.

G. Gaston, MD

Axillary nerve repair by fascicle transfer from the ulnar or median nerve in upper brachial plexus palsy

Haninec P, Kaiser R (Charles Univ, Prague, Czech Republic)

J Neurosurg 117:610-614, 2012

Object.—Nerve repair using motor fascicles of a different nerve was first described for the repair of elbow flexion (Oberlin technique). In this paper, the authors describe their experience with a similar method for axillary nerve reconstruction in cases of upper brachial plexus palsy.

Methods.—Of 791 nerve reconstructions performed by the senior author (P.H.) between 1993 and 2011 in 441 patients with brachial plexus injury, 14 involved axillary nerve repair by fascicle transfer from the ulnar or median nerve. All 14 of these procedures were performed between 2007 and 2010. This technique was used only when there was a deficit of the thoracodorsal or long thoracic nerve, which are normally used as donors.

Results.—Nine patients were followed up for 24 months or longer. Good recovery of deltoid muscle strength was seen in 7 (77.8%) of these 9 patients, and in 4 patients with less follow-up (14–23 months), for an overall success rate of 78.6%. The procedure was unsuccessful in 2 of the 9 patients with at least 24 months of follow-up. The first showed no signs of reinnervation of the axillary nerve by either clinical or electromyographic evaluation in 26 months of follow-up, and the second had Medical Research Council (MRC) Grade 2 strength in the deltoid muscle 36 months after the operation. The last of the group of 14 patients has had 12 months of follow-up and is showing progressive improvement of deltoid muscle function (MRC Grade 2).

Conclusions.—The authors conclude that fascicle transfer from the ulnar or median nerve onto the axillary nerve is a safe and effective method for reconstruction of the axillary nerve in patients with upper brachial plexus injury.

▶ The authors start this article by saying that nerve transfers are controversial. This statement should apply to some transfers more than others. The Oberlin and Modified Oberlin procedures seem to be well accepted and are both predictable and reliable. Likewise, the triceps branch of the radial nerve to axillary nerve transfer would fit into this category and is both reliable and predictable. Others, such as median nerve to radial nerve, do seem to be more controversial since results are not as predictable and the surgery itself is more risky than effective alternatives. This new transfer described by the authors seems to fit more in the second category than the first.

This article's main contribution to the peripheral nerve surgeon's armamentarium is the confirmation of the concept that any nerve or fascicle can be sacrificed to restore function of a more essential nerve. It is not clear in which scenarios transfer of fascicles from the ulna or median nerve will be better spent on deltoid function than for elbow flexion. Additionally, one of the reasons why the Oberlin is so popular is that elbow flexion and wrist flexion are synergistic motions. Triceps branch to the axillary nerve and transfer benefits in a similar fashion. A similar synergism does not seem to exist between the flexor carpi radialis, flexor carpi ulnaris, and the deltoid. This concept is not addressed in the article. Additionally, the authors do not comment on loss of wrist flexion (although hand motor function was not affected and sensory deficits, if they occurred, were transient).

Weaknesses of the article include a lack of clear indications for this particular surgery, a heterogeneous group of patients, and failure to describe how this particular transfer fits into a comprehensive brachial plexus reconstructive paradigm.

Additionally, the excellent results seen in the study may be partially attributed to a relatively short delay between injury and surgery and a relatively young patient population compared with other studies.

The authors should be commended for sharing an interesting idea, but indications for this transfer are probably quite rare, and it is unlikely that this concept will seriously impact many practices.

J. Isaacs, MD

Tendon Transfer Options About the Shoulder in Patients with Brachial Plexus Injury

Elhassan B, Bishop AT, Hartzler RU, et al (Mayo Clinic, Rochester, MN)
J Bone Joint Surg Am 94:1391-1398, 2012

Background.—The purpose of this study was to evaluate the early outcome of shoulder tendon transfer in patients with brachial plexus injury and to determine the factors associated with favorable outcomes.

Methods.—Fifty-two patients with traumatic brachial plexus injury and a paralytic shoulder were included in the study. All patients were evaluated at a mean of nineteen months (range, twelve to twenty-eight months) postoperatively. Twelve patients had a C5-6 injury, twenty-two had a C5-7 injury, five had a C5-8 injury, and thirteen had a C5-T1 injury. Transfer of the lower portion of the trapezius muscle was performed either in isolation or as part of multiple tendon transfers to improve shoulder function. Additional muscles transferred included the middle and upper portions of the trapezius, levator scapulae, upper portion of the serratus anterior, teres major, latissimus dorsi, and pectoralis major.

Results.—All patients had a stable shoulder postoperatively. Shoulder external rotation improved substantially in all patients from no external rotation (hand-on-belly position) to a mean of 20° ($p = 0.001$). Patients who underwent additional transfers had marginal improvement of shoulder flexion, from a mean of 10° preoperatively to 60° postoperatively, and of shoulder abduction, from a mean of 10° to 50° ($p = 0.01$ for each). Mean pain on a visual analog scale improved from 6 points preoperatively to 2 points postoperatively. The mean Disabilities of the Arm, Shoulder and Hand (DASH) score improved from 59 to 47 points ($p = 0.001$). The mean Subjective Shoulder Value improved from 5% to 40% ($p = 0.001$). Greater age, higher body mass index, and more extensive nerve injury were associated with a poorer DASH score in a multivariate analysis ($p = 0.003$).

Conclusions.—Tendon transfers about the shoulder can improve shoulder function in patients with brachial plexus injury resulting in a paralytic shoulder. Significant improvement of shoulder external rotation but only marginal improvements of shoulder abduction and flexion can be achieved. The outcome can be expected to be better in patients with less severe nerve injury.

▶ The authors of this study present a combination of novel tendon transfers used to reconstruct both rotator cuff and deltoid function in the paralyzed shoulder secondary to brachial plexus injury. Their assertion that more favorable results were obtained in patients with less severe brachial plexus injuries, as they had more functioning muscles available for transfer, is somewhat intuitive. Their results indicate that younger patients (younger than age 35 years of age at the time of surgery) have significantly better outcomes. They also note that regardless of the combination of tendons transferred to improve function, external rotation improved significantly, but forward flexion and abduction did not. The gain in external rotation would likely present a significant improvement in daily function for these patients. The tendon transfers described, although well depicted in the accompanying illustrations, are likely best performed by expert surgeons such as the authors of this article. Although their study population and the surgical procedures performed are very heterogeneous, this study does offer data that would be helpful in counseling patients regarding realistic outcomes after surgical intervention for brachial plexus injury resulting in shoulder dysfunction.

F. G. Fishman, MD

8 Microsurgery

Epinephrine, Norepinephrine, Dobutamine, and Dopexamine Effects on Free Flap Skin Blood Flow
Eley KA, Young JD, Watt-Smith SR (Univ of Oxford, UK)
Plast Reconstr Surg 130:564-570, 2012

Background.—The optimal sympathomimetic drug to support blood pressure without adverse vasoconstriction of free flap circulation remains unknown. This study examined the effects of four agents (epinephrine, norepinephrine, dobutamine, and dopexamine) on free flaps following resection of head and neck cancer.

Methods.—Twenty-four patients (25 data sets) were recruited into the study. Each patient received an infusion of the four drugs in a random order, with an intervening washout period between drugs, at four infusion rates. Continuous free flap skin blood flow monitoring was performed using laser Doppler velocimetry, with a second sensor on normal skin acting as a control. Global cardiovascular variables were monitored using the LiDCO Rapid Pulse Contour Analysis System (LiDCO Ltd., Cambridge, United Kingdom).

Results.—Dose-dependent, increased free flap skin blood flow was observed with norepinephrine and dobutamine. Both dopexamine and epinephrine infusions decreased blood flow. Flap skin blood conductance decreased (vasoconstriction) with norepinephrine, but markedly less than in control tissue, so overall the flap skin blood flow increased with increasing arterial blood pressure. Dobutamine increased flap skin conductance, without significantly increasing blood pressure, and modestly increased flap blood flow.

Conclusions.—Both dobutamine and norepinephrine had beneficial effects on flap skin blood flow. The maximal improvement in flow occurred with norepinephrine, making it the optimal pressor to use in patients with hypotension after free flap surgery.

▶ Hand surgeons that perform free tissue transfer are wary of the administration of pressors during surgery because it is thought that these agents can cause detrimental vasoconstriction of the flap itself. There are few data to corroborate this assertion, although many of us have anecdotal observations of their harmful effects. The authors of this article attempt to determine which of 4 vasoactive agents have the most effect on flap blood flow. The authors are, quite frankly, very brave for performing this study.

Twenty-four patients (25 flaps) undergoing head and neck free tissue transfer were recruited into the study, and there are clear inclusion and exclusion criteria listed. Blood flow on the flap and on a control area (deltoid skin) was assessed with laser Doppler. If and when mean arterial pressure went below 80 mm Hg in the immediate postoperative period, each of the 4 drugs was administered in random order with a washout period between.

The results of the study were quite interesting: Norepinephrine, although a vasoconstrictor, caused an increase in blood flow that overpowered the vaso-constrictive effects. Dopexamine (a synthetic analog of dopamine) also caused increased flap blood flow, but often at the expense of tachycardia that required premature termination of the drug. The authors conclude by stating that norepi-nephrine is now their drug of choice when a vasopressor is required during free tissue transfer.

This is a sound study with justifiable conclusions. In the day-to-day practice of free tissue transfer, adequate perfusion can usually be obtained by the use of fluid resuscitation (colloid and crystalloid) rather than pressors. However, there may be instances when a patient requires more than just fluid, in which case the use of norepinephrine is reasonable based on this study.

J. B. Friedrich, MD, FACS

Aesthetic and Functional Reconstruction of Fingertip and Pulp Defects With Pivot Flaps
Ni F, Appleton SE, Chen B, et al (Shanghai Jiaotong Univ School of Medicine, People's Republic of China; Dalhousie Univ, Halifax, Canada)
J Hand Surg 37A:1806-1811, 2012

Purpose.—Sensate reconstruction with glabrous skin is essential for ideal resurfacing of fingertip and pulp defects. The purpose of this study was to examine the palmar pivot flap as a reconstructive option for fingertip and pulp defects.

Methods.—We used the palmar pivot flap to repair fingertip and pulp defects in 21 consecutive patients. Outcomes measured included range of motion of the distal interphalangeal and proximal interphalangeal joints, sensation, pain, cold intolerance, and percussion tenderness. We assessed patient satisfaction with the aesthetic outcome using the Michigan Hand Outcomes Questionnaire.

Results.—All flaps survived. We achieved complete mobility at the distal interphalangeal and proximal interphalangeal joints. Sensory recovery was demonstrated in all flaps within 2 weeks postoperatively. No painful tips were reported at an average follow-up of 11 months. All flaps had mild cold intolerance, and 1 patient reported mild percussion tenderness. All patients were satisfied with the appearance of the reconstructed fingertips.

Conclusion.—The palmar pivot flap can provide sensate glabrous skin for the effective reconstruction of fingertip and pulp defects, resulting in aesthetically pleasing and good functional outcomes (Figs 1 and 2).

▶ There are many forms of reconstruction for fingertip injuries. However, no universal approach to these injuries exists because there is no clear superior flap for each situation. One reason is because the different flaps each have their advantages and disadvantages in terms of reliability, ease of surgery, donor site morbidity, and ultimate result. The second is because many flaps have been described with an emphasis on a surgical technique and flap survival. There is little high-quality data comparing the different flaps with good outcome information.

The authors were not the originators of this flap. It was previously described[1] in a technical paper, which focused on the vascular basis, surgical technique, and its utility in a few clinical cases. There were too few cases and limited outcome information in that study to assess the general utility of the flap for fingertip reconstruction.

This article fills that gap. There are clear inclusion criteria for use of this flap. The maximum dimensions of flap possible are shown (Fig 1), with a clear description of the surgical technique (Fig 2) and postoperative rehabilitation. Most important,

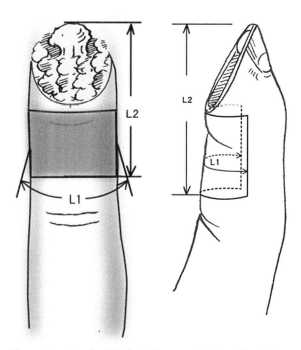

FIGURE 1.—The maximum length of the flap is determined by the midlateral distance of the digital segment proximal to the affected area (L1). This length should be equal to or longer than the distance between distal margin of the fingertip defect and the proximal transverse dissection line (L2). (Reprinted from Ni F, Appleton SE, Chen B, et al. Aesthetic and functional reconstruction of fingertip and pulp defects with pivot flaps. *J Hand Surg.* 2012;37A:1806-1811, with permission from the American Society for Surgery of the Hand.)

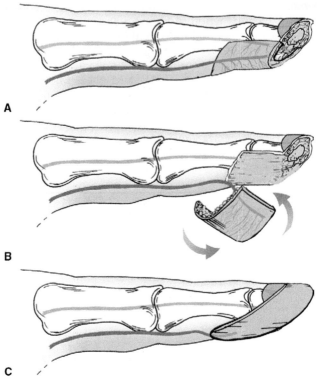

FIGURE 2.—A Diagram of palmar pivot flap. The digital artery and its transverse subcutaneous branches are shown in red. **B** The flap is elevated. **C** The flap is pivoted on the digital neurovascular bundle. The contralateral neurovascular bundle is left intact and is not incorporated into the flap. (Reprinted from The Journal of Hand Surgery. Ni F, Appleton SE, Chen B, et al. Aesthetic and functional reconstruction of fingertip and pulp defects with pivot flaps. *J Hand Surg.* 2012;37A:1806-1811, Copyright 2012, with permission from the American Society for Surgery of the Hand.)

there is a good description of the outcome measures allowing some comparison with other flaps used for fingertip reconstruction.

The pivot flap appears reliable with reasonable aesthetic, functional, and patient outcomes. Although it does not replace the need for further comparison studies, this work allows surgeons some basis to assess the utility of this flap for inclusion in their armamentarium.

A. Chong, MD

Reference

1. Yam A, Peng YP, Pho RW. "Palmar pivot flap" for resurfacing palmar lateral defects of the fingers. *J Hand Surg Am.* 2008;33:1889-1893.

The Effectiveness of Pedicled Groin Flaps in the Treatment of Hand Defects: Results of 49 Patients

Goertz O, Kapalschinski N, Daigeler A, et al (Ruhr-Univ Bochum, Germany)
J Hand Surg 37A:2088-2094, 2012

Purpose.—Despite the growing number of free and local flaps used for repairing defects of the hand, groin flaps are also still widely used. The aims of this study were to evaluate the outcome of a large series of patients whose defects were covered by pedicled groin flaps, and to find out whether it is still indicated in replacing damaged soft tissue of the hand in the era of microsurgery.

Methods.—From 1982 to 2009, we treated 85 patients with soft tissue defects on the hand and distal forearm with pedicled groin flaps in our department and recorded them in a prospective database. We interviewed and examined 49 patients in this cohort.

Results.—The mean age of the 85 patients was 33 years, the male/female ratio was 4:1, the mean hospital stay was 29 ± 13 days, and the mean follow-up was 9 years. The duration to flap division was 24 ± 5 days. Altogether, we performed a mean of 4.6 operations per patient, including thinning of the flap, deepening of the interdigital fold, and stump and flap revisions. One flap loss occurred. Of the 49 patients, results were mostly classified as good, and 82% of patients would undergo the procedure again. The mean Disabilities of the Arm, Shoulder, and Hand score value was 23 ± 17. The Vancouver Scar Scale showed nearly normal height and vascularity of the groin flap (0.2 ± 0.4 and 0.3 ± 0.6, respectively), pigmentation was slightly abnormal (0.8 ± 0.6), and pliability was evaluated between "supple" and "yielding" (1.5 ± 1.2).

Conclusions.—Results achieved with the groin flaps were positive. Most patients were satisfied with the results, and the operation was easily performed when McGregor's recommendations were followed. Nevertheless, considering the high number of secondary operations, the long hospital stay, and immobilization of the arm, groin flaps should be used only when free flaps or regional pedicle flaps are either not feasible or not indicated.

Type of Study/Level of Evidence.—Therapeutic III.

▶ This article directs our attention to the pedicled groin flap. This flap has been tremendously popular for several decades and is still frequently used as a last-resort flap, especially in the emergency setting. Because of increasing refinements in microsurgery, this truly useful flap is now regarded as old fashioned by many surgeons.

Although the title of the article suggests a study on 49 groin flaps transferred to the hand, this article actually deals with 85 patients with groin flaps to the hand and forearm. Of these, 70 are hand cases and 15 are forearm cases. The term "49 patients" actually refers to the number of patients that were reexamined for this study out of a total of 85. The number of patients with groin flaps to the hand (excluding the forearm) that were reexamined remains unclear.

Except for this uncertainty, the study design is well thought out. A significant difference in DASH (Disabilities of the Arm, Shoulder and Hand) score was found depending on the site of the lesion: Patients with groin flaps to the fingers scored much better than those with flaps to the forearms. The authors attribute this finding to the fact that to necessitate flap coverage on the forearm, a higher degree of trauma is required compared with the sparsely covered finger area. Another reason for less morbidity after flap surgery could be the fact that pedicled groin flaps exert a lower degree of motion restriction when applied to the fingers as the most distal part of the upper extremity as compared to the forearm, allowing more shoulder motion before pedicle division.

Patient satisfaction is high, and more than 80% of patients would undergo the procedure again.

High scar quality is found with the Vancouver Scar Scale. The average number of operations per patient is 4.6. Looking at this high number, I agree with the authors that free flap surgery could be a smarter solution than the pedicled groin flap in indicated cases.

Nevertheless, the pedicled groin flap is a useful tool for the reconstructive surgeon in carefully selected cases, especially as a last-resort flap.

M. S. S. Choi, MD

Primary free functioning muscle transfer for fingers with accompanying tendon transfer for thumb provide one-stage upper extremity composite reconstruction in acute open wound

Lin C-H, Zhu Z-S, Lin C-H, et al (Chang Gung Memorial Hosp, Taiwan)
J Trauma Acute Care Surg 72:737-743, 2012

Background.—Upper limb trauma may present as both soft tissue and muscle defects necessitating a free skin flap to effect a repair. The limb's core (basic) functionality can be returned with a secondary tendon transfer or a functioning muscle transfer. A functioning muscle flap can provide for soft tissue repair and functional restoration in a single procedure, but the success of such procedures requires further clarification.

Material.—From 1997 to 2006, nine patients underwent free functioning muscle transfer performed for upper extremity composite structure and functional defects, including four flexor digitorum profundus muscle and three extensor digitorum comminis muscle defects. Seven thumb tendon defects were managed with simultaneous tendon and free functioning muscle transfer. In addition, two opponensplasties and one thumb basal joint arthrodesis were performed for thumb function revision.

Result.—In all nine patients, procedures were completed without complications, the flaps surviving, enabling the patients to achieve opposable hand function. The muscle strength accomplished M4.2 (M3–5). The grip power was 41.7, and pinch power 55.3%, when compared with the other hand.

Conclusion.—Primary functioning muscle transfer can provide a one-stage composite functional restoration in an open wound. The thumb can be reconstructed with tendon transfer followed by opponensplasty to achieve a satisfactory range of opposable function.

▶ Traumatic injuries to the upper extremity are difficult to manage without the consideration of the overlying soft tissues. The authors address one of the most complex issues of returning function with a soft tissue deficit when dealing with upper extremity trauma. As noted by the authors, it has been classically thought that complex functional reconstruction should not be undergone in the acute phase of an injury. The authors aim to debunk this philosophy by presenting their experience with 9 complex upper extremity reconstructions with free-functioning muscle transfers (FFMT) in the acute phase. The acute phase of an injury is defined as a period when the initial wounds and injuries are not completely healed; in their examples, it ranges up to 30 days after the injury. As with all retrospective reviews, it is sometimes difficult to place the patients into well-organized groups, and the authors have the same difficulty. Because of the wide range of initial traumatic injuries treated, it is difficult to compare outcomes of these patients. The authors used several different free-functioning graft donors, including gracilis, sartorius, and rectus femoris, in differing constructs for finger flexion or extension based on the initial deficit. They also discuss the use of free-functioning graft for thumb opposition as well as concomitant opponensplasty during the FFMT. As reported by the authors, 6 of the 9 FFMTs achieved 5/5 muscle strength as recorded by the British Medical Council Grading System, although this specific finding is curious, as the average power grip was 41.7% and pinch grip was 55.3% of the contralateral side. The authors should be commended on presenting these 9 complex cases in a succinct and clear structure. Although limited by its small series numbers and retrospective nature, I do believe this article does provide 2 important findings; First, that all of the free-functioning muscle graft survived when performed in the acute setting with only one requiring a second look, and second, the authors' outcomes and lack of complications help revisit the notion of complex reconstruction in the acute traumatic window.

J. M. Froelich, MD

9 Tendon

The Effects of Oblique or Transverse Partial Excision of the A2 Pulley on Gliding Resistance During Cyclic Motion Following Zone II Flexor Digitorum Profundus Repair in a Cadaveric Model
Moriya T, Thoreson AR, Zhao C, et al (Mayo Clinic, Rochester, MN)
J Hand Surg 37A:1634-1638, 2012

Purpose.—To compare the gliding resistance of flexor tendons after oblique versus transverse partial excision of the A2 pulley in a human cadaveric model, to determine the effect of the angle of pulley trimming.

Methods.—We obtained 36 human flexor digitorum profundus tendons from the index through the little finger and repaired them with a modified Massachusetts General Hospital suture using 4-0 FiberWire. We repaired all tendons with a similar epitendinous stitch. We randomly assigned the tendons to 1 of 3 groups: intact pulley, transverse partial excision, or oblique partial excision. We measured peak and normalized peak gliding resistance between the repairs and the A2 pulley during 1,000 cycles of simulated motion.

Results.—There was no significant difference in the peak or normalized peak gliding resistance at any cycle among the 3 groups.

Conclusions.—Both transverse and oblique trimming of the A2 pulley had similar effects on the peak and normalized gliding resistance after flexor tendon repair.

Clinical Relevance.—When partial pulley resection is needed after flexor tendon repair, the transverse or oblique trimming of pulley edge does not affect repaired tendon gliding resistance.

▶ The partial venting of the A2 pulley is now practiced more frequently when the repair sites of the flexor tendons have to glide under the A2 pulley and the tendons are too tight under this pulley. The investigation by Moriya et al was intended to answer the question: Does a transverse partial excision or oblique partial excision make a difference in terms of gliding resistance to the flexor tendon? The results indicate that the gliding resistance to the flexor tendon is not affected by a transverse or oblique partial excision of the pulley. It is surprising to note the gliding resistance did not decrease after 100 or even 1000 cycles of motion. The small changes in resistance likely relate to the test model, in which only the A1 and A2 pulleys were left, with all subcutaneous tissue, skin, and other pulleys and the sheath stripped off. Of course, these loading conditions are not seen clinically. Resistance to tendon motion in vivo usually decreases after cyclic digital motion.

Clinically, several methods of venting are available: incision, excision (ie, pulley shortening), enlargement plasty with an interpositional graft, etc. In my practice, I incise part of the A2 pulley along the volar midline longitudinally if the tendons are repaired primarily or have not been delayed beyond 1 week after injury. When the repair is delayed more than 2 weeks, the pulley collapses and scar forms around the pulley. In that situation, I perform partial excision of the pulley. During tenolysis, partial excision is more common if venting is necessary because of scars in the pulley and tendons. I do not perform pulley plasty in primary or delayed primary repairs, and I believe that additional reconstruction after incision or excision is not necessary.

I agree that the shapes of the vented pulley have the potential to affect the resistance to tendon gliding. Triggering of the repair sites against the pulley edge poses the greatest risk of repair rupture. I consider a simple incision the best in avoiding triggering of the tendon repair site against the pulley rims because the longitudinal incision transforms the tight tunnel to a funnel, in which no sharp rim is present along the route of tendon gliding. Excision of the pulley creates a sharp pulley rim, against which the repair site can be snagged. To avoid this, I sometimes trim the pulley rim to an oval shape.

J. B. Tang, MD

Surface Modification Counteracts Adverse Effects Associated with Immobilization after Flexor Tendon Repair

Zhao C, Sun Y-L, Jay GD, et al (Mayo Clinic, Rochester, MN; Brown Univ, Providence, RI)
J Orthop Res 30:1940-1944, 2012

Although post-rehabilitation is routinely performed following flexor tendon repair, in some clinical scenarios post-rehabilitation must be delayed. We investigated modification of the tendon surface using carbodiimide derivatized hyaluronic acid and lubricin (cd-HA-Lub) to maintain gliding function following flexor tendon repair with postoperative immobilization in a in vivo canine model. Flexor digitorum profundus tendons from the 2nd and 5th digits of one forepaw of six dogs were transected and repaired. One tendon in each paw was treated with cd-HA-Lub; the other repaired tendon was not treated. Following tendon repair, a forearm cast was applied to fully immobilize the operated forelimb for 10 days, after which the animals were euthanized. Digit normalized work of flexion (nWOF) and tendon gliding resistance were assessed. The nWOF of the FDP tendons treated with cd-HA-Lub was significantly lower than the nWOF of the untreated tendons ($p < 0.01$). The gliding resistance of cd-HA-Lub treated tendons was also significantly lower than that of the untreated tendons ($p < 0.05$). Surface treatment with cd-HA-Lub following flexor tendon repair provides an opportunity to improve outcomes for patients in whom the post-operative therapy must be delayed after flexor tendon repair.

▶ Great advances have been made in the treatment of flexor tendon injuries. However, postrepair complications, such as repair rupture and stiffness from adhesions, are still common. Immobilization after flexor tendon repair continues to have a place in rehabilitation in certain clinical situations. The ability to reduce flexor tendon adhesions after immobilization will have clinical value.

Attempts to modify the tendon surface to prevent adhesions and improve function are not new. What is novel in this approach is that this work uses a compound containing hyaluronic acid and lubricin, 2 substances shown to have beneficial effects on flexor tendon healing. According to the authors, the combination of hyaluronic acid and lubricin with the carbodiimide crosslinking reagent improves the binding efficiency and half-life of the agents.

This in vivo study using a well-established model of flexor tendon injury and repair shows that modification of the tendon surface using a new gelatin compound can reduce work of flexion and tendon gliding resistance at a single time point.

The findings are promising but still very preliminary. As the authors discuss, the work has several limitations. It remains to be shown that the effect is sustained and whether tendon healing is affected by this approach. Future studies are planned, which will better clarify whether this approach will be useful in the clinical setting.

A. Chong, MD

A Biomechanical Comparison of 3 Loop Suture Materials in a 6-Strand Flexor Tendon Repair Technique
Gan AWT, Neo PY, He M, et al (Singapore General Hosp; Natl Univ Hosp, Singapore)
J Hand Surg 37A:1830-1834, 2012

Purpose.—The braided polyblend (FiberWire) suture is recognized for its superiority in tensile strength in flexor tendon repair. The purpose of this study was to compare the biomechanical performance of 3 loop-suture materials used in a locking 6-strand flexor tendon repair configuration: braided polyblend (FiberLoop 4-0), cable nylon (Supramid Extra II 4-0), and braided polyester (Tendo-Loop 4-0). We hypothesized that, using this technique, the braided polyblend suture would give superior tensile strength compared with the other 2 suture materials.

Methods.—We divided 30 fresh porcine flexor tendons transversely and repaired each with 1 of the 3 suture materials using a modified Lim-Tsai 6-strand suture technique. We loaded the repaired tendons to failure using a materials testing machine and collected data on the mechanism of failure, ultimate tensile strength, gap strength, and stiffness.

Results.—Failure mechanisms for the repaired specimens were as follows: the braided polyblend had 50% suture breakage and 50% suture pullout; the cable nylon had 100% suture breakage; and the braided polyester had 80% suture breakage and 20% suture pullout. Specimens repaired with the braided polyblend suture had the highest mean ultimate tensile strength (97 N; standard deviation, 22) and the highest mean gap force (35 N; standard deviation, 7).

Conclusions.—This study supports the findings of previous studies showing superior strength of the braided polyblend suture.

Clinical Relevance.—We were able to achieve up to 124 N in ultimate tensile strength and 48 N of gap force with this suture in porcine tendons. This gives greater confidence in starting immediate controlled passive or active rehabilitation after repair of flexor tendon injuries.

▶ This is a well-performed in vitro study of using FiberWire in making a 6-strand repair in a porcine tendon model. The experimental setup and assessment are standard. The findings again showed that FiberWire has superior strength compared with cable nylon and braided polyester. All sutures were 4-0. However, in interpreting results using FiberWire, we should be mindful that these sutures are generally greater in diameter than those of other sutures labeled with the same size (in other words, 4-0 FiberWire is larger than 4-0 Ethilon). The difference in the diameter adds strength. The strength gained by using FiberWire can easily be overestimated. Although I believe FiberWire is stronger than a few other sutures, the difference may not be as great, as we read in these reports, if all suture materials are of the same diameter.

Other reports have documented the poor knot security of FiberWire sutures and concluded that at least 5-throw knots are necessary to ensure knot unraveling.[1,2] The present authors also used 5-throw knots in their study. Technically, the flexibility of FiberWire is a concern, especially in the digital sheath area. Here, I draw the reader's attention to a few recent reports in which the investigators continued to voice concerns about the knot security of FiberWire and the need for a large number of throws of the knots in securing the repair.

Clinically, although this suture has been used in tendon repair, the mainstream suture materials remain nylon and braided polyester. Absorbable sutures are used occasionally. I have used FiberWire in repairing tendons in the palm and forearm but not within the digital sheath because of reservations about the security and bulkiness of knots.

J. B. Tang, MD

References

1. Le SV, Chiu S, Meineke RC, Williams P, Wongworawat MD. Number of suture throws and its impact on the biomechanical properties of the four-strand cruciate locked flexor tendon repair with FiberWire. *J Hand Surg Eur Vol.* 2012;37: 826-831.

2. Waitayawinyu T, Martineau PA, Luria S, Hanel DP, Trumble TE. Comparative biomechanic study of flexor tendon repair using FiberWire. *J Hand Surg Am.* 2008;33:701-708.

Effect of Bone Morphogenetic Protein 2 on Tendon-to-Bone Healing in a Canine Flexor Tendon Model

Thomopoulos S, Kim HM, Silva MJ, et al (Washington Univ, St Louis, MO)
J Orthop Res 30:1702-1709, 2012

Tendon-to-bone healing is typically poor, with a high rate of repair-site rupture. Bone loss after tendon-to-bone repair may contribute to poor outcomes. Therefore, we hypothesized that the local application of the osteogenic growth factor bone morphogenetic protein 2 (BMP-2) would promote bone formation, leading to improved repair-site mechanical properties. Intrasynovial canine flexor tendons were injured in Zone 1 and repaired into bone tunnels in the distal phalanx. BMP-2 was delivered to the repair site using either a calcium phosphate matrix (CPM) or a collagen sponge (COL) carrier. Each animal also received carrier alone in an adjacent repair to serve as an internal control. Repairs were evaluated at 21 days using biomechanical, radiographic, and histologic assays. Although an increase in osteoid formation was noted histologically, no significant increases in bone mineral density occurred. When excluding functional failures (i.e., ruptured and gapped repairs), mechanical properties were not different when comparing BMP-2/CPM groups with carrier controls. A significantly higher percentage of BMP-2 treated specimens had a maximum force < 20 N compared to carrier controls. While tendon-to-bone healing can be enhanced by addressing the bone loss that typically occurs after surgical repair, the delivery of BMP-2 using the concentrations and methods of the current study did not improve mechanical properties over carrier alone. The anticipated anabolic effect of BMP-2 was insufficient in the short time frame of this study to counter the post repair loss of bone.

▶ Negative results sometimes send even more powerful messages than reports of positive findings. This report by Thomopoulos et al is one such example! This study once again illustrates the difficulty in achieving gains in mechanical strength of the healing tendon by means of biological therapy. The authors reported that use of bone morphogenetic protein 2 (BMP-2) failed to promote tendon-to-bone healing at postoperative 21 days in a canine model. Over the last few years, enhancement of the healing strength of the flexor tendon (including the tendon-to-bone junction) has been attempted and was found difficult. Many factors can affect the results, and optimizing the effect of treatments is both arduous and hardly comprehensive.

Theoretically, the choice of BMP-2 is reasonable, as its major biological effects are mineralization and bone formation. At the bone-tendon junction, mineralization is a basic biological requirement of healing and restoration of strength. Practically, biological effects such as cellular proliferation and changes in growth factor expression are more easily achievable than gains in mechanical healing strength, the latter remaining an ultimate measure of the effectiveness of treatment. A few years ago, the same group reported that a basic fibroblast growth factor–loaded controlled release system failed to enhance the healing strength of the digital flexor tendon after end-to-end repair in a canine model.[1] Other groups have tested sutures loaded with growth factors or stem cells; while some of the investigations showed positive and promising results, most investigations produced more difficulties than optimism. Biological modulation has been attractive to my group as well, and my laboratory has undertaken an arduous multiyear journey toward using gene therapy to achieve faster healing and increased strength. I expect to see exciting findings in this challenging area in the years to come.

J. B. Tang, MD

Reference

1. Thomopoulos S, Kim HM, Das R, et al. The effects of exogenous basic fibroblast growth factor on intrasynovial flexor tendon healing in a canine model. *J Bone Joint Surg Am.* 2010;92:2285-2293.

Percutaneous Release of the A1 Pulley: A Cadaver Study
Habbu R, Putnam MD, Adams JE (Univ of Minnesota, Minneapolis; Inst for Hand&Upper Extremity Surgery, Mumbai, India)
J Hand Surg 37A:2273-2277, 2012

Purpose.—Percutaneous release of the A1 pulley has been used for treatment of trigger fingers with success. However, lack of direct visualization raises concerns about the completeness of the release and about potential injury to the tendons or neurovascular structures. The purpose of this study was to assess the efficacy and safety of percutaneous release of the A1 pulley in a cadaveric model using a commonly available instrument, a #15 scalpel blade.

Methods.—Fourteen fresh frozen cadaveric hands (54 fingers, thumbs excluded) were used. Landmarks were established for the A1 pulley based upon cutaneous features. Percutaneous release was performed using a #15 blade. The specimens were then dissected and examined for any tendon or neurovascular injury, and completeness of A1 pulley release was evaluated.

Results.—There were 39 (72%) complete releases of the A1 pulley with 14 partial and 1 missed (failed) release. There was a 22% incidence of release of the proximal edge of the A2 pulley. However, there was no case of release of more than 25% of the A2 pulley length, nor was bowstringing of flexor tendons seen in these specimens. Eleven digits showed longitudinal scoring of the flexor tendons and 3 had partial tendon lacerations. No neurovascular injuries were noted.

Conclusions.—Percutaneous release of the A1 pulley using a #15 blade was associated with good efficacy and an acceptable margin of safety in this series.

Clinical Relevance.—Percutaneous release of trigger digits may assume a greater role in the treatment of patients with trigger finger because of cost containment pressures. The data from this study suggest that the technique used in this study is both safe and effective. With use of proper anatomical guidelines, risk to neurovascular structures is low, although longitudinal scoring of the tendon can occur.

▶ Trigger finger is one of the most common clinical problems that hand surgeons treat. Although it is a simple procedure, the logistics of organizing an operating room to perform open trigger release seems to be more involved than the technical aspects of the surgery. In this article by Habbu et al, the authors use a cadaver model to outline a percutaneous release using a #15 blade. Because the topographical landmarks of the A1 pulley have been well documented in previous studies, this procedure was performed without risk to the neurovascular bundles.

However, the authors report that there was a complete release of the A1 pulley using this technique in only 72% of cases. Additionally, 14 of the 54 fingers had some evidence of partial flexor tendon laceration or longitudinal scoring of the flexor tendons. Certainly, these results do not warrant immediate adoption of the technique. The open procedure itself continues to be a simple procedure with good results. It is hoped that authors such as these will find a streamlined and effective method of release in clinic that will lead to cost savings in terms of time and expense for both the patient and surgeon.

J. Chang, MD

Effect of Platelet-Rich Plasma With Fibrin Matrix on Healing of Intrasynovial Flexor Tendons

Sato D, Takahara M, Narita A, et al (Yamagata Univ School of Medicine, Japan; Izumi Orthopedic Hosp, Miyagi, Japan; Yamagata Saisei Hosp, Japan)
J Hand Surg 37A:1356-1363, 2012

Purpose.—To investigate the effects of platelet-rich plasma (PRP) with fibrin matrix on the healing of intrasynovial flexor tendons in a rabbit model *in vivo*.

Methods.—We transected and repaired 156 toe flexors of 73 rabbits using the technique of Tsuge et al and a simple running epitendinous suture. We randomly assigned Repaired tendons to groups that recieved no additional treatment (control) or to which we applied PRP, fibrin (F), or PRP with fibrin matrix (PRP-F) at the repair site. We scored edema and adhesion at 2, 3, and 6 weeks after surgery, and linearly tested repaired tendons for load to failure. We also histologically evaluated tendons at 2 and 3 weeks.

Results.—Edema scores and adhesion scores did not significantly differ among the 4 groups at any time point. Mean load to failure in the PRP-F group (14.7 N) was the highest among the 4 groups at 2 weeks after surgery, and was significantly higher than in the control group (10.0 N). Median histological scores in the PRP-F group (3.3 points) were significantly higher than in the control group (1.0 point). Mean load to failure in the PRP-F group (16.1 N) was highest, and median histological scores in the PRP-F group (3.5 points) were higher than in the control group (2.4 points) at 3 weeks, although there were no significant differences at 3 or 6 weeks.

Conclusions.—In a rabbit model of cut flexor tendons, PRP with fibrin matrix significantly increased healing strength within 2 weeks after surgery. Side effects such as increases in toe edema or adhesions around the tendons did not arise.

Clinical Relevance.—Platelet-rich plasma with fibrin matrix might help reduce the risk of repeated rupture after flexor tendon surgery, and lead to early rehabilitation.

▶ In this article by our colleagues in Yamagata, Japan, the authors investigate the effect of platelet-rich plasma with fibrin matrix on healing of intrasynovial flexor tendons. This work was done in a rabbit model of flexor tendon wound healing. The hypothesis was that platelet-rich plasma would contain growth factors and other proteins that would enhance healing without increasing adhesion formation. This would have good clinical translation because the platelet-rich plasma could be produced from the same patient at the time of flexor tendon surgery. This approach seems simpler than utilizing exogenously produced growth factors.

The authors found that the load to failure with the platelet-rich plasma with fibrin matrix addition was greater in this experimental group. The highest effect was 2 weeks after surgery, a critical time in clinical flexor tendon postoperative therapy protocols. By week 6, however, the effect was not significantly different.

The authors also attempted to evaluate adhesion formation by histologic measures, such as edema score and adhesion scores. However, these are subjective measurements at best. The authors did not attempt more quantitative measures of adhesion formation, such as range of motion or gliding potential.

Platelet-rich plasma with fibrin matrix resulted in a short-term increase in tendon healing strength. This strategy of increasing early strength must be weighed against any contradictory effects of increased adhesion formation. We look forward to more work from this group investigating the mechanisms of increased tendon repair strength.

J. Chang, MD

The Impact of Fiberwire, Fiberloop, and Locking Suture Configuration on Flexor Tendon Repairs

Haimovici L, Papafragkou S, Lee W, et al (Univ of Medicine and Dentistry of New Jersey, Newark; Stony Brook Univ, NY)
Ann Plast Surg 69:468-470, 2012

Purpose.—Suture technique, suture material, and the number of strands all play critical roles in achieving optimal strength of flexor tendon repairs. We evaluated the contribution to the tensile strength of flexor tendon repair using the strongest suture material, Fiberwire, and the best surgical technique (locking configuration) using 2- and 4-strand core repair to see what factor played the most important role in tendon repair.

Methods.—Human cadaver flexor tendons were harvested and repaired in a randomized fashion using locking configuration as derived from

Pennington's report. Ten tendons per group were repaired using either 4-0 Fiberloop, 4-0 Fiberwire, or 2-0 Fiberwire. During load-to-failure testing, visible gap force and maximum tensile strength were statistically analyzed. *Results.*—All flexor tendon repairs failed by suture pullout. The 4-strand 4-0 Fiberwire double-Pennington repair was found to be significantly stronger than the 4-strand 4-0 Fiberloop single-Pennington repair. When the 2-strand repair (2-0 Fiberwire) was compared to the 4-strand single-Pennington repair (4-0 Fiberloop), there was no significant difference found.

Conclusions.—The suture strand configuration rather than the strict number of strands or the strength of the suture material yielded the maximum tensile strength with reduced gapping at the repair site (Fig 1).

▶ There are several important factors that contribute to flexor tendon repair strength, including suture size, suture configuration, number of suture strands across the repair, peripheral suture, and motion and tension at the repair. Many different suture configurations have been proposed, including 2-strand, 4-strand, 6-strand, and 8-strand repairs. To facilitate increasing the number of strands across the repair site, looped sutures have been developed allowing 2 strands of material per pass.

In this cadaver study, the authors evaluate whether there is a difference in strength between a 4-strand repair and a nonlooped 4-0 Fiberwire suture passed in a double Pennington configuration compared with a 4-0 Fiberloop in a single Pennington repair (Fig 1). They also looked at the effect of suture size by testing a 2-0 Fiberwire single Pennington repair. During load-to-failure suture testing, although the 2-0 Fiberwire demonstrated the highest tensile strength, all sutures ruptured at the knot, whereas in the tendon repair testing, all failures occurred by

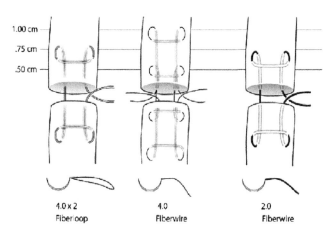

FIGURE 1.—A, Pennington repair. Note the critical relationship between the transverse and the longitudinal intratendinous parts of the suture. B, Four-strand 4-0 Fiberloop single-Pennington repair. C, Four-strand 4-0 Fiberwire double-Pennington repair. D, Two-strand 2-0 Fiberloop single-Pennington repair. (Reprinted from Haimovici L, Papafragkou S, Lee W, et al. The impact of Fiberwire, Fiberloop, and locking suture configuration on flexor tendon repairs. *Ann Plast Surg.* 2012;69:468-470, with permission from Lippincott Williams & Wilkins.)

suture pullout. This suggests that the repair configuration is more important than the suture size. This was further supported by the comparison between repairs that found the double Pennington repair with 4-0 Fiberwire was significantly stronger than the 4-0 Fiberloop repair and had a significantly higher resistance to 2-mm gap than either the 4-0 Fiberloop or 2-0 Fiberwire repair.

The key point to remember from this study is that it is not simply the number of strands across a repair that matters but, more importantly, the configuration of the repair. Based on this study and other recent literature on flexor repairs, in my opinion, the current minimum gold standard for flexor tendon repair in zone 2 is a 4-strand repair with a configuration that includes more than 2 locking loops in each tendon end. My current preferred technique is the Winters-Gelberman et al[1] repair utilizing a 4-0 looped Supramid suture passed in a configuration similar to the double-Pennington described in this article, followed by a 6-0 Prolene epitendinous suture.

F. T. D. Kaplan, MD

Reference

1. Winters SC, Gelberman RH, Woo SL, Chan SS, Grewal R, Seiler JG 3rd. The effects of multiple-strand suture methods on the strength and excursion of repaired intrasynovial flexor tendons: a biomechanical study in dogs. *J Hand Surg Am.* 1998;23:97-104.

Flexor Tendon Rehabilitation
Matarrese MR, Hammert WC (Univ of Rochester Med Ctr, NY)
J Hand Surg 37A:2386-2388, 2012

Background.—Given a patient who has cut the nondominant ring and small fingers and cannot bend the fingers at the proximal interphalangeal (PIP) or distal interphalangeal (DIP) joints, repair is done and a postoperative splint applied, usually a dorsal extension block splint with the wrist in neutral or slight flexion, the metacarpophalangeal (MCP) joints flexed, and the interphalangeal (IP) joints in full extension. Determining the best exercise program after repair of such a zone II flexor tendon laceration is challenging. The current course is to begin postoperative exercises within 5 days of operation under the supervision of a certified hand therapist (CHT). Both passive flexion and active extension with rubber bands and passive flexion and passive extension are commonly used approaches. With stronger tendon repairs, place-and-active-hold or active flexion may be used. The evidence was reviewed to determine the best approach.

Evaluation of Current Evidence.—Most of the studies focus on a specific technique and use no control subjects. Even if controls are used, the trials differ in important areas such as suture repairs, splinting positions, days until therapy is initiated, and outcome measures. If children are involved, few protocols include exercise. It is known that practitioners with specialized training in hand rehabilitation achieve better combined active flexion of injured digits, less PIP and DIP joint contracture, and greater patient satisfaction with care than practitioners skilled in general rehabilitation. Some support has been found for allowing patients unrestricted use of their injured hand after 8 weeks rather than waiting 10 weeks, with no adverse effects on function, rupture rates, grip strength, or subjective analysis. However, overall it is difficult to compare the various studies because of their inconsistent parameters.

Recommendations.—Exercises can be initiated under the direction of a CHT within 4 days of surgery. The wrist is splinted in neutral, then the therapist progresses through passive flexion exercises using the other hand, active extension, place-and-active-hold activities, and then full, unrestricted use of the hand 8 weeks postoperatively. The progression of the program depends on good patient compliance, which must be assessed when designing the approach.

Conclusions.—Future research should include focusing on the splinted position of the wrist, the number of days that elapse between surgery and exercise commencement, how to perform passive digit flexion, the use of active and passive extension, place-and-active-hold activities, active flexion uses, and when it is best to allow the patient unrestricted use of the injured hand. Randomization should help manage known and unknown confounding factors and limit bias in the study design, which should also include blinded independent evaluators.

▶ This article gives a nice summary of the history and outcomes of the various rehabilitation protocols for zone 2 flexor tendon injuries. The various passive (Duran and Houser), combination of active and passive (Kleinert), and newer early active protocols are compared.

The literature to date suggests that early active motion protocols result in better overall range of motion than when passive protocols are used. However, further randomized studies are needed to determine the following: "the splinted position of the wrist; number of days between surgery and initiation of exercises; methods for passive digit flexion; active versus passive extension; place and active hold; active flexion and when to allow the patient unrestricted use of the hand."

The authors also point out that studies have shown that results from a certified hand therapist are superior to those of a general rehabilitation consultant. Overall, this is a good refresher article and will hopefully serve as an inspiration for outcomes studies.

J. Frankenhoff, MD

Ultrasound-guided Injections for de Quervain's Tenosynovitis
McDermott JD, Ilyas AM, Nazarian LN, et al (Thomas Jefferson Univ, Philadelphia, PA)
Clin Orthop Relat Res 470:1925-1931, 2012

Background.—Nonsurgical management of de Quervain's tenosynovitis often includes corticosteroid injections. If the injection does not enter the compartment, or all subcompartments, response to the injection is variable. To ensure proper location of injections we evaluated the role of ultrasound.

Questions/Purposes.—We determined (1) the incidence of two or more subcompartments, (2) the incidence of anatomic variations during surgical release after failed injections, and (3) the relief of pain after ultrasound-guided injections.

Patients and Methods.—A prospective series of 40 consecutive patients (42 wrists) diagnosed with de Quervain's tenosynovitis by clinical examination were referred to a radiologist for an ultrasound-guided injection. The radiologist injected the first dorsal compartment and noted any septations. Patients returned for followup where outcomes, DASH, and VAS scores were calculated. The treating surgeon was blinded to any anatomic variations. Followup was at 6 weeks and a minimum of 6 months (mean, 6 weeks, range, 3—17 months; mean, 11 months, range, 7—18 months). Four patients were lost to followup.

Results.—Multiple subcompartments were noted in 22 of 42 (52%) wrists. At the 6-week followup, 36 of the 37 wrists examined in 36 patients (97%) had at least partial resolution of symptoms. Multiple subcompartments were identified in 52% of cases. At last followup, the mean DASH and VAS scores were 18.4 and 2.2, respectively. However 14% of wrists had recurrence of symptoms, all of which had subcompartments on ultrasound. No adverse effects from the injections were noted.

Conclusion.—We found ultrasound-guided injections to be useful for treatment of de Quervain's tenosynovitis. Our success with ultrasound-guided injections was slightly better than that reported in the literature and without adverse reactions.

▶ The authors present a series of patients that underwent ultrasound-guided injections of the first dorsal compartment for de Quervain's tenosynovitis. It demonstrated the incidence of septation of the first compartment in 52% of the patients. Unfortunately, the authors did not provide a control of normal patients. Although this percentage is lower than in other previous anatomic studies, the true incidence of this anatomic variant is unclear. In particular, it is important to know the incidence in normals because it speaks to the accuracy of ultrasound in determining the number of compartments.

The study does confirm that there is some connection between separate compartments and the intensity or persistence of this disease process. All 3 patients that eventually underwent surgical treatment had ultrasound evidence of 2 compartments, which was confirmed at the time of surgery. However, of the 5 people with recurrent symptoms, 2 did not have separate compartments for the abductor pollicis longus and extensor pollicis brevis.

The other control the study lacks is that of patients injected without the aid of ultrasound guidance. It would be beneficial to know, with direct comparison, how the addition of this imaging modality affects treatment success. Obviously, using the methods described in the article, there is a significant addition to the cost of the care provided. Without adequate data demonstrating superiority of the ultrasound-guided injection, adding that cost has to be carefully considered.

T. Hughes, MD

Exploring the Application of Stem Cells in Tendon Repair and Regeneration
Ahmad Z, Wardale J, Brooks R, et al (Addenbrooke's Hosp, Cambridge, UK; et al)
Arthroscopy 28:1018-1029, 2012

Purpose.—To conduct a systematic review of the current evidence for the effects of stem cells on tendon healing in preclinical studies and human studies.

Methods.—A systematic search of the PubMed, CINAHL (Cumulative Index to Nursing and Allied Health Literature), Cochrane, and Embase databases was performed for stem cells and tendons with their associated terminology. Data validity was assessed, and data were collected on the outcomes of trials.

Results.—A total of 27 preclinical studies and 5 clinical studies met the inclusion criteria. Preclinical studies have shown that stem cells are able to survive and differentiate into tendon cells when placed into a new tendon environment, leading to regeneration and biomechanical benefit to the tendon. Studies have been reported showing that stem cell therapy can be enhanced by molecular signaling adjunct, mechanical stimulation of cells, and the use of augmentation delivery devices. Studies have also shown alternatives to the standard method of bone marrow—derived mesenchymal stem cell therapy. Of the 5 human studies, only 1 was a randomized controlled trial, which showed that skin-derived tendon cells had a greater clinical benefit than autologous plasma. One cohort study showed the benefit of stem cells in rotator cuff tears and another in lateral epicondylitis. Two of the human studies showed how stem cells were successfully extracted from the humerus and, when tagged with insulin, became tendon cells.

Conclusions.—The current evidence shows that stem cells can have a positive effect on tendon healing. This is most likely because stem cells have regeneration potential, producing tissue that is similar to the preinjury state, but the results can be variable. The use of adjuncts such as molecular signaling, mechanical stimulation, and augmentation devices can potentially enhance stem cell therapy. Initial clinical trials are promising, with adjuncts for stem cell therapy in development.

▶ This article reviewed reports dealing with stem cell therapy for tendon engineering. There are several problems to be solved before clinical application of stem cells to tendon surgery. First, the role of transplanted stem cells in the recipient site should be clarified. Plenty of articles describe transplantation of some sorts of stem cells in tendon tissue that facilitates tenocyte proliferation and tendon tissue maturation. However, it is not clearly understood whether the stem cells seeded in the tendon tissue would transform to tenocytes or just produce some growth factors to facilitate expansion of the primary tenocytes in the recipient tendon tissue.

The kind of growth factors or hormones that function in the process of proliferation of tendon tissue should also be investigated. A previous in vitro study found that platelet-derived growth factor-BB, insulin-like growth factor-1, and basic fibroblast growth factor worked synergistically to promote proliferation of 3 different cell groups of tendon tissue (cells of the synovial sheath, endotenon, and epitenon) and that the cells in each group proliferated maximally in the presence of one of the growth factors, which was specific to each cell group.[1] It is still not fully understood how transplanted stem cells work with the growth factors to form tendon tissue. Further investigation for stem cell function is needed to promote cell therapy in tendon tissue engineering.

R. Kakinoki, MD

Reference

1. Costa MA, Wu C, Pham BV, Chong AK, Pham HM, Chang J. Tissue engineering of flexor tendons: optimization of tenocyte proliferation using growth factor supplementation. *Tissue Eng.* 2006;12:1937-1943.

Fractional Fowler Tenotomy for Chronic Mallet Finger: A Cadaveric Biomechanical Study

Hiwatari R, Kuniyoshi K, Aoki M, et al (Chiba Univ, China; Sapporo Daiichi Hosp, Hokkaido, Japan)
J Hand Surg 37A:2263-2268, 2012

Purpose.—The Fowler tenotomy, adjusting the balance of the extensor mechanism by central slip and lateral band detachment, is a common surgical technique for chronic mallet finger. The purpose of this study was to determine how much tendon to detach from the middle phalanx by measuring the extensor lag of the distal interphalangeal (DIP) joint following the procedure and to quantify how often a boutonniere deformity occurred as a consequence of the procedure.

Methods.—Sixteen fingers were obtained from 8 fresh-frozen cadaver hands. We made mallet finger deformity models by terminal tendon elongation. We detached the central slip and lateral band from the middle phalanx by one-third, one-half, and two-thirds of the phalangeal length and measured extensor lag of the DIP and proximal interphalangeal joints before and after this procedure.

Results.—In these models, the average extensor lag of the DIP joint was 44° (range, 40° to 50°). After central slip and lateral band detachment over one-third of the phalangeal length, the average residual extensor lag of the DIP joint was 19° (range, 0° to 40°). With one-half detachment, the average lag was 13° (range, 0° to 35°), and with two-thirds detachment, the average

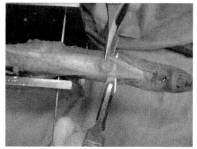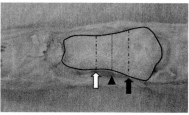

A   B

FIGURE 2.—A Chao et al[1] reported a cadaveric study of the Fowler central slip tenotomy in a model of chronic mallet finger of 45°. The same model was used in our study. The central slip insertion has been detached from the middle phalanx, and subsequently, the transverse retinacular ligament was sectioned. **B** The definition of the range of detachment. The black arrow indicates one-third of the length of the middle phalanx, the arrowhead indicates half of the phalangeal length, and the white arrow indicates two-thirds of the phalangeal length. The central slip and lateral bands were detached to these lines. *Editor's Note:* Please refer to original journal article for full references. (Reprinted from The Journal of Hand Surgery. Hiwatari R, Kuniyoshi K, Aoki M, et al. Fractional fowler tenotomy for chronic mallet finger: a cadaveric biomechanical study. *J Hand Surg.* 2012;37A:2263-2268, Copyright 2012, with permission from the American Society for Surgery of the Hand.)

lag was 6° (range, 0° to 15°). Extensor lag at the proximal interphalangeal joint occurred in 4 fingers, with an average lag of 8° (range, 5° to 15°).

Conclusions.—In the Fowler tenotomy models, detachment of the central slip and lateral band from the middle phalanx reduced extensor lag of the DIP joint. Detachment of up to two-thirds of the phalangeal length was effective in this model and did not cause any boutonniere deformity.

Clinical Relevance.—Controlled clinical application of our cadaveric results might yield improved active motion for chronic mallet extensor lag (Fig 2).

▶ Fowler central slip tenotomy as a treatment for chronic mallet deformity is an important option for hand surgeons to remember. Although most patients who appropriately treat their injury with true 24-hour per day splinting in full extension for 6 to 8 weeks will do well, with residual lag less than 10°, not all patients obtain a successful result. Opposed to more complex methods of reconstruction, the Fowler tenotomy is a simple, straightforward technique that can greatly reduce or eliminate the residual lag seen at the distal interphalangeal (DIP) joint.

This study tries to determine over what length of the middle phalanx the central slip and lateral bands should be detached for optimal correction of the DIP joint lag, and at what point, if any, there is an increased risk of developing a lag at the proximal interphalangeal joint. The study is limited by the fact that it is uses a cadaver model and tested a relatively inconsistent small number of digits (3 index, 4 middle, 3 ring, and 6 small). Despite small numbers, the authors were able to demonstrate that there was a statistically significant decrease in the amount of extensor lag at the DIP joint between each level of detachment. The average lag before tenotomy was 44 ± 3°, which improved to 19 ± 9° after one-third detachment, 13 ± 8° after one-half detachment, and 6 ± 5° after two-thirds detachment (see Fig 2 for graphic of level of detachment).

Concern over too aggressive release was the development of a lag at the PIP joint. Four digits in the study developed a PIP lag—2 with a one-third release and 2 with one-half release. The authors conclude that the development of a lag was more related to differences among individuals rather than the amount of release.

When performing the Fowler tenotomy in practice, it is beneficial to do the procedure under local anesthesia, ideally without a tourniquet, so that the amount of release can be carefully titrated. After each incremental release, the patient is asked to actively flex and extend his or her finger, and further release is performed as needed, until adequate improvement is achieved or a PIP lag begins developing.

F. T. D. Kaplan, MD

10 Trauma

The use of bone morphogenic protein-7 (OP-1) in the management of resistant non-unions in the upper and lower limb
Papanna MC, Al Hadithy N, Somanchi BV, et al (Salford Royal Hosp, UK; Lister General Hosp, Stevenage, UK)
Injury 43:1135-1140, 2012

The aim of the present study was to investigate the safety and efficacy of local implantation of BMP-7 for the treatment of resistant non-unions in the upper and lower limb. Fifty-two patients (30 males, mean age 52.8 years; range 20—81) were treated with local BMP-7 implantation in a bovine bone-derived collagen paste with or without revision of fixation. Thirty-six patients had closed injuries, ten had open injuries and six had infected non-unions. Patients had undergone a mean of 2 (1—5) operations prior to implantation of BMP-7. Clinical and radiological union was achieved in 94% at a mean time of 5.6 months (3—19). Two patients with subtrochanteric femoral fractures failed to achieve union secondary to inadequate fracture stabilisation, persistent unfavourable biological environment and systemic co-morbidities. One patient developed synostosis attributed to the BMP-7 application. This study demonstrates BMP-7 implanted in a bovine-derived collagen paste is an effective adjunctive treatment for resistant non-unions in the upper and lower limb.

▶ The authors present an interesting article that adds to the growing literature about using bone morphogenic proteins (BMPs) in nonunions. Classically, most reports are focused on lower extremity long bone injuries or spine procedures, but the authors add their experience with atrophic diaphyseal nonunions of the upper extremity as well. Specifically, the authors mention their experience with clavicle, humerus, ulna, and radius nonunions. This report involves 52 cases, with 17 of those being upper extremity. This article helps to provide a foundation for growing discussions on the appropriate use of BMPs in the upper extremity. The inclusion of whether autologous bone graft was used in previous surgeries as well as the number of previous procedures helps add strength to this study. The appropriate use of BMPs as well as the associated safety profile is of concern in our profession, and the authors openly and intelligently discuss these concerns. The data are presented in a concise and clean format that allows this article to be an easy review and adds important safety and healing rate data for lower and upper extremity atrophic nonunions, but I believe that based on the limited data available, hesitation should still be used when considering use of BMPs in upper extremity nonunions.

J. M. Froelich, MD

Intermediate Outcomes Following Percutaneous Fixation of Proximal Humeral Fractures

Harrison AK, Gruson KI, Zmistowski B, et al (Mount Sinai School of Medicine, NY; Barnes-Jewish Hosp, St Louis, MO, Univ of Pennsylvania Health System, Philadelphia)

J Bone Joint Surg Am 94:1223-1228, 2012

Background.—Mini-open reduction and percutaneous fixation of proximal humeral fractures historically results in good outcomes and a low prevalence of osteonecrosis reported with short-term follow-up. The purpose of this study was to determine the midterm results of our multicenter case series of proximal humeral fractures treated with percutaneous fixation.

Methods.—Between 1999 and 2006, thirty-nine patients were treated with percutaneous reduction and fixation for proximal humeral fractures at three tertiary shoulder referral centers. Twenty-seven of these patients were available for intermediate follow-up at a minimum of three years (mean, eighty-four months; range, thirty-seven to 128 months) after surgery; the follow-up examination included use of subjective outcome measures and radiographic analysis to identify osteonecrosis and posttraumatic osteoarthritis on radiographs.

Results.—Osteonecrosis was detected in seven (26%) of the total group of twenty-seven patients at a mean of fifty months (range, eleven to 101 months) after the date of percutaneous fixation. Osteonecrosis was observed in five (50%) of the ten patients who had four-part fractures, two (17%) of the twelve patients who had three-part fractures, and none (0%) of the five patients who had two-part fractures. Posttraumatic osteoarthritis, including osteonecrosis, was present on radiographs in ten (37%) of the total group of twenty-seven patients. Posttraumatic osteoarthritis was observed in six (60%) of the ten patients who had four-part fractures, four (33%) of the twelve patients who had three-part fractures, and none (0%) of the five patients who had two-part fractures.

Conclusions.—Intermediate follow-up of patients with percutaneously treated proximal humeral fractures demonstrates an increased prevalence of osteonecrosis and posttraumatic osteoarthritis over time, with some patients with these complications presenting as late as eight years postoperatively. Development of osteonecrosis did not have a universally negative impact on subjective outcome scores.

▶ The authors have described the intermediate results (minimum 3 years' follow-up) of minimally invasive fixation of proximal humeral fractures using percutaneous screw fixation. They found about 26% incidence of osteonecrosis, with higher incidence in more complex fractures. Also, they found changes of arthritis in high number of patients. However, these findings are not surprising. As in other fractures, higher incidence of complication is usually seen with higher complexity of fracture pattern. The authors have failed to provide the adequacy of reduction and compression achieved at the time of surgery. This may play a role in increasing the complication rate, similar to that in femur neck fractures. A discussion on the same topic would strengthen the study. Almost 10 patients (nearly 25%) refused to be included in the study. The incidence of complication may have changed if these patients were included. Percutaneous fixation of proximal humeral fracture is a standard procedure used by orthopedic surgeons across the world, and the literature has shown this to be a good method. I would not hesitate to use this method for a well-indicated fracture pattern. As with other minimally invasive procedures, surgeons have started expanding the indications for this procedure. While achieving a percutaneous fixation, we tend to forget 2 important principles: reduction and compression. This may give rise to higher complications seen. Hence, I am a little hesitant to broaden the indications for this procedure. The authors have described them very well. This study does help me in an important aspect: It made me more aware of what to expect a few years down the line after I have achieved a beautiful postoperative radiograph. This will help surgeons have a better discussion with patients about the incidence of complications years after surgery.

R. A. Habbu, MS, MBBS

Thermoplastic Hinges: Eliminating the Need for Rivets in Mobilization Orthoses
Schwartz DA (Orfit Industries America, Leonia, NJ)
J Hand Ther 25:335-341, 2012

Simplifying orthotic fabrication in the clinic is of value to both therapists and patients. This author describes a technique of using thermoplastic material to create a hinge, thus eliminating the task of lining up hinges with the joint axis of motion. Three different orthotic designs using this technique are described in this article.

▶ Thermoplastic orthoses required to be hinged for the purpose of achieving motion can be accomplished by the described method in this article. Three thermoplastic hinge designs were used on 3 different splints. The structure of the article was good, spending a significant portion describing the process and use of specific material. Case examples placed before the summary section described use of the thermoplastic hinge. It would have been helpful to have a comparison case example of the average length of time it took a practitioner to fabricate the thermoplastic hinge vs a standard method of hinged static progressive splints. The article cited the case examples of success with static progressive splinting and ease of fabrication, yet it did not mention cost. It was also interesting that the turnbuckle (Figs 10 and 11 in the original article) was used as a static progressive stretch splint, adding to cost and complexity of such splints. Further studies could result from this article, which is an added benefit. The concept of cost containment and using clinic-available resources is well described. However, it does make assumptions in the initial paragraph, "Hinging two-piece orthoses together at the joint axis of motion can be challenging, time consuming, and difficult to do correctly," that the article directs from by stating that a one-piece design is most efficient, and the reader should consider this with orthosis.

S. Kranz, OTR/L, CHT

Influence of Screw Design, Sex, and Approach in Scaphoid Fracture Fixation

Meermans G, Verstreken F (Lievensberg Hosp, Berchem, The Netherlands; Monica Hosp, Deurne, Belgium)
Clin Orthop Relat Res 470:1673-1681, 2012

Background.—Screw fixation of scaphoid fractures has gained popularity. A long central screw has been shown to be biomechanically advantageous.

Questions/Purposes.—We compared the ability of different screw designs to obtain this goal and determined the influence of sex and approach on screw length.

Methods.—We performed all measurements on three-dimensional reconstructions of 20 CT scans of normal scaphoids (10 men and 10 women) with the use of software. The three-dimensional computer models were analyzed, the central axis was defined, and the screws were placed along this axis. We compared 15 different available screw designs and volar and dorsal screw placement.

Results.—The length of the scaphoid along its central axis was longer in men (mean, 27.14 mm; standard error of the mean, 0.97 mm) than in women (mean, 23.86 mm; standard error of the mean, 0.37 mm). The screw length that can be used was longer in the volar approach (mean, 23.72 mm; standard error of the mean, 0.19 mm) than in the dorsal approach (mean, 23.31 mm; standard error of the mean, 0.19 mm) regardless of the screw design. Screws with a trailing thread diameter greater than 3.9 mm and leading thread diameter greater than 3.0 mm were shorter.

Conclusions.—Scaphoids in women are smaller than in men. Theoretically, fixation of scaphoid fractures through a volar approach will allow the surgeon to use longer screws. The screw design has a significant influence on the screw length that can be used in scaphoid fracture fixation. We recommend using a differential pitch screw with a thread diameter of 3.9 mm or less.

▶ The authors use 3-dimensional imaging data of 20 computed tomography scans to calculate maximum lengths for different screw designs placed in the perfect virtual central axis from volar and dorsal approaches. They also compare the dimensions of male and female scaphoid bones. They find that male bones are larger than female ones and that different screw designs lead to different maximum lengths, whereas the volar approaches allow longer screw lengths.

This is a rather theoretical article that is of limited practical relevance. As the authors state themselves, "perfect" screw placements are virtually impossible to achieve because of positioning issues and adjacent bones, especially the trapezium. It is also questionable whether statistically significant differences of less than 1 mm really have an impact on maximum compression forces and, ultimately, osseous union. However, this publication beautifully illustrates that the margin of error for percutaneous screw placement is quite narrow. Operative treatment, especially of displaced fractures, is not easy, and although it may be performed in minutes by experts, it requires a considerable level of experience. Although not in clinical practice yet, navigation systems may be of great value in the future.

K. Megerle, MD

Economic Impact of Hand and Wrist Injuries: Health-Care Costs and Productivity Costs in a Population-Based Study

de Putter CE, Selles RW, Polinder S, et al (Erasmus MC Rotterdam, The Netherlands; Consumer and Safety Inst, Amsterdam, The Netherlands)
J Bone Joint Surg Am 94:e56.1-e56.7, 2012

Background.—Injuries to the hand and wrist account for approximately 20% of patient visits to emergency departments and may impose a large economic burden. The purpose of this study was to estimate the total health-care costs and productivity costs of injuries to the hand and wrist and to compare them with other important injury groups in a nationwide study.

Methods.—Data were retrieved from the Dutch Injury Surveillance System, from the National Hospital Discharge Registry, and from a patient follow-up survey conducted between 2007 and 2008. Injury incidence, health-care costs, and productivity costs (due to absenteeism) were calculated by age group, sex, and different subgroups of injuries. An incidence-based cost model was used to estimate the health-care costs of injuries. Follow-up data on return to work rates were incorporated into the absenteeism model for estimating the productivity costs.

Results.—Hand and wrist injuries annually account for $740 million (in U.S. dollars) and rank first in the order of most expensive injury types, before knee and lower limb fractures ($562 million), hip fractures ($532 million), and skull-brain injury ($355 million). Productivity costs contributed more to the total costs of hand and wrist injuries (56%) than did direct health-care costs. Within the overall group of hand and wrist injuries, hand and finger fractures are the most expensive group ($278 million), largely due to high productivity costs in the age group of twenty to sixty-four years ($192 million).

Conclusions.—Hand and wrist injuries not only constitute a substantial part of all treated injuries but also represent a considerable economic burden, with both high health-care and productivity costs. Hand and wrist injuries should be a priority area for research in trauma care, and further research could help to reduce the cost of these injuries, both to the health-care system and to society.

▶ de Putter et al have written an interesting article supporting an impression that many upper-extremity surgeons have had but one that to date has not been rigorously demonstrated. They investigate if the economic impacts of hand- and wrist-level injuries on a societal level are larger than injuries in other anatomic regions. The strengths of this article are that it was done on a national level (The Netherlands) and that it was an incidence-based model accounting for both direct costs to the health care system and lost productivity costs. This article demonstrates that the economic impact is largest on a societal level for injuries to the hand and wrist. The 2 main drivers of this difference are (1) the lost productivity of the injured patients (largely men of working age) and (2) the volume of these injuries. Hand and wrist injuries represented 28% of the total number of injuries seen. Hip fractures, in contrast, were individually much more expensive in terms of direct health care costs but accounted for only 1.6% of injuries in this series. The quantitative details of a study of this type will vary by nation studied, the methods of calculating the economic impact of injury, the health care and workers compensation system, and worker protection laws. However, the qualitative finding that these types of injuries represent an enormous economic burden on modern societies suggests that research into methods to speed recovery from these injuries should be a research funding priority.

P. Blazar, MD

Comparison of three types of treatment modalities on the outcome of fingertip injuries

van den Berg WB, Vergeer RA, van der Sluis CK, et al (Univ of Groningen, The Netherlands)

J Trauma Acute Care Surg 72:1681-1687, 2012

Background.—In this retrospective study, we analyzed the outcomes of different types of treatment of fingertip injuries and compared them after a mean follow-up of 4.5 years.

Methods.—A total of 53 patients (59 injuries) were included in this study. The fingertip injuries were classified according to Allen classification. The patients were categorized into three groups based on the treatment: reconstructive group, bone-shortening group, and conservative group. As objective assessments, strength, sensibility, and goniometry were measured; as subjective assessments, cold intolerance, nail deformation, and aesthetics were measured.

Results.—The mean reduction in strength, the Semmes-Weinstein monofilament test, and the reduction in mobility for the injured fingers compared with those of the uninjured finger were not significantly different between the groups. Cold intolerance was reported in 50 (84.7%) of the 59 fingers, and in almost 90% of all the cases, there was some kind of nail distortion.

For the cold intolerance and nail distortions, there was no difference between the groups. The aesthetic outcomes judged by patients and surgeon were comparable.

Conclusion.—In conclusion, the outcome of treatment of Allen II, III, and IV fingertip injuries was irrespective of the treatment chosen. In an era where the enormous variety of surgical options suggests that treatment with a flap is the best, this outcome is at least surprising.

▶ This study has the same shortcomings of any retrospective study, and there is potential selection bias as the surgeon chose what was felt to be the most appropriate method, so a true comparison between the techniques cannot be made. It does demonstrate, however, that outcomes for treatment of fingertip injuries can be successful using a variety of techniques. It was interesting that the patient's perception of aesthetic appearance of the fingertip following healing was substantial, with ratings between 0 and 10 in both the bone shortening and reconstructive groups and range between 5 and 10 in the secondary healing group. Return to work, cold intolerance, and nail deformities were similar between groups. With the lack of high-quality, prospective, randomized clinical trials, the physician is left to choose treatment based on personal experience or preferences, and this study suggests that reasonable outcomes can be obtained with multiple treatments.

W. C. Hammert, DDS, MD

Mechanical Comparison of Novel Bioabsorbable Plates with Titanium Plates and Small-Series Clinical Comparisons for Metacarpal Fractures
Sakai A, Oshige T, Zenke Y, et al (Univ of Occupational and Environmental Health, Kitakyushu, Japan)
J Bone Joint Surg Am 94:1597-1604, 2012

Background.—The use of bioabsorbable implants to negate the need for subsequent removal could offer major clinical advantages for the fixation of fractures. The aims of this study were to compare the mechanical properties of novel bioabsorbable plates with those of titanium plates in a fracture model and to demonstrate the clinical results of the use of these new plates for metacarpal fractures.

Methods.—The first set of experiments compared the mechanical properties of bioabsorbable and titanium plates. Two types of bioabsorbable plates (one-third tubular and semi-tubular in cross-section) made of hydroxyapatite/poly-L-lactide and two types of titanium plates (for 1.5 and 2.0-mm screws) were tested. Each plate was fixed on a polyether ether ketone (PEEK) rod, which was transversely cut at its midsection. The second part of the study compared the clinical results associated with the bioabsorbable and titanium plates that were used in sixteen non-randomized consecutive patients with metacarpal fractures.

Results.—The bending strength and stiffness of one-third tubular bioabsorbable plate constructs were comparable with those of titaniumplates for 1.5-mm screws, and those of one-half tubular bioabsorbable plates were comparable with those of titanium plates for 2.0-mm screws. The mean torsional strength (and standard deviation) of the semi-tubular bioabsorbable plates (79.0 ± 7.9 N·cm) was significantly greater than that of titanium plates for 2.0 mm screws (56.7 ± 4.0 N·cm) ($p < 0.05$). There were no significant differences in six-month postoperative clinical results between patients who received bioabsorbable plates and those who received titanium plates (total range of active motion, 267.0° ± 6.0° compared with 250.0° ± 28.3°; grip strength, 92.7% ± 19.7% compared with 86.4% ± 28.6% of that on the contralateral side).

Conclusions.—The bending strength, stiffness, and torsional strength of novel one-third or semi-tubular bioabsorbable plates, when fixed on a PEEK rod, were comparable with those for titanium plates for 1.5 or 2.0-mm screws. There were no significant differences in clinical results between these two types of plates in a small group of patients after short-term follow-up.

▶ This article is significant in that it presents both biomechanical and pilot data on novel bioabsorbable plate and screw constructs for the repair of metacarpal fractures.

Strengths of the study are the well-designed comparison model between bioabsorbable plates and the commonly used titanium plates of the same curvature (one-third tubular and semitubular in cross-section) and their screws (1.5 mm and 2.0 mm), the specific parameters that were measured (bending strength, stiffness, and torsional strength), and the discussion of a novel material (unsintered hydroxyapatite/poly-L-lactide) of which the bioabsorbable implants were made. A weakness of the study (which was also pointed out by the authors) is that the actual shape and size of the bioabsorbable plates that were used clinically varied from case to case, depending on the fracture configuration, making it difficult to make direct comparisons clinically to the standard titanium plates that were used in the other group.

I believe the findings of this study are very important for future treatment. It is only a matter of time before metal implants for fracture fixation become a thing of the past, to be replaced by a durable material such as used here that will disappear over time. The appeal of such a material to both surgeons and patients alike will be great.

I do not have any personal experience with bioabsorbable plates, only pins and screws. However, I look forward to the day when these plates will become a viable option for surgeons in the United States. If locking technology can somehow be incorporated into these plates, then they will be that much more appealing.

S. S. Shin, MD, MMSc

Selective and Non-Selective Cyclooxygenase Inhibitors Delay Stress Fracture Healing in the Rat Ulna
Kidd LJ, Cowling NR, Wu AC, et al (The Univ of Queensland, Gatton, Australia; Griffith Univ, Gold Coast, Queensland, Australia)
J Orthop Res 31:235-242, 2013

Anti-inflammatory drugs are widely used to manage pain associated with stress fractures (SFxs), but little is known about their effects on healing of those injuries. We hypothesized that selective and non-selective anti-inflammatory treatments would retard the healing of SFx in the rat ulna. SFxs were created by cyclic loading of the ulna in Wistar rats. Ulnae were harvested 2, 4 or 6 weeks following loading. Rats were treated with non-selective NSAID, ibuprofen (30 mg/kg/day); selective COX-2 inhibition, [5,5-dimethyl-3-3 (3 fluorophenyl)-4-(4 methylsulfonal) phenyl-2 (5H)-furanone] (DFU) (2.0 mg/kg/day); or the novel c5a antagonist PMX53 (10 mg/kg/day, 4 and 6 weeks only); with appropriate vehicle as control. Quantitative histomorphometric measurements of SFx healing were undertaken. Treatment with the selective COX-2 inhibitor, DFU, reduced the area of resorption along the fracture line at 2 weeks, without affecting bone formation at later stages. Treatment with the non-selective, NSAID, ibuprofen decreased both bone resorption and bone formation so that there was significantly reduced length and area of remodeling and lamellar bone formation within the remodeling unit at 6 weeks after fracture. The C5a receptor antagonist PMX53 had no effect on SFx healing at 4 or 6 weeks after loading, suggesting that PMX53 would not delay SFx healing. Both selective COX-2 inhibitors and non-selective NSAIDs have the potential to compromise SFx healing, and should be used with caution when SFx is diagnosed or suspected.

▶ The authors investigated the effects of anti-inflammatory medications (conventional, COX-2 inhibitors, and C5a inhibitors) on bone healing of stress fractures. The ulna rat model was studied.

Stress fractures were induced in the rats, and 80 were treated with ibuprofen; 60 with COX-2 inhibitor, 5,5-dimethyl-3-3 (3 fluorophenyl)-4-(4 methylsulfonal) phenyl-2 (5H)-furanone; and 30 with an investigational C5a inhibitor, PMX-53.

Results showed that COX-2 inhibitors reduced the area of resorption along the fracture line at 2 weeks and had no effect on bone formation at later stages. Treatment with ibuprofen decreased both bone resorption and bone formation at 6 weeks after fracture. Although ibuprofen reduced remodeling to a greater extent than COX-2 inhibitors, the differences may be secondary to differences in administration and dose between the 2 drugs. The C5a receptor antagonist had no negative effect on fracture healing at 4 or 6 weeks after loading.

M. Rizzo, MD

Treatment and Outcomes of Fingertip Injuries at a Large Metropolitan Public Hospital

Weichman KE, Wilson SC, Samra F, et al (New York Univ Langone Med Ctr; Univ of Pennsylvania Hosp, Philadelphia)
Plast Reconstr Surg 131:107-112, 2013

Background.—Fingertip injuries are the most common hand injuries presenting for acute care. Treatment algorithms have been described based on defect size, bone exposure, and injury geometry. The authors hypothesized that despite accepted algorithms, many fingertip injuries can be treated conservatively.

Methods.—A prospectively collected retrospective review of all fingertip injuries presenting to Bellevue Hospital between January and May of 2011 was conducted. Patients were entered into an electronic database on presentation. Follow-up care was tracked through the electronic medical record. Patients lost to follow-up were questioned by means of telephone. Patients were analyzed based on age, mechanism of injury, handedness, occupation, wound geometry, defect size, bone exposure, emergency room procedures performed, need for surgical intervention, and outcome.

Results.—One hundred fingertips were injured. Injuries occurred by crush (46 percent), laceration (30 percent), and avulsion (24 percent). Sixty-four percent of patients healed without surgery, 18 percent required operative intervention, and 18 percent were lost to follow-up. Patients requiring operative intervention were more likely to have a larger defect ($3.28 \, cm^2$ versus $1.75 \, cm^2$, $p < 0.005$), volar oblique injury (50 percent versus 8.8 percent, $p < 0.005$), exposed bone (81.3 percent versus 35.3 percent, $p < 0.005$), and an associated distal phalanx fracture (81.3 percent versus 47.1 percent, $p < 0.05$). Patients requiring surgical intervention had a longer average return to work time when compared with those not requiring surgical intervention (4.33 weeks versus 2.98 weeks, $p < 0.001$).

Conclusion.—Despite current accepted algorithms, many fingertip injuries can be treated nonoperatively to achieve optimal sensation, fine motor control, and earlier return to work.

Clinical Question/Level of Evidence.—Therapeutic, III (Table 1).

▶ There are many articles on the various surgical flaps that can cover the fingertip. Recently, fingertip replantation has also been the subject of a number of articles as it has grown in popularity. Understanding which patients will benefit from surgery and which will do fine with nonoperative treatment would be useful information.

Unfortunately, this article does not adequately provide this. A great deal of raw data are presented and nicely summarized in Table 1. The stratification of injuries into crush vs laceration vs avulsion mechanism was interesting although not highlighted in the article. The number of crush injuries that healed without surgery was surprising (15 of 16 patients), and a more in-depth discussion of this result would have been interesting.

The written results and discussion sections do not synthesize the information or conclude which patients may benefit from nonoperative treatment. Hopefully,

TABLE 1.—Characteristics of Those Who Healed Without Surgery Versus with Surgery

	Healed with Surgery (%)	Healed Without Surgery (%)	*p*
No. of patients	16	68	
Mean age, yr	31 ± 10.8	32 ± 18.2	0.86
Manual labor	9 (56.3)	25 (36.7)	0.14
Sex			
Male	11 (68.8)	50 (73.5)	0.704
Female	5 (31.2)	18 (26.4)	0.698
Crush mechanism	1 (6.25)	15 (22.1)	0.146
Laceration mechanism	8 (50)	22 (32.3)	0.183
Avulsion mechanism	7 (43.7)	31 (45.5)	0.896
Orientation			
A	0 (0)	29 (42.6)	0.0013
B	8 (50)	6 (8.8)	<0.001
C	7 (43.7)	25 (36.7)	0.652
D	1 (6.25)	8 (11.7)	0.525
Exposed bone	13 (81.3)	24 (35.3)	0.0009
Fracture	13 (81.3)	32 (47.1)	0.013
Average soft-tissue defect, cm^2	3.28	1.75	<0.001

the authors will take these data and go forward with a prospective, randomized trial, which could provide a guide for which patients to treat with nonoperative intervention.

J. Frankenhoff, MD

11 Distal Radius Fractures

Fibulo-scapho-lunate arthrodesis after resection of the distal radius for giant-cell tumor of the bone
Jaminet P, Rahmanian-Schwarz A, Pfau M, et al (Eberhard Karls Univ Tübingen, Germany)
Microsurgery 32:458-462, 2012

Background.—Giant-cell tumors of the distal radius are rare. They have a high-risk of local recurrence and a risk of pulmonary metastasis. Curettage alone or combined with adjunctive agents is often associated with local recurrence.

Methods.—Three patients with giant-cell tumor of the distal radius are presented. All patients showed Campanacci grade 3 lesions. All patients underwent complete distal radius resection and reconstruction with a vascularized fibular graft distally fused with the scaphoid and the lunate, allowing midcarpal motion.

Results.—The follow up period ranged from 6 to 60 months. For all three patients, emotional acceptance was excellent. The postoperative motion of the wrist was good, with a range of motion of 30-0-30°, 40-0-0°, and 30-0-10° (extension—flexion). There was neither tumor recurrence nor pulmonary metastasis.

Conclusion.—Fibulo-scapho-lunate fusion is an elegant method of distal radius reconstruction with good functional outcome and low risk of pulmonary metastasis.

▶ The authors present their outcomes in 3 cases of advanced giant cell tumors of the distal radius following resection and vascularized fibula flap with arthrodesis to the scapholunate joint, with follow-up ranging from 6 months to 5 years. They report good flexion and extension in spite of the fact they did not excise the distal pole of the scaphoid, as has been described to improve motion, by unlocking the midcarpal joint following radio scapholunate arthrodesis. They did not report any complications.

This technique has been previously described, so this article does not add a new form of management, but it does confirm that reasonable results can be obtained in treating this condition.

W. C. Hammert, DDS, MD

Incidence and Clinical Outcomes of Tendon Rupture Following Distal Radius Fracture

White BD, Nydick JA, Karsky D, et al (Univ of South Florida, Tampa, FL; Florida Orthopaedic Inst, Tampa; Foundation for Orthopaedic Res and Education, Tampa, FL)

J Hand Surg 37A:2035-2040, 2012

Purpose.—To evaluate the incidence of tendon rupture after nonoperative and operative management of distal radius fractures, report clinical outcomes after tendon repair or transfer, and examine volar plate and dorsal screw prominence as a predictor of tendon rupture.

Methods.—We performed a retrospective chart review on patients treated for tendon rupture after distal radius fracture. We evaluated active range of motion, Disabilities of Arm, Shoulder, and Hand score, grip strength, and pain score, and performed radiographic evaluation of volar plate and dorsal screw prominence in both the study group and a matched control group.

Results.—There were 6 tendon ruptures in 1,359 patients (0.4%) treated nonoperatively and 8 tendon ruptures in 999 patients (0.8%) treated with volar plate fixation. At the time of final follow-up, regardless of treatment, we noted that patients had minimal pain and excellent motion and grip strength. Mean Disabilities of the Shoulder, Arm, and Hand scores were 6 for patients treated nonoperatively and 4 for those treated with volar plating.

Conclusions.—We were unable to verify volar plate or dorsal screw prominence as independent risk factors for tendon rupture after distal radius fractures. However, we recommend continued follow-up and plate removal for symptomatic patients who have volar plate prominence or dorsal screw prominence. In the event of tendon rupture, we report excellent clinical outcomes after tendon repair or tendon transfer.

Type of Study/Level of Evidence.—Therapeutic IV.

▶ This is an underpowered retrospective study with a relative paucity of both collected and reported data. The authors did not effectively or accurately accomplish any of the 3 stated purposes in the abstract, in part because the study design did not adequately lend itself to answer the questions.

Patients were identified initially by the International Classification of Diseases, Ninth Revision (ICD-9) search for distal radius fractures followed up for at least 22 months then further narrowed by the Current Procedural Terminology code for surgical tendon repair. Not identifiable with this search method are patients who may have elected nonoperative management for tendon ruptures, those who were treated and discharged before 22 months, and those that may have sought treatment at another institution (a limitation cited by the authors). This is, thus, a poor study design, as it likely underestimates the true incidence of tendon ruptures.

The authors' report [of] clinical outcomes after tendon repair or transfer is limited to a small cohort of only 14 patients with no control group (or mention of historic controls) and only unilateral grip score (no comparison with uninjured or nonoperative extremity) reported.

Additionally, I'm not clear if the 999 patients who underwent open reduction and internal fixation were all approached volarly (as stated in Results) or a mix of dorsal and volar (as stated in Materials and Methods), but they only report on 8 patients fixed with volar plates with subsequent tendon ruptures. They appropriately note a lack of adequate power to detect differences in volar plate position or dorsal screw prominence between patients with tendon ruptures and matched controls and, thus, cannot implicate either as a predictor of tendon rupture. Finally, it would have been useful to itemize the surgically treated 999 fractures by plate manufacturer, rather than solely those that experienced tendon rupture. The study was nonetheless underpowered to detect differences between manufactures. Despite the fact that the authors acknowledge some of these shortcomings, I find this report to be of minimal impact to my practice.

R. Chris Chadderdon, MD

Early Initiation of Bisphosphonate Does Not Affect Healing and Outcomes of Volar Plate Fixation of Osteoporotic Distal Radial Fractures
Gong HS, Song CH, Lee YH, et al (Seoul Natl Univ Bundang Hosp, South Korea)
J Bone Joint Surg Am 94:1729-1736, 2012

Background.—Bisphosphonates can adversely affect fracture-healing because they inhibit osteoclastic bone resorption. It is unclear whether bisphosphonates can be initiated safely for patients who have sustained an acute distal radial fracture. The purpose of this randomized study was to determine whether the early use of bisphosphonate affects healing and outcomes of osteoporotic distal radial fractures treated with volar locking plate fixation.

Methods.—Fifty women older than fifty years of age who had undergone volar locking plate fixation of a distal radial fracture and had been diagnosed with osteoporosis were randomized to Group I (n = 24, initiation of bisphosphonate treatment at two weeks after the operation) or Group II (n = 26, initiation of bisphosphonate treatment at three months). Patients were assessed for radiographic union and other radiographic parameters (radial inclination, radial length, and volar tilt) at two, six, ten, sixteen, and twenty-four weeks, and for clinical outcomes that included Disabilities of the Arm, Shoulder and Hand (DASH) scores, wrist motion, and grip strength at twenty-four weeks. The two groups were compared with regard to the time to radiographic union, the radiographic parameters, and the clinical outcomes.

Results.—No significant differences were observed between the two groups with respect to radiographic or clinical outcomes after volar locking plate fixation. All patients obtained fracture union, and the mean times to radiographic union in Groups I and II were similar (6.7 and 6.8 weeks, respectively; $p = 0.65$). Furthermore, the time to radiographic union was not related to osteoporosis severity or fracture type.

Conclusions.—In patients with an osteoporotic distal radial fracture treated with volar locking plate fixation, the early initiation of bisphosphonate treatment did not affect fracture-healing or clinical outcomes.

Level of Evidence.—Therapeutic Level I. See Instructions for Authors for a complete description of levels of evidence.

▶ Distal radius fractures continue to be the most common fracture in the upper extremity. Many of these occur in patients with osteopenia or osteoporosis. These fragility fractures portend a higher risk of subsequent fracture and should stimulate us to either initiate therapy for osteoporosis ourselves or ensure appropriate referral. Because bisphosphonates are the most commonly used medication for the treatment of osteoporosis, this study provides important guidance on the safety of early treatment.

This was a well-designed study that was powered to determine a 2-week difference in the time to union in patients with acute distal radius fractures treated with volar locked plating. Strengths of the study are its prospective, randomized design and objective criteria defining radiographic healing assessed by blinded orthopedists. Limitations include the relatively low κ coefficient of the interobserver reliability of determining cortical bridging, indicating only moderate agreement on the primary endpoint, a 6-month follow-up period, the low patient number, which limited the ability to detect complications such as nonunion, and the study of only one bisphosphonate—alendronate.

The important take-home message for upper extremity surgeons is that patients with osteoporosis can begin treatment with alendronate 2 weeks after volar plate fixation, without delaying the time to union. This should encourage us to have our patients with distal radius fragility fractures screened as soon as possible for osteoporosis and referred for appropriate treatment in the hopes that addressing the risk of osteoporosis earlier in treatment will increase the likelihood that screening will be ordered and patients will comply with the recommendation.

F. T. D. Kaplan, MD

Clinical and Radiographic Factors Associated With Distal Radioulnar Joint Instability in Distal Radius Fractures
Kwon BC, Seo BK, Im H-J, et al (Hallym Univ Sacred Heart Hosp, Dongan-gu, Anyang-si, Gyeonggi-do, South Korea; et al)
Clin Orthop Relat Res 470:3171-3179, 2012

Background.—Distal radioulnar joint (DRUJ) instability is an important cause of ulnar-sided wrist pain in distal radius fractures. However, instability is frequently undiagnosed and the clinical and radiographic factors associated with instability are not well understood.

Questions/Purposes.—We therefore identified clinical and radiographic factors associated with DRUJ instability in distal radius fractures.

Patients and Methods.—We retrospectively reviewed all 221 patients who underwent surgical treatment for unstable distal radius fractures from 2007 to 2010. Ten patients (five men and five women) had DRUJ instability by intraoperative manual testing (Group I); these patients had a median age of 52 years. The other 211 patients (81 men and 130 women) (Group II) had a median age of 55 years. Clinical and radiographic data were compared between the groups.

Results.—The incidence of open wounds at the wrist and the relative ulnar length measured on the prereduction radiograph were greater in Group I. An open wound at the wrist and positive ulnar variance of 6 mm or greater on the prereduction radiograph increased the risk of DRUJ instability (relative risks = 45 and 17, respectively) in distal radius fractures.

Conclusions.—An open wound at the wrist or positive ulnar variance of 6 mm or greater observed on the prereduction radiograph in patients with distal radius fractures should alert the physician to the possibility of DRUJ instability.

Level of Evidence.—Level II, prognostic study. See the Guidelines for Authors for a complete description of levels of evidence.

▶ To take plain x-ray films of normal wrists in a constant and reproducible manner, we use a special item invented for fixing the wrist, elbow and shoulder joints to project the x-ray to the wrist at a fixed angle. Radiographic parameters measured on the x-ray films taken in that way deserve statistical analysis. It is impossible to take plain x-ray films of deformed wrists with fractures in such a constant and reproducible manner. Radiographic parameters of the wrists measured on films without fixed x-ray trajectories may be erroneous. Parameters measured on the x-ray films, which are the least influenced by the x-ray trajectory, should be chosen when we perform radiographic assessment on the wrists with pretreated wrist fractures.

Recently, several investigators have attempted to find out the predicting factors of triangular fibrocartilage complex (TFCC) injuries associated with distal radial fractures from several radiographic parameters on plain x-ray films taken just after the injuries. In this report, the authors found that positive ulnar variance more than 6 mm and open fracture were significantly related to the distal radioulnar joint (DRUJ) instability. Fujitani et al assessed the radial or sagittal translation of the fracture fragments using the radial and sagittal translation ratios, respectively, and concluded that the radial translation ratio was a significant risk factor of the DRUJ instability.[1] Ulnar variance may be a radiographic parameter, which might be less influenced by the x-ray trajectory than the sagittal or radial translation ratios.

Is the prediction of the DRUJ instability associated with distal radius fractures beneficial to hand surgeons? Keeping in mind that 10 of 231 (4.5% in this article) or 11 of 163 (6.7% by Fujitani et al) of distal radius fractures were associated with DRUJ instability is more important than predicting DRUJ instability before treatment. After reduction of the radius fracture, the DRUJ stability must be checked. If the fracture is repaired and there is associated DRUJ instability, the TFCC must be repaired.

R. Kakinoki, MD

Reference

1. Fujitani R, Omokawa S, Akahane M, Iida A, Ono H, Tanaka Y. Predictors of distal radioulnar joint instability in distal radius fractures. *J Hand Surg Am.* 2011;36:1919-1925.

The Natural Course of Traumatic Triangular Fibrocartilage Complex Tears in Distal Radial Fractures: A 13–15 Year Follow-up of Arthroscopically Diagnosed But Untreated Injuries

Mrkonjic A, Geijer M, Lindau T, et al (Lund Univ and Skåne Univ Hosp, Sweden; Pulvertaft Hand Centre, Derby, UK)
J Hand Surg 37A:1555-1560, 2012

Purpose.—To evaluate the long-term results of a prospective, longitudinal case series of untreated, traumatic triangular fibrocartilage complex (TFCC) tears found in displaced distal radial fractures.

Methods.—Between 1995 and 1997, 51 patients (24 men, 27 women; age, 20–57 y) with a displaced distal radius fracture had wrist arthroscopy to identify associated injuries. Forty-three patients had complete or partial tears of the TFCC, which were not treated. All patients were contacted in 2010, 13–15 years after the injury. One patient had had a TFCC reattachment due to painful distal radioulnar joint instability and was excluded. Thirty-eight patients returned for a radiographic and clinical follow-up that recorded strength, distal radioulnar joint laxity, range of motion, pain scale score, and subjective and objective outcome scores.

Results.—After 13–15 years, 17/38 patients were lax in the distal radioulnar joint. The mean grip strength was worse in the patients with a lax distal radioulnar joint (83%, SD 15 of the contralateral side vs 103%, SD 33). The median Gartland and Werley score was 5 (good; range, 0–15) in the lax group compared to 1 (excellent; range, 0–9) in the non-lax group, and the median Disabilities of the Arm, Shoulder, and Hand scores were 14 (range, 0–59) and 5 (range, 0–70) respectively.

Conclusions.—In this 13–15 year, prospective, longitudinal outcome study of the natural course of TFCC tears associated with distal radius fracture, only 1 patient had been operated on for painful instability since the injury. The subjective and objective results did not provide evidence that a TFCC injury would influence the long-term outcome. However, trends were found and, by speculation, the low number of patients in the series and the risk for a type II error could be the cause of absent statistically significance. Larger, preferably prospective, randomized studies are needed to find out whether a more aggressive treatment is beneficial.

Type of Study/Level of Evidence.—Diagnostic I.

▶ This study attempts to answer an important question: Do tears of the triangular fibrocartilage complex (TFCC) need to be addressed at the time of a distal radius fracture? With long-term follow-up of 13 to 15 years, 17 of the 38 patients who participated in the study exhibited laxity in the distal radioulnar joint on clinical examination. Of these 17 cases, 6 had complete peripheral tears of the TFCC, 10 had partial peripheral or central tears, and 1 patient had no tear at all. Only 1 patient underwent a surgical TFCC reattachment because of painful distal radio-ulnar joint instability. Although 8 patients had developed mild-to-medium grade osteoarthritis in the distal radioulnar joint, it is not clear how much of this can be attributed to the healing alignment of the distal radius or the aging process. Nevertheless, there was no statistically significant relationship between arthroscopically diagnosed TFCC injury and osteoarthritis development.

There was also no statistically significant link between TFCC injury and long-term outcomes. However, there appeared to be trends indicating that the cohort with a partial or no TFCC tear was superior to the cohort with complete tears in the objective and subjective domains. Though statistical significance was not achieved in showing these differences, the findings may be clinically relevant and point to the need to study a larger series of patients. Although the authors find "no support for aggressive surgical management when TFCC tears are diagnosed in association with distal radius fractures," the study's trends hint at an opposite truth that may come to light with a better-powered study.

E. Shin, MD

Open Reduction Internal Fixation Versus Percutaneous Pinning With External Fixation of Distal Radius Fractures: A Prospective, Randomized Clinical Trial

Grewal R, MacDermid JC, King GJW, et al (Univ of Western Ontario, London, Ontario, Canada)
J Hand Surg 36A:1899-1906, 2011

Purpose.—The purpose of this randomized clinical trial was to investigate the functional outcomes of the surgical treatment of distal radius fractures, comparing treatment by external fixation and percutaneous pinning to open reduction and internal fixation (ORIF) using a plate.

Methods.—We randomized 53 patients with distal radius fractures that failed closed reduction and casting to ORIF (n = 27) or external fixation (n = 26). For pragmatic reasons, the choice of ORIF was left to the surgeon's discretion (early recruitment, dorsal plates [n = 9]; later recruitment, volar locked plates [n = 18]). Outcomes were measured before surgery, at 6 weeks, and at 3, 6, and 12 months and included the Patient-Rated Wrist Evaluation (PRWE); Disabilities of the Arm, Shoulder, and Hand; range of motion; grip strength; and serial radiographic analysis. Generalized linear modeling using repeated measures was used to identify differences in outcome scores between fixation types over time. Other continuous variables were analyzed using the Student *t*-test or one-way analysis of variance for multiple groups.

Results.—There were no differences in the demographic characteristics or fracture severity between groups. Based on generalized linear modeling, on average, the ORIF group scored 11 points lower on the PRWE across all time points compared to the external fixation group. The PRWE detected higher pain and disability with external fixation before surgery, at 6 weeks, and at 3 months. Using generalized linear modeling, a post hoc subgroup analysis identified significantly better (15-point advantage) PRWE scores averaged across all time points with volar locking plates compared to both external fixation and dorsal plating.

Conclusions.—The PRWE scores were significantly lower for patients treated with ORIF compared to those with external fixation, with the best outcomes observed with volar locking plates. These advantages were observed in the early postoperative period, and overall scores equalized at 1 year. A higher mean initial preoperative PRWE score was seen with external fixation, perhaps indicating a more severe initial injury. Given this difference, the interpretation of these results is not clear.

▶ Grewal et al present an article that sounds like a significant contribution to the literature comparing 2 common operations for distal radius fractures: open reduction and internal fixation (ORIF) with volar locked plates (VLP) and external fixation. They found a difference of 15 points in Patient-Rated Wrist Evaluation (PWRE) scores across all time points between the 2 groups. However, as the authors state in the last sentence of their abstract, "the interpretation of these results is not clear." There are several reasons that the study is hard to interpret. First, the baseline PRWE scores (the main outcome variable for this study) before surgery was 11 points different between the 2 groups. Second, the ORIF group of this study was actually 2 groups. Early on, second-generation dorsal "pi" plates were used (8 patients) but later on VLP was used (18 patients). Third, despite this trial being conducted at a busy hand/upper limb trauma center with patients from the practices of 3 surgeons, the total number of patients was 53 in a study that lasted long enough for the surgeons to have a significant shift in practice. Based on the inclusion and exclusion criteria, most readers would wonder why the numbers were so small. The reader is left to speculate that there was a much larger number of patients who declined to be randomized, which although understandable, is a potential source of significant bias. As the authors state, this issue remains unresolved and a multicenter trial is the next logical step in trying to answer this complex question.

P. Blazar, MD

Distal Radius Fracture Risk Reduction With a Comprehensive Osteoporosis Management Program
Harness NG, Funahashi T, Dell R, et al (Univ of California Irvine, Orange; Downey Med Ctr, CA; Kaiser Permanente Southern California, Pasadena)
J Hand Surg 37A:1543-1549, 2012

Purpose.—To study risk factors associated with osteoporotic distal radius fractures and evaluate the effectiveness of the screening and treatment components of a comprehensive osteoporosis program.

Methods.—We retrospectively identified a cohort of patients aged 60 years or older from a large health maintenance organization. For the period 2002 to 2008, information on age, race, sex, diabetes status, osteoporosis diagnosis, osteoporosis screening activity, medications dispensed, and fracture events, including distal radius, proximal humerus, and hip fractures were recorded. We compared demographic and clinical characteristics for patients with and without distal radius fractures. We estimated multivariable estimates of the associations between pharmacologic treatment, and osteoporosis screening and distal radius fracture risk using Cox proportional hazards methods, and adjusted them for age, sex, race, diabetes status, and prior history of hip or proximal humerus fractures.

Results.—Overall, 1.7% of the cohort (n = 8,658) of the study population (N = 524,612) sustained a new distal radius fracture during 2002 to 2008. In the multivariable model, we found that patients who received pharmacological intervention were 48% less likely to sustain a distal radius fracture. Similarly, patients who were screened for osteoporosis were 83% less likely to sustain a distal radius fracture. Patients with osteoporosis were 8.9 times more likely to have a distal radius fracture than patients without osteoporosis. White subjects had a 1.6 times higher risk of distal radius fracture than non-whites, and women had a 3.8 times higher risk than men.

Conclusions.—White race, female sex, and a diagnosis of osteoporosis are high risks for distal radius fracture. Screening for and pharmacologic management of osteoporosis using a multidisciplinary team approach in a comprehensive osteoporosis management program resulted in a statistically significant decrease in the risk of distal radius fracture.

Type of Study/Level of Evidence.—Therapeutic III.

▶ This study provides the preliminary data from a large health maintenance organization to support the concept and institution of a comprehensive osteoporosis management program, one that begins to provide the statistics related to comorbidity, pharmacologic intervention/prevention, related fragility fractures, and, importantly, differences between men and women. The retrospective analysis suggests that intervention equates with prevention that may ultimately provide cogent arguments for institutional cost-savings, which is the current sticky wicket for most hospitals that are reluctant to adopt such programs. Furthermore, the data indicate that patients with osteoporosis have an almost 9 times higher rate of distal radius fracture than those without. This represents a nice continuum of the questions raised with the Fitzpatrick article published in the *Journal of Hand Surgery* (October 2012).[1]

The numbers collected may represent the most expansive of an American study—more heterogeneous than studies of Northern European countries with socialized medicine—and perhaps hold a wealth of data untapped. Further discussion, and perhaps further investigation, is warranted regarding the incidence and screening of men in this cohort. Less than 20% of men underwent screening: What happened to the ones who did? Who had distal radius fractures and subsequent fragility fractures? The literature supports higher morbidity/

comorbidity and mortality in men with osteoporosis in general as well as related to fragility fractures; insight into their outcome would be valuable information.

A. Ladd, MD

Reference

1. Fitzpatrick SK, Casemyr NE, Zurakowski D, Day CS, Rozental TD. The effect of osteoporosis on outcomes of operatively treated distal radius fractures. *J Hand Surg Am.* 2012;37:2027-2034.

Salvage of Failed Resection Arthroplasties of the Distal Radioulnar Joint Using an Ulnar Head Prosthesis: Long-term Results

van Schoonhoven J, Mühldorfer-Fodor M, Fernandez DL, et al (Klinik für Handchirurgie, Bad Neustadt, Germany; Lindenhof Hosp, Berne, Switzerland; St Lukes Hosp, Sydney, Australia)

J Hand Surg 37A:1372-1380, 2012

Purpose.—The aim of this prospective multicenter study was to evaluate the long-term outcome of the Herbert ulnar head prosthesis for painful instability of the distal radioulnar joint (DRUJ) following resection of the ulnar head.

Methods.—Twenty-three patients were treated with a Herbert ulnar head prosthesis in 3 international hand centers. One patient was excluded from the study because a septic prosthesis had to be removed after 3 months. Sixteen of the remaining 22 patients could be assessed at 2 follow-up times, 28 months (range, 10—43 mo) and 11 years and 2 months (range, 97—158 mo) after surgery, for DRUJ stability, forearm rotation, grip strength, pain level (0—10), and satisfaction (0—10). Standardized radiographs of the wrist were evaluated for displacement of the ulnar head and loosening or bony reactions at the sigmoid notch or the ulna shaft.

Results.—All patients demonstrated a clinically stable DRUJ at the latest examination, and no patient required further surgery at the DRUJ since the short-term evaluation in 1999. Average pain measured 3.7 before surgery, 1.7 at the short-term follow-up, and 1.7 at the long-term follow-up; patients' satisfaction, 2.2, 8.2, and 8.9; pronation, 73°, 86°, and 83°; supination, 52°, 77°, and 81°; and grip strength, 42%, 72%, and 81% of the unaffected side. All clinical parameters improved significantly from before surgery to the short-term follow-up, with no further statistically significant change between the short-term and long-term follow-up. Radiographs demonstrated no signs of stem loosening or incongruity of the DRUJ.

Conclusions.—The previously reported short-term results with the Herbert prosthesis did not deteriorate in the long term. Reconstruction of the DRUJ with this prosthesis in painful radioulnar impingement following ulnar head resection is a reliable and reproducible procedure with lasting results.

▶ This study evaluates the long-term outcomes of the Herbert ulnar head prosthesis. It is one of the few studies that reports on the long-term follow-up (mean 11 years) of ulnar prostheses. Other strengths of this study include a comprehensive clinical assessment with comparison to previous midterm results in the same cohort. There are also some weaknesses that should be noted. The sample size is quite small (n = 16), the follow-up rate is less than 80%, and there was no standardized validated measure used to assess outcomes. Despite these shortcomings, this study adds valuable information to the literature because it demonstrates continued successful results with this prosthesis in the long term, with no evidence of stem loosening or other radiographic signs of failure. Because this procedure is not typically performed in high volumes, a sample size of 16 is still reasonable and adds to the existing literature. In the future, a joint registry for hand and wrist prosthesis would be valuable to allow hand surgeons to study the long-term effects of various prostheses in larger cohorts.

R. Grewal, MD

Assessment of Pronator Quadratus Repair Integrity Following Volar Plate Fixation for Distal Radius Fractures: A Prospective Clinical Cohort Study
Swigart CR, Badon MA, Bruegel VL, et al (Yale School of Medicine, New Haven, CT; Univ of Massachusetts Med Ctr, Worcester; Univ of Vermont College of Medicine, Burlington)
J Hand Surg 37A:1868-1873, 2012

Purpose.—To assess prospectively the integrity of pronator quadratus (PQ) muscle repair following volar plate fixation of distal radius fractures and to compare the clinical and radiographic outcomes of durable versus failed repairs in 24 subjects. In addition, by grading the degree of PQ injury, an attempt was made to correlate failure of repair with the PQ injury severity.

Methods.—The extent of PQ injury was graded for each fracture. After fracture fixation, the PQ muscle was repaired along its radial and distal borders. Radiopaque hemoclips were attached to each side of the PQ repair, 2 radially and 2 distally. The distance between these markers at time 0 versus x-rays taken at approximately 2 weeks, 6 weeks, and 3 months was recorded. Clip displacement of 1 cm or more compared to time 0 indicated repair failure.

Results.—One of 24 repairs (4%) failed at 3 months. No statistical difference was noted between the type of PQ injury and wrist flexion/extension, pronation/supination, and grip strength.

Conclusions.—Pronator quadratus repairs after volar plate fracture fixation are generally durable. They withstand forces that occur at the distal radius during the healing process with a 4% failure rate. No correlation was shown between type of PQ injury and radiographic failure of the repair.

▶ This well-performed level II study by Swigart et al evaluated pronator quadratus repair in a cohort of 31 patients. Twenty-four patients completed the study, with all 24 patients followed up with serial radiographs for 3 months postoperatively. The authors report on pronator quadratus muscle injury at surgery, with more than 50% exhibiting some degree of pronator quadratus (PQ) muscle damage. Using radiopaque markers, the authors found no change in the position of the markers in 23 of 24 patients 3 months after surgery. There were no flexor tendon ruptures, and 2 different low-profile plating systems were utilized. This study shows that PQ repairs hold up over time, and I agree that PQ repair should be performed restoring normal anatomy as best as possible. However, I still believe that the keys to preventing attritional flexor tendon injury are primarily restoration of normal volar tilt and plate placement proximal to the watershed line.

D. Zelouf, MD

Predictors of Distal Radioulnar Joint Instability in Distal Radius Fractures
Fujitani R, Omokawa S, Akahane M, et al (Affiliated Hosp of Nara Med Univ, Osaka; Nara Med Univ, Kashihara, Japan)
J Hand Surg 36A:1919-1925, 2011

Purpose.—A tear of the triangular fibrocartilage complex (TFCC) is the most frequent soft tissue injury associated with fractures of the distal radius, and repair of the deep ligamentous portion of the TFCC is considered when the tear contributes to instability of the distal radioulnar joint (DRUJ). The purpose of this prospective cohort study was to identify predictors of DRUJ instability accompanying unstable distal radius fractures.

Methods.—Between 2002 and 2007, we prospectively treated 163 consecutive patients with unstable distal radius fractures with the volar locking plating system. Complete radioulnar ligament tears representing DRUJ instability were present in 11 of 163 distal radius fractures. We tested univariate associations between DRUJ instability and potential predictors and conducted multivariate analysis to establish independent predictors of instability. We applied receiver operating characteristics curves within the significant risk factors to determine threshold values.

Results.—In univariate analyses, only the radial and sagittal translation ratios of the fracture site were significant predictors of DRUJ instability. Multivariate logistic regression analysis confirmed that the radial translation ratio, which corresponds to a normalized DRUJ gap, was a significant risk factor. According to the receiver operating characteristics curve for the radial translation ratio, the area under the curve was 0.89. A cutoff value of 15% for the radial translation ratio showed the highest diagnostic accuracy rate.

Conclusions.—A radiographic finding of a normalized DRUJ gap on posteroanterior views was the most important predictor to identify DRUJ instability accompanying unstable distal radius fractures. The relative risk of instability increases by 50% when the ratio of DRUJ widening increases by 1%.

▶ This retrospective study identified predictors of distal radioulnar joint (DRUJ) instability after fractures of the distal radius treated with volar plate fixation. The authors examined demographic as well as fracture characteristics and determined that radial and sagittal translations of fracture fragments were independent predictors of DRUJ instability.

The study is valuable in that it provides objective criteria to identify DRUJ instability. Indeed, undiagnosed instability can result in significant morbidity for patients with distal radius fractures. When confronted with large amounts of radial or sagittal translation in distal radius fractures, treating surgeons will now have an increased index of suspicion for associated injuries to the DRUJ. The study weaknesses lie in the subjective assessment of DRUJ instability initially used to identify cases as well as the small numbers of patients with instability included. Furthermore, the authors do not discuss their operative indications in detail, and it is not clear whether the detected DRUJ instability would have resolved with temporary pinning of the joint rather than open ligamentous repair. Finally, the calculated ratios of translation are not practical for use in a clinical setting and, as mentioned by the authors, identification of a clinically significant threshold of DRUJ gapping would be more meaningful in accurately identifying patients with DRUJ instability after fixation of distal radius fractures.

My current practice is to assess the DRUJ at the time of surgery, both clinically and with fluoroscopy, after reduction of the main fracture fragments. Subjective laxity or significant residual incongruity are indications for pinning the DRUJ in the acute setting. As of yet, there is no better scientific method of assessing DRUJ pre- or intraoperatively. A threshold of DRUJ gapping would thus be helpful in identifying patients who require additional treatment for DRUJ instability.

T. D. Rozental, MD

Dynamic versus static external fixation for unstable distal radius fractures: An up-to-date meta-analysis
Cui Z, Yu B, Hu Y, et al (Southern Med Univ, Guangzhou, China)
Injury 43:1006-1013, 2012

Objects.—Whether dynamic or static external fixation is more appropriate for distal radius fractures is still being debated, our aim is to determine the effect of dynamic versus static external fixation for unstable distal radius fractures in terms of postoperative complication, clinical results and radiological outcomes.

Methods.—We selected PubMed, Cochrane Library, EMBASE, BIOSIS, Ovid and the relevant English orthopaedic journals and pooled data from eligible trials including six eligible randomised controlled trials and two comparative studies containing 998 patients comparing dynamic and static external fixation for unstable distal radius fractures to conduct a sub-group analysis according to different periods of follow-up, aiming to summarise the best available evidence.

Results.—The results showed there was an increased risk for pin-track infection in dynamic external fixation group than that in static external fixation group, however, there was the trend of obtaining better clinical effect towards less malunion in dynamic external fixation group, although the results were not statistically significant. With regard to clinical results, range of motion such as extension, supination and pronation were superior in dynamic external fixation group than that in static external fixation group at 6 weeks postoperatively. And there were the trend of obtaining better clinical effect in dynamic external fixation group towards pronation at one year follow-up and grip strength at six weeks, six months and one year follow-up, although no significant differences were viewed. With regard to radiological outcomes, better clinical result was obtained in terms of radial length in dynamic external fixation group immediately after surgery and at six weeks, one year follow-up postoperatively.

Conclusions.—The final results show that there are some evidences supporting the use of dynamic external fixation, which may also have practical advantages over static fixation by allowing earlier limb mobility during the fixation period and enabling such patients to maintain their independence. Limitations remain, a cost-effectiveness analysis and DASH-score assessments at all follow-up evaluations should be more carefully considered and reported in a reliable, consistent and standardised manner.

▶ The potential advantages of dynamic external fixators reported include early mobilization of the wrist, stimulation of cartilage repair, molding of articular fragments, and diminished periarticular osteopenia. Smaller comparative studies have been conducted, but a large, pooled, meta-analysis has not. The authors present a meta-analysis of all comparative studies evaluating static vs dynamic external fixators. They analyzed and graded each study using a valid, systematic method; they searched all relevant databases and included a large number of pooled patients (n = 998). Weaknesses of this meta-analysis include the heterogeneity, underlying publication bias, and lack of validated outcome measures in the included studies.

The pooled results of this meta-analysis show an increased pin-tract infection risk with dynamic external fixation, with no significant difference in malunion rate, range of motion after 6 weeks, or other long-term clinical differences. There was better maintenance of radial length with the dynamic external fixator; however, no significant differences were viewed with regard to radial inclination and volar tilt in both groups at any periods of follow-up. Like most comparative studies evaluating different fixation methods in the distal radius, there were no long-term differences seen between groups. Therefore, I feel that it is important for surgeons to study the fracture pattern and determine in their own hands which fixation technique affords the best outcomes.

R. Grewal, MD

A Biomechanical Comparison of Volar Locked Plating of Intra-Articular Distal Radius Fractures: Use of 4 Versus 7 Screws for Distal Fixation
Moss DP, Means KR Jr, Parks BG, et al (Union Memorial Hosp, Baltimore, MD)
J Hand Surg 36A:1907-1911, 2011

Purpose.—To determine whether the number of distal locking screws significantly affects stability of a cadaveric simulated distal radius fracture fixed with a volar locking plate.

Methods.—We created AO/ASIF type C2 fractures in 10 matched pairs of human fresh-frozen cadaveric wrists and then fixed them using volar locking plates. The number of distal locking screws used was 4 screws or 7 screws in each wrist of the matched pair. We loaded the stabilized fractures cyclically to simulate 6 weeks of postoperative stressing during a therapy protocol and then loaded them to failure. Failure was defined as 2 mm or more of displacement of any fracture fragment as recorded by differential variable reluctance transducers.

Results.—No wrists failed during the cyclic loading portion for either the 4- or 7-screw construct. The average initial stiffness of the 7-screw construct was 69 N/mm ($\pm$38) versus 48 N/mm ($\pm$14) for the 4-screw construct. The average failure load for the 7-screw construct was 139 N ($\pm$78) versus 108 N ($\pm$18) for the 4-screw construct. Neither of these differences was statistically significant.

Conclusions.—Although there was a trend toward increased initial stiffness and higher failure load in fractures fixed distally with 7 locking screws, the results were not statistically significant compared with fractures fixed with only 4 screws. Both constructs can withstand forces likely encountered in early therapy protocols.

Clinical Relevance.—The use of extra distal locking screws when fixing distal radius fractures increases expense and may increase the risk of complications, such as extensor tendon irritation or rupture.

▶ This cadaveric study compares construct stability in intra-articular distal radius fractures treated with volar locking plates with the use of either 4 or 7 distal bicortical locking screws. The authors report that the 7-screw construct had higher initial stiffness and load to failure, although the average values did not reach statistical significance.

The results presented reinforce our current clinical practice of initiating early range of motion in patients treated with volar locking plates. Indeed, no specimens failed during the loading portion of the study simulating 6 weeks of postoperative stress. Early range of motion for distal radius fractures treated with volar locking plates appears safe regardless of the number of distal screws used in the construct.

The study limitations include the small number of specimens analyzed as well as a homogenous cadaveric model. As the authors correctly point out, it is difficult to determine whether their findings can be extrapolated to osteoporotic bone or more comminuted fracture patterns. For simple fractures in healthy bone, however, limited use of distal screws may provide adequate fixation at a lower cost and with fewer potential complications.

T. D. Rozental, MD

An Economic Analysis of Outcomes and Complications of Treating Distal Radius Fractures in the Elderly
Shauver MJ, Clapham PJ, Chung KC (Univ of Michigan Health System, Ann Arbor; Michigan State Univ College of Human Medicine, East Lansing)
J Hand Surg 36A:1912-1918.e3, 2011

Purpose.—There is a lack of scientific data regarding which treatment provides the best outcome for distal radius fractures (DRFs) in the elderly. Currently, casting is used to treat the majority of these fractures, although open reduction and internal fixation (ORIF) has been used increasingly in recent years. Given the recent emphasis on the wise use of medical resources, we conducted a cost–utility analysis to assess which of 4 common DRF treatments (casting, wire fixation, external fixation, or ORIF) optimizes the cost–to–patient preference ratio.

Methods.—We created a decision tree to model the process of choosing a DRF treatment and experiencing a final outcome. Fifty adults aged 65 and older were surveyed in a time trade-off, one-on-one interview to obtain utilities for DRF treatments and possible complications. We gathered Medicare reimbursement rates and calculated the incremental cost–utility ratio for each treatment.

Results.—Participants rated DRF treatment relatively high, assigning utility values close to perfect health to all treatments. The ORIF was the most preferred treatment (utility, 0.96), followed by casting (utility, 0.94), wire fixation (utility, 0.94), and external fixation (utility, 0.93). The ORIF was the most expensive treatment (reimbursement, $3,516), whereas casting was the least expensive (reimbursement, $564). The incremental cost–utility ratio for ORIF, when compared to casting, was $15,330 per quality-adjusted life years, which is less than $50,000 per quality-adjusted life year, thereby indicating that, from the societal perspective, ORIF is considered a worthwhile alternative to casting.

Conclusions.—There is a slight preference for the faster return to minimally restricted activity provided by ORIF. Overall, patients show little preference for one DRF treatment over another. Because Medicare patients pay similar out-of-pocket costs regardless of procedure, they are not particularly concerned with procedure costs. Considering the similar long-term outcomes, this study adds to the uncertainty surrounding the choice of

DRF treatment in the elderly, further indicating the need for a high-powered, randomized trial.

▶ With the elderly population representing one of the fastest-growing population demographics today, the economic impact of fragility fractures represents an important health care concern, and this study does an excellent job of tackling this important subject. The methodology used was very thorough and included a consideration of potential complications. The cost-utility analysis assessed the optimal cost-to-patient preference ratio and not the outcome, and the decision tree methodology is inherently based on assumptions. This study was able to demonstrate that elderly individuals might not feel strongly that one treatment is superior to any others because the quality-adjusted life year difference found between the most and least preferred treatment was only 0.3. The authors found that elderly patients most preferred the open reduction and internal fixation treatment option, presumably because of its allowance of quick return to everyday activities, but this was not proven. Whether any of these interventions have an impact on outcome will likely influence patient preferences; this question needs to be addressed with a large, randomized, controlled trial on the subject.

R. Grewal, MD

Correction of dorsally-malunited extra-articular distal radial fractures using volar locked plates without bone grafting

Mahmoud M, El Shafie S, Kamal M (Kasr Al Ainy Hosp, Cairo, Egypt)
J Bone Joint Surg Br 94-B:1090-1096, 2012

Malunion is the most common complication of the distal radius with many modalities of treatment available for such a problem. The use of bone grafting after an osteotomy is still recommended by most authors. We hypothesised that bone grafting is not required; fixing the corrected construct with a volar locked plate helps maintain the alignment, while metaphyseal defect fills by itself. Prospectively, we performed the procedure on 30 malunited dorsally-angulated radii using fixed angle volar locked plates without bone grafting. At the final follow-up, 22 wrists were available. Radiological evidence of union, correction of the deformity, clinical and functional improvement was achieved in all cases. Without the use of bone grafting, corrective open wedge osteotomy fixed by a volar locked plate provides a high rate of union and satisfactory functional outcomes.

▶ This study investigates the use of volar locking plates in the correction of distal radius malunion without the addition of supplemental bone graft. This is a common practice among hand surgeons, and this study addresses the feasibility of this technique. Strengths of this study include its prospective design, follow-up to 18 months, and the use of validated, standardized, patient-rated outcome measures. The follow-up rate, unfortunately, is less than 80% (22/30, 73%), and there were several patients excluded for various reasons that are not made clear (ie, dorsal scarring). This study was able to demonstrate excellent union rates following 4-to-6 weeks of immobilization in a cohort that included a significant number of smokers (14/19). Personally, I tend to reserve the use of bone graft in cases that require a significant lengthening or in those with higher risk of nonunion (ie, smokers, diabetics). However, this study gives support to proceeding with corrective osteotomies without the use of supplemental bone graft, greatly reducing the morbidity associated with this procedure.

R. Grewal, MD

Early Initiation of Bisphosphonate Does Not Affect Healing and Outcomes of Volar Plate Fixation of Osteoporotic Distal Radial Fractures
Gong HS, Song CH, Lee YH, et al (Seoul Natl Univ Bundang Hosp, Seongnam, South Korea)
J Bone Joint Surg Am 94:1729-1736, 2012

Background.—Bisphosphonates can adversely affect fracture-healing because they inhibit osteoclastic bone resorption. It is unclear whether bisphosphonates can be initiated safely for patients who have sustained an acute distal radial fracture. The purpose of this randomized study was to determine whether the early use of bisphosphonate affects healing and outcomes of osteoporotic distal radial fractures treated with volar locking plate fixation.

Methods.—Fifty women older than fifty years of age who had undergone volar locking plate fixation of a distal radial fracture and had been diagnosed with osteoporosis were randomized to Group I (n = 24, initiation of bisphosphonate treatment at two weeks after the operation) or Group II (n = 26, initiation of bisphosphonate treatment at three months). Patients were assessed for radiographic union and other radiographic parameters (radial inclination, radial length, and volar tilt) at two, six, ten, sixteen, and twenty-four weeks, and for clinical outcomes that included Disabilities of the Arm, Shoulder and Hand (DASH) scores, wrist motion, and grip strength at twenty-four weeks. The two groups were compared with regard to the time to radiographic union, the radiographic parameters, and the clinical outcomes.

Results.—No significant differences were observed between the two groups with respect to radiographic or clinical outcomes after volar locking plate fixation. All patients obtained fracture union, and the mean times to radiographic union in Groups I and II were similar (6.7 and 6.8 weeks, respectively; $p = 0.65$). Furthermore, the time to radiographic union was not related to osteoporosis severity or fracture type.

Conclusions.—In patients with an osteoporotic distal radial fracture treated with volar locking plate fixation, the early initiation of bisphosphonate treatment did not affect fracture-healing or clinical outcomes.

Level of Evidence.—Therapeutic Level I. See Instructions for Authors for a complete description of levels of evidence.

▶ This randomized trial by Gong et al concludes that early initiation of bisphosphonate treatment has no effect on the clinical or radiographic outcomes of distal radius fractures treated with volar plate fixation. Because bisphosphonates suppress both bone resorption and formation, controversy surrounds their use in the immediate postfracture period. The majority of patients with distal radius fractures have osteopenia or osteoporosis at the time of injury and benefit from treatment for their low bone mineral density.[1-3]

This study is important in that it examines bisphosphonate treatment in the setting of fracture healing in a clinical setting. The authors demonstrated that bisphosphonates can safely be started in the immediate postoperative period without any deleterious effects. This is important in ensuring that orthopedic surgeons do not miss a valuable opportunity to initiate treatment for osteoporosis immediately after a fracture occurs. The definition of fracture healing continues to be debated in the orthopedic literature, with some studies categorizing radiographic healing and some focusing on clinical factors. This study adopts a comprehensive definition of fracture healing, including both radiographic parameters and clinical outcome scores, further strengthening its conclusions.

Weaknesses include relatively small numbers and a limited assessment of complications because of short follow-up. Also, the authors only included patients with a known diagnosis of osteoporosis, although most patients with distal radius fractures will have a diagnosis of osteopenia. The study thus fails to provide treatment guidelines in the most common patient population with fragility fractures of the distal radius. Despite these limitations, this study reveals that bisphosphonates are safe after fixation for fractures of the distal radius. Treating surgeons should thus consider initiating treatment in the immediate postoperative period.

T. D. Rozental, MD

References

1. Li C, Mori S, Li J, et al. Long-term effect of incadronate disodium (YM-175) on fracture healing of femoral shaft in growing rats. *J Bone Mine Res.* 2001;16: 429-436.
2. Amanat N, Brown R, Bilston LE, Little DG. A single systemic dose of pamidronate improves bone mineral content and accelerates restoration of strength in a rat model of fracture repair. *J Orthop Res.* 2005;23:1029-1034.
3. Rozental TD, Makhni EC, Day CS, Bouxsein ML. Improving evaluation and treatment for osteoporosis following distal radial fractures. A prospective randomized intervention. *J Bone Joint Surg Am.* 2008;90:953-961.

Functional Results of the Darrach Procedure: A Long-Term Outcome Study

Grawe B, Heincelman C, Stern P (Univ of Cincinnati, OH)
J Hand Surg 37A:2475-2480.e2, 2012

Purpose.—To assess long-term functional outcome after ulnar head excision for distal radioulnar joint dysfunction with prior or concomitant wrist trauma. We hypothesized that long-term outcomes would reflect good functional results with satisfactory pain relief.

Methods.—A retrospective chart review identified patients who had undergone the Darrach procedure for traumatic or posttraumatic distal radioulnar joint (DRUJ) pathology. We assessed subjective outcomes using a visual analog scale questionnaire to assess pain, wrist stability, and overall satisfaction. We evaluated objective functional outcomes using the Quick Disabilities of the Shoulder, Arm, and Hand and Patient-Rated Wrist Evaluation measures. Final radiographs were compared with preoperative x-rays to investigate the effect of possible ulnar impingement syndrome (convergent instability).

Results.—A total of 98 patients with 99 wrists met our predetermined inclusion criteria. Of these, 27 patients with a total of 27 wrists were available for final follow-up, 15 of whom were available for final in-office follow-up with radiographs (6–20 y). Patients displayed an average Quick Disabilities of the Shoulder, Arm, and Hand score of 17 and a Patient-Rated Wrist Evaluation score of 14. Final average visual analog scale scores for pain (0–4), pain with activity (0–4), overall satisfaction (0–4), and wrist stability (0–10) were 0.1, 0.6, 3.7, and 1.5, respectively. Final average wrist range of motion was 85°/78° and 41°/45° for pronation-supination and flexion-extension, respectively. A total of 7 patients displayed radioulnar impingement based on dynamic radiography. This ulnar impingement was not associated with clinical reports of pain and did not affect outcome measures in a statistically significant manner.

Conclusions.—The Darrach procedure provides reliably good long-term subjective and objective results for the treatment of a symptomatic DRUJ after a distal radius fracture. Patients can expect to have excellent forearm range of motion at long-term follow-up. Nearly one-half of patients had dynamic convergence of the DRUJ when stressed radiographically; however, the presence of radiographic dynamic convergence did not influence clinical outcomes.

▶ The Darrach procedure is one of those time-tested procedures in hand surgery for which classic teaching is that all patients do well. That is, until they don't. Problems after the Darrach procedure, most commonly pain and mechanical symptoms secondary to radioulnar impingement and instability, have been highlighted in more recent literature. The authors of this study bring more evidence to the debate, providing long-term follow-up for patients undergoing distal ulnar resection for posttraumatic arthritis.

The main strengths of the study are its average 13-year follow-up, evaluation of functional results, and focus on a single indication—post-traumatic distal radioulnar joint arthrosis. In the patients who chose to participate in the study, the average patient was satisfied and functional, and only one had further surgery on their distal ulna despite radiographic radioulnar impingement in half the patients. There were patients who reported poor outcomes; however, we do not know how many, as the study only lists the range of scores and the average but does not specify cutoffs or group patients into good/excellent or fair/poor results based on the Quick DASH (Disability of the Arm, Shoulder, and Hand), PRWE (Patient-Rated Wrist Evaluation), or VAS (Visual Analogue Scale) scores. Other weaknesses include the study's retrospective nature, limited patient population of 27 patients, and the fact that less than 30% of patients meeting the inclusion criteria participated.

This study is important because it supports the argument that the Darrach procedure should be the primary procedure for patients with posttraumatic distal radioulnar joint arthrosis. Although implants are now available for reconstruction of the distal ulna and distal radioulnar joint, these can be reserved as secondary options for patients in whom the Darrach procedure fails, while we await prospective studies comparing the Darrach with implant arthroplasty.

F. T. D. Kaplan, MD

Arthroscopic Resection Arthroplasty for Malunited Intra-Articular Distal Radius Fractures
del Piñal F, Klausmeyer M, Thams C, et al (Hosp Mutua Montañesa, Santander, Spain)
J Hand Surg 37A:2447-2455, 2012

Purpose.—Cartilage damage of the carpals is a contraindication for corrective osteotomy of the malunited intra-articular distal radius fracture and typically is treated in the symptomatic patient with a salvage procedure. Here, we present our experience and early results with arthroscopic resection arthroplasty of the radiocarpal joint.

Methods.—We treated 10 patients (age, 17–68 y; average, 53 y) who had intra-articular malunion of the distal radius with mirror erosion on the carpals. The original fracture occurred 4 to 36 months (average, 9 mo) before our intervention. We performed arthroscopic arthrolysis and resected the offending portion of the radial malunited fragment, eliminating the stepoff and creating a smoother joint surface. Range of motion was started immediately after the operation, except in 2 patients.

Results.—The locations of the malunions were evenly distributed between the scaphoid fossa, the lunate fossa, or both. Stepoffs varied from 2 to 6 mm. We resected up to 60% of the entire radial articular surface to obtain a smooth surface (average, 28%; range, 20% to 60%). All patients reported immediate relief of pain and improvement in motion (particularly extension). At the latest follow-up (average, 28 mo; range, 13–42 mo), average extension improved from 24° to 54°, average grip strength improved from 47% to 89% of the contralateral wrist, average Disabilities of the Arm, Shoulder, and Hand score improved from 74 to 18, and average Patient-Rated Wrist Hand Evaluation score improved from 79 to 15.

Conclusions.—The aim of the operation was to relieve patients' pain by providing a smooth, although fibrocartilaginous, surface for the carpus to glide on the radius. The follow-up was short and the results may be short-lived. However, for the younger patient, it may provide a temporary alternative to partial wrist arthrodesis with minimal morbidity, and for the less demanding patients, it may be a definitive procedure.

▶ The authors of this article present a novel case series of arthroscopic resection arthroplasty for the treatment of posttraumatic osteoarthrosis of the radiocarpal joint in the setting of intra-articular distal radius malunion. The short-term results of 10 patients are well described, and the patient-reported outcome scores were dramatically improved at final follow-up. Conceptually, temporary pain relief would be expected from the removal of impinging bony surfaces, which create progressive erosive changes with wrist use. Although the transfer of increased loads to a smaller surface area of healthy articular cartilage may lead to accelerated wear in the long term, the authors counter with the favorable outcomes achieved by proximal row carpectomy in which the same biomechanical argument can be made. The advantage of this method, of course, is the minimally invasive approach compared with more traditional salvage procedures for posttraumatic radiocarpal osteoarthrosis, all of which remain future options as a next line of treatment. Many previous reports have questioned the overall contribution of posterior interosseous nerve denervation to postoperative pain relief when performed in conjunction with fusion or arthroplasty procedures in this clinical setting. However, the elimination of this variable as part of this described procedure is a notable strength in my opinion. In my experience, the younger and more active population has a strong desire for motion-sparing options that reliably relieve pain but do not risk further progressive joint damage as they return to vocational and avocational activities. It remains to be seen just how long this temporizing measure may hold up for the initial cohort before secondary surgery becomes inevitable. I expect that this method will gain in popularity for a select group of patients, as many of us look for expanded applications of wrist arthroscopy that can realistically meet the intended goals of surgery.

L. M. Brunton, MD

Incidence and Clinical Outcomes of Tendon Rupture Following Distal Radius Fracture
White BD, Nydick JA, Karsky D, et al (Univ of South Florida, Tampa)
J Hand Surg 37A:2035-2040, 2012

Purpose.—To evaluate the incidence of tendon rupture after nonoperative and operative management of distal radius fractures, report clinical outcomes after tendon repair or transfer, and examine volar plate and dorsal screw prominence as a predictor of tendon rupture.

Methods.—We performed a retrospective chart review on patients treated for tendon rupture after distal radius fracture. We evaluated active range of motion, Disabilities of Arm, Shoulder, and Hand score, grip strength, and pain score, and performed radiographic evaluation of volar plate and dorsal screw prominence in both the study group and a matched control group.

Results.—There were 6 tendon ruptures in 1,359 patients (0.4%) treated nonoperatively and 8 tendon ruptures in 999 patients (0.8%) treated with volar plate fixation. At the time of final follow-up, regardless of treatment, we noted that patients had minimal pain and excellent motion and grip strength. Mean Disabilities of the Shoulder, Arm, and Hand scores were 6 for patients treated nonoperatively and 4 for those treated with volar plating.

Conclusions.—We were unable to verify volar plate or dorsal screw prominence as independent risk factors for tendon rupture after distal radius fractures. However, we recommend continued follow-up and plate removal for symptomatic patients who have volar plate prominence or dorsal screw prominence. In the event of tendon rupture, we report excellent clinical outcomes after tendon repair or tendon transfer.

▶ These authors reviewed a number of distal radius fractures comparing nonoperatively and operatively treated fractures. Their purpose was to evaluate the incidence of tendon rupture after nonoperative and operative management of distal radius fractures, report the clinical outcomes after tendon repair or tendon transfer, and look at the role of hardware as a predictor of tendon rupture. The primary strength of the study is the large number of patients from a single institution, and there were multiple treaters and techniques, including multiple types of hardware, used. They culled this set of patients from an 8-year review of charts looking at codes for distal radius fracture and tendon rupture. They obtained a 4-to-1 match for controls to patients to compare tendon ruptures to patients who did not have tendon ruptures.

The principal weaknesses are that it is possible they did not consider patients who did not undergo operative repair of a tendon rupture. Their use of Current Procedural Terminology codes to look for surgically treated tendon ruptures at the wrist may understate the total number of tendon ruptures diagnosed. It also does not take into account tendon ruptures that were not diagnosed. Despite their large number of patients, they were unable to get statistical significance in most of the variables they examined, but they present an organized review of a large number of cases by looking at propensity toward tendon rupture, results of repair, and predisposing factors to tendon rupture. This article has significance for its contribution to a difficult complication after a common fracture. The authors leave us more work to do in the area but have contributed to our understanding of the frequency of the problem. They correctly point out that attention should be paid to patients who have prominence of volar hardware. In our own practice, patient education is a critical factor in preventing tendon rupture by indicating hardware removal when tendon symptoms occur and allowing the patient to realize that late complication is a possibility.

An additional limitation of this study is a conflict of interest, with several of the authors having financial interests in the hardware discussed. They did, however, correctly identify that potential for conflict.

D. Mastella, MD

The Effect of Osteoporosis on Outcomes of Operatively Treated Distal Radius Fractures
Fitzpatrick SK, Casemyr NE, Zurakowski D, et al (Harvard Med School, Boston, MA; Boston Children's Hosp, MA)
J Hand Surg 37A:2027-2034, 2012

Purpose.—We hypothesized that postmenopausal osteoporotic women with distal radius fractures treated with open reduction internal fixation had worse functional outcomes than women without osteoporosis sustaining similar injuries.

Methods.—We retrospectively reviewed prospectively collected data for 64 postmenopausal women treated with open reduction internal fixation for distal radius fractures between 2006 and 2010 with known bone mineral density measured by dual-energy x-ray absorptiometry at the time of injury (osteopenia, n = 44; osteoporosis, n = 20). Data collected included age, mechanism of injury, fracture severity, and associated comorbidities. Outcomes included range of motion, Disabilities of the Arm, Shoulder, and Hand (DASH) scores, and radiographic parameters of fracture reduction. We calculated patients' Charlson Comorbidity Index and tabulated complications. The primary outcome was DASH score at 12 months after injury. We applied multiple linear regression to determine whether bone mineral density status was predictive of functional outcomes 12 months after injury. We used logistic regression analysis to identify factors independently associated with poor outcomes and applied likelihood estimation to determine predictors of a high DASH score at 12 months.

Results.—At 1 year postoperatively, women with osteoporosis had average DASH scores 15 points higher than those with osteopenia. Both osteoporosis and the Charlson Comorbidity Index were strong positive independent predictors of higher DASH scores (ie, poorer functional outcomes). There were no significant differences in range of motion or radiographic data between groups. Patients with osteoporosis had a higher rate of major complications.

Conclusions.—Osteoporosis had a negative impact on functional outcomes for women with distal radius fractures treated with open reduction internal fixation. Surgeons should identify high-risk patients, ensure close monitoring, and initiate appropriate preventative measures in this patient population.

Type of Study/Level of Evidence.—Prognostic II (Fig 1).

▶ This article substantiates and refines what we inherently know (or suspect)—that osteoporosis has greater morbidity than osteopenia as it relates to surgical

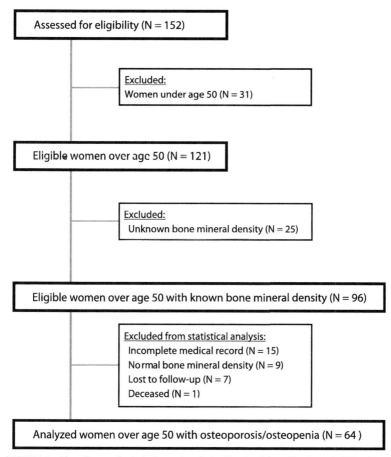

FIGURE 1.—Flow diagram for inclusion and analysis. (Reprinted from The Journal of Hand Surgery. Fitzpatrick SK, Casemyr NE, Zurakowski D, et al. The effect of osteoporosis on outcomes of operatively treated distal radius fractures. *J Hand Surg*. 2012;37A:2027-2034, Copyright 2012, with permission from the American Society for Surgery of the Hand.)

intervention—using criteria defined by the World Health Organization (WHO). The purpose is somewhat misleading because the hypothesis states that patients with osteoporosis would have "worse functional outcomes than women without osteoporosis," which, at least to my read, suggests normal patients. In fact, they have dual-energy x-ray absorptiometry—classified osteopenia, which represents a lesser degree on the WHO continuum of bone density loss and, therefore, not a normal subject cohort. Only 9 subjects met the normal criteria, and these were excluded (Fig 1). Although it is a retrospective analysis, the article introduces the utility of a prospective bone mineral density screening program as well as the importance of global assessment instruments to assess the impact of osteoporosis on general health, and vice versa. In this study, the authors used the Charlson Comorbidity Index. The limitations are readily pointed out, including the lack of stratifying bisphosphonate treatment and hormone replacement therapy. This article, however, provides preliminary evidence of the importance of scrutinizing the common osteoporotic distal radius fracture, especially the need for concerted institutional bone health programs.

A. Ladd, MD

External Fixation Versus Internal Fixation for Unstable Distal Radius Fractures: A Systematic Review and Meta-Analysis of Comparative Clinical Trials
Wei DH, Poolman RW, Bhandari M, et al (Columbia Univ Med Ctr, NY; Onze Lieve Vrouwe Gasthuis, Amsterdam, The Netherlands; McMaster Univ, Hamilton, Ontario, Canada)
J Orthop Trauma 26:386-394, 2012

Objectives.—There is no consensus on the surgical management of unstable distal radius fractures. In this systematic review and meta-analysis, we pool data from trials comparing external fixation and open reduction and internal fixation (ORIF) for this injury.

Data Sources.—We searched electronic databases (including MEDLINE, EMBASE, and SCOPUS) and conference proceedings from 1950 to 2009 in the English literature.

Study Selection.—We pooled data from 12 trials totaling 1011 patients (491 fractures treated with external fixation and 520 with ORIF). All randomized studies of external fixation to ORIF for unstable distal radius fractures were considered, and nonrandomized trials were included if and only if they directly compared external fixation with ORIF.

Data Extraction.—Two authors independently extracted data from all eligible studies, including patient characteristics, sample size, fracture type, length of follow-up, intervention, and outcomes.

Data Synthesis.—Continuous variables were pooled across studies using the method of standard mean differences (SMD) or effect size. ORIF demonstrated significantly better Disabilities of the Arm, Shoulder, and Hand scores (SMD, 0.28; 95% confidence interval, 0.03–0.53; $P = 0.03$), recovery of forearm supination (SMD, 0.23; 95% CI, 0.08–0.38; $P = 0.003$), and restoration of volar tilt (SMD, 0.53; 95% CI, 0.34–0.72; $P < 0.00001$). However, external fixation resulted in significantly better grip strength (SMD, -10.32; 95% CI, -16.36 to -4.28; $P = 0.0008$), and subgroup analyses of randomized studies showed external fixation yielded better wrist flexion (SMD, -0.38; 95% CI, -0.58 to -0.17; $P = 0.0004$).

Conclusions.—For surgical fixation of unstable distal radius fractures, ORIF yields significantly better functional outcomes, forearm supination, and restoration of anatomic volar tilt. However, external fixation results in better grip strength, wrist flexion, and remains a viable surgical alternative (Fig 1, Table 2).

▶ This article deserves scrutiny from anyone who wishes to learn the merits of a robust systematic review. It has all the critical parts: the authors have used more than 1 database; 2 independent reviewers did the search and defined criteria (Table 2), a flow diagram presents their screening and selection of the articles (Fig 1); and they compared reviewer statistics. Little reproducible evidence to compare fixation methods exists in the literature, if their original pool of 1537

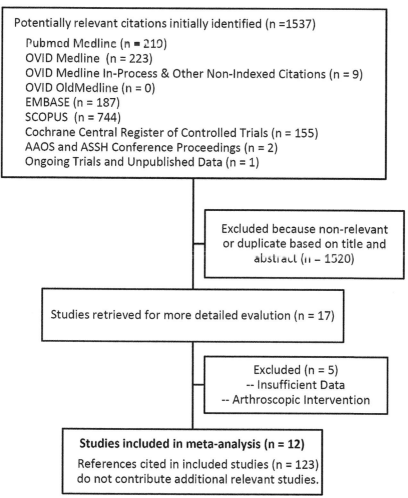

FIGURE 1.—Study flow diagram. A summary of the search process and study identification. Twelve studies were included in the final analysis. (Reprinted from Wei DH, Poolman RW, Bhandari M, et al. External fixation versus internal fixation for unstable distal radius fractures: a systematic review and meta-analysis of comparative clinical trials. *J Orthop Trauma*. 2012;26:386-394, with permission from Lippincott Williams & Wilkins.)

TABLE 2. —Characteristics of Included Trials*

Study Author	Year	Study Design	Number of Patients			Mean Age	Percent Female	Fracture Types
			Total	Ex-Fix	Plate			
Abramo	2009	RCT	50	24	26	48	72	OTA A2, A3, C1, C2, C3
Egol	2008	RCT	88	44	44	51	53	OTA A,B,C
Grewal	2005	RCT	62	33	29	45	48	OTA C1, C2, C3
Kapoor	2000	RCT	57	28	29	—‡	28	Frykman III, IV, VII, VIII
Kreder	2005	RCT	179	88	91	40	39	OTA B, C
Leung	2008	RCT	144	74	70	42	38	OTA C1, C2, C3
Rozental	2009	RCT	45	22	23	52	75	A2, A3, C1, C2
Schmelzer-Schmied	2009	Retrospective	45	15	30	60	—	OTA C1, C2
Wei	2009	RCT	46	22	24	58	72	OTA A3, C1, C2, C3
Westphal	2005	Combined†	237	118	119	60	52	OTA A3, C2
Wright	2005	Combined†	32	11	21	50	56	OTA A2, A3, C2, C3
Zamzuri	2004	Pro	26	12	14	—‡	19	OTA C1, C2, C3
Total number of patients			1011	491	520			

Ex-Fix, external fixation; RCT, randomized clinical trial; OTA, Orthopaedic Trauma Association.

*The 12 trials included in this review are shown with publication year, study design, baseline characteristics of the study population, and types of fractures included.

†Combined retrospective and prospective study design.

‡Some studies did not report the age or number of female patients.

potential articles refined to 12 is any indication. The authors' conclusions, however, are meaningful, because they provide statistical evidence that supports operative intervention, especially as it relates to functional recovery. Because external fixation has largely fallen out of favor in the United States, a more relevant comparison would be to nonoperative treatment; however, given the paucity of comparable references for this current study, finding a similar cohort of nonoperative treatment articles seems unlikely.

A. Ladd, MD

A Biomechanical Comparison of Volar Locked Plating of Intra-Articular Distal Radius Fractures: Use of 4 Versus 7 Screws for Distal Fixation
Moss DP, Means KR Jr, Parks BG, et al (Union Memorial Hosp, Baltimore, MD)
I Hand Surg 30A.1907-1911, 2011

Purpose.—To determine whether the number of distal locking screws significantly affects stability of a cadaveric simulated distal radius fracture fixed with a volar locking plate.

Methods.—We created AO/ASIF type C2 fractures in 10 matched pairs of human fresh-frozen cadaveric wrists and then fixed them using volar locking plates. The number of distal locking screws used was 4 screws or 7 screws in each wrist of the matched pair. We loaded the stabilized fractures cyclically to simulate 6 weeks of postoperative stressing during a therapy protocol and then loaded them to failure. Failure was defined as 2 mm or more of displacement of any fracture fragment as recorded by differential variable reluctance transducers.

Results.—No wrists failed during the cyclic loading portion for either the 4- or 7-screw construct. The average initial stiffness of the 7-screw construct was 69 N/mm ($\pm$ 38) versus 48 N/mm ($\pm$ 14) for the 4-screw construct. The average failure load for the 7-screw construct was 139 N ($\pm$ 78) versus 108 N ($\pm$ 18) for the 4-screw construct. Neither of these differences was statistically significant.

Conclusions.—Although there was a trend toward increased initial stiffness and higher failure load in fractures fixed distally with 7 locking screws, the results were not statistically significant compared with fractures fixed with only 4 screws. Both constructs can withstand forces likely encountered in early therapy protocols.

Clinical Relevance.—The use of extra distal locking screws when fixing distal radius fractures increases expense and may increase the risk of complications, such as extensor tendon irritation or rupture.

▶ This study adds to a sizable body of literature trying to answer the question of how locking screws or pegs should be placed in the distal fragment using a volar locking plate. This is the first study to try to determine how many screws are necessary in an intra-articular fracture model. As with many cadaveric biomechanical studies, this model simplifies the forces across a distal radius fracture (they assessed a cantilever bending moment) compared with in vivo conditions.

Moreover, the investigators examine only 1 manufacturer's volar locking plate. There is significant variability in different volar locking plates, such as the diameter of the distal screws, the splay of the fixed angle screw pattern, or the capacity of variable-angle screws to achieve different splays within the distal fragments. Whether the findings in this study are applicable to all volar locking plates is unknown. Another inherent weakness is that different fracture patterns, such as a smaller lunate facet fragment or a more distal fracture variant, may respond differently.

However, this is a well-conceived and nicely executed study, and it supports the concept that more distal screws are not necessarily better. It suggests that in an AO C2 fracture, 2 points of fixation for each the scaphoid and lunate facet fracture fragments are likely adequate. For intra-articular fractures that meet surgical criteria and are amenable to isolated volar locking plate fixation, I have found it imperative to achieve at least 2 screws just shy of bicortical length in each of the lunate facet and radial styloid fragments. Depending on fracture characteristics, bone quality, and available screw holes (often dependent on plate selection), I will occasionally augment fixation of 1 fragment with a third. It is uncommon for me to fill the plate (including this particular manufacturer's plate) with screws.

R. C. Chadderdon, MD

Do Traction Radiographs of Distal Radial Fractures Influence Fracture Characterization and Treatment?

Goldwyn E, Pensy R, O'Toole RV, et al (Univ of Maryland School of Medicine, Baltimore)

J Bone Joint Surg Am 94:2055-2062, 2012

Background.—Our center evaluates all distal radial fractures with traction radiographs before splinting. Although investigations of various imaging modalities to evaluate distal radial fractures have been presented in the literature, to our knowledge the use of traction radiographs has not been well described. We hypothesized that the addition of traction radiographs to standard radiographs increases interobserver and intraobserver reliability for injury descriptions, affects the choice of treatment plan, and decreases the perceived need for computed tomography.

Methods.—Radiographs for fifty consecutive eligible patients with distal radial fractures that were treated at a level-1 trauma center were used to create two image sets for each patient. Set 1 included injury and splint radiographs, and Set 2 included the images from Set 1 plus traction radiographs. The image sets were stripped of all demographic data and were presented in random order to seven fellowship-trained orthopaedic surgeons. The surgeons independently reviewed each of the 100 image sets and answered ten questions regarding the description and treatment of the injury. Analyses were conducted with kappa statistics to evaluate interobserver reliability. Intraobserver variability was assessed with the McNemar test after adjusting for clustering.

Results.—Traction radiographs improved interobserver reliability for four of ten questions. With regard to intraobserver variability, responses to two questions were significantly changed. With the addition of traction radiographs, the observation of intra-articular fragments requiring reduction increased from 38.3% to 53.1% ($p < 0.05$) and the perceived need to order computed tomography for further evaluation decreased from 21.7% to 5.1% ($p < 0.001$). No other changes reached significance.

Conclusion.—The addition of traction radiographs appeared to affect surgeons' interobserver reliability in the evaluation of distal radial fractures. In addition, traction radiographs changed the rate of detection of intra-articular fragments requiring reduction and the perceived need for computed tomography. These data indicate that traction radiographs may provide some of the same information as computed tomographic scans at a lower cost and argue for additional research comparing computed tomographic scans and traction radiographs of the distal part of the radius.

▶ The authors attempted to determine the value of traction radiographs in patients with distal radius fractures. Fifty consecutive distal radius fractures were studied. Standard and standard plus traction x-rays were performed. The authors recruited 7 orthopedic surgeons to review the films and answer 10 questions ranging from descriptive aspects, additional study recommendations, treatment recommendations, and preferred surgical techniques.

Although the authors noted that traction views did not improve reliability of identifying intra-articular fracture extension, they did improve reliability of assessing intra-articular displacement of the fracture. In addition, there was greater agreement regarding the need (or lack of need) for computed tomography (CT) scans.

The addition of stress x-rays is easy and inexpensive and could reduce the need for additional imaging such as CT scans. This would result in decreased health care costs for the patient.

M. Rizzo, MD

12 Elbow: Trauma

A New Fracture Model for "Terrible Triad" Injuries of the Elbow: Influence of Forearm Rotation on Injury Patterns

Fitzpatrick MJ, Diltz M, McGarry MH, et al (VA Long Beach Healthcare System, CA)
J Orthop Trauma 26:591-596, 2012

Objective.—The purpose of this study was to evaluate the influence of forearm rotation on failure patterns of the elbow under axial loads.

Methods.—Fourteen upper extremities were resected mid-humerus and mounted on a custom apparatus, which allowed rotation of the ulna, radius, and humerus about a fixed wrist while loading in axial compression. Seven specimens were loaded to failure with the forearm in pronation and 7 in supination.

Results.—Six of the 7 elbows axially loaded in pronation resulted in fractures of the radial head and coronoid with posterior dislocation (terrible triad). Six of the 7 elbows loaded in supination dislocated without fracture. One of the 7 elbows tested in supination had a terrible triad—type elbow injury. Five of the 6 specimens with ulna external rotation had damage to the lateral ligaments; all 8 specimens with internal rotation had damage to the medial ligaments. There were no significant differences in biomechanical parameters between pronation and supination.

Conclusions.—The forearm position during axial load was the primary determinant of fracture—dislocation pattern. When the forearm was pronated, a terrible triad injury pattern most often occurred. When the forearm was supinated, a dislocation without fracture most often occurred. In both forearm rotation positions, when the ulna internally rotated during failure, the medial structures were the first to be disrupted. When the ulna externally rotated, the lateral structures were the first to be disrupted. Understanding the pathomechanics of elbow dislocation may improve diagnosis and treatment of these injuries.

▶ This original biomechanical cadaveric study of elbow injury patterns disputes the long-standing assumption that the lateral ligament complex fails first in the progression to elbow dislocation or fracture dislocation. Instead, the authors present novel evidence that forearm position and ulna rotation predict the failure sequence of static soft-tissue restraints and osseous structures about the elbow. Study limitations are adequately addressed and discussed. The conclusions of the study would be strengthened by the testing of more specimens or by the reproduction of the findings by another investigating group elsewhere. Clearly, this study will not change the treatment of high-energy elbow injuries once the pattern is recognized, characterized, and understood by the treating surgeon. The results of these types of studies are more likely to end up on in-training or board-certifying examinations than on the minds of surgeons who are confronted with either the inconvenient midnight call from the emergency department or the unreduced elbow that shows up unexpectedly in Friday afternoon clinic.

L. M. Brunton, MD

Short- to mid-term results of metallic press-fit radial head arthroplasty in unstable injuries of the elbow
Flinkkilä T, Kaisto T, Sirniö K, et al (Oulu Univ Hosp, Finland)
J Bone Joint Surg Br 94-B:805-810, 2012

We assessed the short- to mid-term survival of metallic press-fit radial head prostheses in patients with radial head fractures and acute traumatic instability of the elbow.

The medical records of 42 patients (16 males, 26 females) with a mean age of 56 years (23 to 85) with acute unstable elbow injuries, including a fracture of the radial head requiring metallic replacement of the radial head, were reviewed retrospectively. Survival of the prosthesis was assessed from the radiographs of 37 patients after a mean follow-up of 50 months (12 to 107). The functional results of 31 patients were assessed using range-of-movement, Mayo elbow performance score (MEPS), Disabilities of the Arm, Shoulder and Hand (DASH) score and the RAND 36-item health survey.

At the most recent follow-up 25 prostheses were still well fixed, nine had been removed because of loosening, and three remained implanted but were loose. The mean time from implantation to loosening was 11 months (2 to 24). Radiolucent lines that developed around the prosthesis before removal were mild in three patients, moderate in one and severe in five. Range of movement parameters and mass grip strength were significantly lower in the affected elbow than in the unaffected side. The mean MEPS score was 86 (40 to 100) and the mean DASH score was 23 (0 to 81). According to RAND-36 scores, patients had more pain and lower physical function scores than normal population values.

Loosening of press-fit radial head prostheses is common, occurs early, often leads to severe osteolysis of the proximal radius, and commonly requires removal of the prosthesis.

▶ This is the first study to report the medium-term clinical and radiographic results of press-fit radial head arthroplasty in the setting of acute fracture. Modern radial head implants are usually manufactured from cobalt-chrome or titanium alloys and are modular to allow independent sizing of the head and stem. The stem can be press fit, cemented, or intentionally left loose. Loose-fitting polished stems allow the head to settle into the patients' anatomy, where it essentially acts as a spacer. Press-fit stems, in contrast, attempt to recreate the normal anatomy (elliptical head and offset neck) and need to be well fixed into the radius to maintain the proper anatomy. As observed in this report, they do not appear to show adequate bony ingrowth. Press-fit stems that loosen are often symptomatic, in contrast to what has been reported in loose, smooth-stemmed prostheses. Furthermore, loose, press-fit stems also often lead to severe osteolysis and forearm pain. According to the authors, loose-fitting or cemented bipolar prostheses have better midterm radiographic results and should be considered superior to press-fit prostheses.

E. Cheung, MD

Treatment of Mason Type II Radial Head Fractures Without Associated Fractures or Elbow Dislocation: A Systematic Review

Kaas L, Struijs PAA, Ring D, et al (Amphia Hosp, Breda, The Netherlands; Academic Med Ctr, Amsterdam, The Netherlands; Massachusetts General Hosp, Boston)
J Hand Surg 37A:1416-1421, 2012

Purpose.—There is no consensus as to the best treatment of Mason type II fractures without concomitant elbow fractures or dislocation. The aim of this systematic review was to compare the results of operative and nonoperative treatment of these injuries.

Methods.—We systematically screened the databases of PubMed, EMBASE, and Cochrane Library until September 2011 for studies on nonoperative or operative treatment of Mason type II fractures. We defined successful treatment as an excellent or good result according to the Broberg and Morrey score, Mayo Elbow Performance Score, or Radin score. Exclusion criteria were duration of follow-up of less than 6 months, an improperly described therapy or combination of therapies, skeletal immaturity, and articles written in languages other than English.

Results.—Among 717 studies, 9 retrospective case series (level IV) describing 224 patients satisfied our inclusion criteria. Nonoperative treatment was successful in 114 of 142 patients (80%) pooled from the studies (42% to 96% success in individual studies). Open reduction and internal fixation was successful in 76 of 82 patients (93%) (81% to 100% success in individual studies).

Conclusions.—Only a few studies with a low level of evidence address the treatment of isolated, displaced, partial articular fractures. There is a need for sufficiently powered randomized, controlled trials.

Clinical Relevance.—There is insufficient evidence to draw firm conclusions on the optimal treatment of isolated, displaced, partial articular Mason type II fractures.

▶ The best treatment (operative vs nonoperative) of isolated Mason type II radial head fractures is debated. In this review, the rate of success was significantly higher in the open reduction and internal fixation group compared with the nonoperative group. However, most of the studies included in this systematic review were low level of evidence studies with small numbers and large heterogeneity in study design. The mean range of motion decreased with both operative and nonoperative treatment. The mean follow-up periods of most of the studies included in this review were short, and clinical outcomes may decline over time. There is room for debate about the indications for surgery and the risks and benefits for Mason type II radial head fractures. Complications such as persistent pain and failed initial treatment with subsequent revision surgery may not have been adequately reported. Other data regarding development of arthrosis, motion, pain, and mechanical symptoms were presented in different ways. Combined with the variety in classification systems, treatments, and outcome measures, it is difficult to compare results among studies. Clinical results are often positive for both nonoperative and operative treatment.

E. Cheung, MD

A New Fracture Model for "Terrible Triad" Injuries of the Elbow: Influence of Forearm Rotation on Injury Patterns
Fitzpatrick MJ, Diltz M, McGarry MH, et al (VA Long Beach Healthcare System, CA)
J Orthop Trauma 26:591-596, 2012

Objective.—The purpose of this study was to evaluate the influence of forearm rotation on failure patterns of the elbow under axial loads.

Methods.—Fourteen upper extremities were resected mid-humerus and mounted on a custom apparatus, which allowed rotation of the ulna, radius, and humerus about a fixed wrist while loading in axial compression. Seven specimens were loaded to failure with the forearm in pronation and 7 in supination.

Results.—Six of the 7 elbows axially loaded in pronation resulted in fractures of the radial head and coronoid with posterior dislocation (terrible triad). Six of the 7 elbows loaded in supination dislocated without fracture. One of the 7 elbows tested in supination had a terrible triad—type elbow injury. Five of the 6 specimens with ulna external rotation had damage to the lateral ligaments; all 8 specimens with internal rotation had damage to the medial ligaments. There were no significant differences in biomechanical parameters between pronation and supination.

Conclusions.—The forearm position during axial load was the primary determinant of fracture—dislocation pattern. When the forearm was pronated, a terrible triad injury pattern most often occurred. When the forearm was supinated, a dislocation without fracture most often occurred. In both forearm rotation positions, when the ulna internally rotated during failure, the medial structures were the first to be disrupted. When the ulna externally rotated, the lateral structures were the first to be disrupted.

Understanding the pathomechanics of elbow dislocation may improve diagnosis and treatment of these injuries.

▶ The authors present a well-designed cadaveric biomechanical study to evaluate the position of the forearm when a patient suffers an associated elbow dislocation, radial head fracture, and coronoid fracture. The authors make an important distinction in this biomechanical study over previously published projects in that they specifically evaluated the influence of supination and pronation of the forearm on the injury pattern. Specifically noted by the authors is the increased prevalence of a classic terrible triad elbow injury with the forearm in pronation compared with loading the arm in supination, which created a simple posterior dislocation. The most compelling portion of this article is the finding that the direction of rotation of the ulna during axial loading influences the pattern of the ligamentous injury to the elbow. Despite popular belief in the essential lesion of injury to the lateral collateral ligament as described originally by Osborne and Cotterill, the authors note that in their model, with openly discussed limitations, with internal rotation of the ulna at the ulnohumeral joint, the medial structures failed first. This article is significant because it adds new biomechanical understanding to the injury patterns experienced by individuals with elbow dislocations. The finding of initial medial ligamentous failure in a reproducible model may help to explain the patients that have a dislocation and persistent medial pain and evidence of instability with intact lateral ligamentous structures.

J. M. Froelich, MD

Biomechanical Comparison of Parallel Versus 90-90 Plating of Bicolumn Distal Humerus Fractures With Intra-Articular Comminution
Got C, Shuck J, Hiercevicz A, et al (Brown Univ, Providence, RI)
J Hand Surg 37A:2512-2518, 2012

Purpose.—To compare the biomechanical properties of 90-90 versus mediolateral parallel plating of C-3 bicolumn distal humerus factures.

Methods.—We created intra-articular AO/Orthopaedic Trauma Association C-3 bicolumn fractures in 10 fresh-frozen matched pairs of cadaveric elbows. We determined bone mineral density of the metaphyseal region with dual-energy x-ray absorptiometry. The matched pairs of elbows were randomly assigned to either 90-90 or parallel plate fixation. We tested anteroposterior displacement at a rate of 0.5 mm/s to a maximum load of ± 100 N for both the articular and entire distal humerus segments. We tested torsional stability at a displacement rate of 0.1 Hz to a maximum torque of ± 2.5 Nm. After cyclical testing, we loaded the specimens in torsion to failure.

Results.—There was no significant difference in the bone density of the paired specimens. Compared with parallel fixation, 90-90 plate fixation had significantly greater torque to failure load. Both plating constructs were equally sensitive to bone density. Both techniques had the same

TABLE.—Results of Testing Modalities

| | 90/90 | | Parallel | | |
	Mean	SD	Mean	SD	P Value
Maximum deflection (fragment) (mm)	1.29	0.42	1.20	0.27	.581
Maximum deflection (entire segment) (mm)	0.67	0.08	0.70	0.08	.312
Delta deflection (mm)	0.62	0.39	0.50	0.24	.439
Stiffness fragment cycle 120 (N/mm)	150.61	47.69	156.74	32.58	.727
Stiffness entire segment cycle 120 (N/mm)	278.81	37.41	269.32	34.16	.400
Torque to failure (Nm)	44.07	16.87	31.92	16.23	.047
Maximum deflection at maximum torque (°)	22.14	10.58	14.92	10.84	.179

mode of failure in torsion, a spiral fracture extending from the medial plate at the metaphyseal-diaphyseal junction. There was no significant difference in the stiffness of fixation of the articular fragment or the entire distal segment in anteroposterior loading.

Conclusions.—This study demonstrated that 90-90 and parallel plating had comparable biomechanical properties for fixation of comminuted intra-articular distal humerus fractures, and that 90-90 plating had greater resistance to torsional loading (Table).

▶ There has been continued controversy regarding treatment options for humeral factures and optimal plate configuration. This important series investigated biomechanics of parallel vs 90-90 plate configurations.

A total of 20 matched cadaver humeri underwent creation of a simulated C3 fracture; right and left arms of each specimen were randomized to parallel vs 90-90 plate configurations. Anteroposterior displacement of the articular segment and the entire distal humerus, as well as torsional stiffness, were assessed (Table).

The results are in contradistinction to several prior studies that have suggested that 90-90 plating is inferior to parallel plating, particularly in resisting torsional loads. This series found the opposite: that 90-90 plating was superior to parallel plating to resist torsional loads. The authors conclude either parallel or 90-90 plating is appropriate for fixation of distal humerus fractures, and the data suggest similar biomechanical properties.

J. E. Adams, MD

13 Pediatric Trauma

Risk Factors for Redisplacement of Pediatric Distal Forearm and Distal Radius Fractures
McQuinn AG, Jaarsma RL (Flinders Med Centre, Bedford Park, South Australia, Australia)
J Pediatr Orthop 32:687-692, 2012

Background.—Fractures of the distal forearm and distal radius represent the most common types of fracture in the pediatric population, with the majority treated by closed reduction and cast. Redisplacement has been known to occur in up to 39% of cases. There have been numerous risk factors and radiologic indices put forward as methods of predicting redisplacement, but this topic remains a matter of debate. This retrospective study aims to further assess the significance of the many factors in redisplacement after treatment with closed reduction.

Methods.—This retrospective study included 155 children with distal radius and forearm fractures. Age, sex, location of fracture, angulation, displacement, an associated ulna fracture, obliquity of fracture, and accuracy of reduction were measured for assessment as potential risk factors. In addition, the cast index, padding index, Canterbury index, second metacarpal-radius index, gap index, and 3-point index were measured on postreduction radiographs.

Results.—Redisplacement occurred in 33 of the 155 cases (21.3%). Initial displacement and accuracy of the reduction were identified as significant risk factors for redisplacement. Initial displacement of >50% (of the radius width) was significantly associated with redisplacement (odds ratio of 5.4). Failure to achieve anatomic reduction was significantly higher in the redisplacement group (odds ratio 3.9). The only radiologic index that differed significantly between groups was the cast index, with more patients without redisplacement meeting the cut-off value (60% vs. 32%, $P = 0.010$).

Discussion.—Initial displacement of >50% and inability to achieve anatomic reduction are major risk factors for redisplacement. Given its effectiveness and ease of clinical application, the cast index remains the most useful measure of cast molding.

Level of Evidence.—Level II—Retrospective prognostic study.

▶ There is a common misconception among clinicians who care for pediatric distal radius and forearm fractures that the remodeling potential of the immature skeleton will overcome a poor reduction in all cases. Remodeling cannot correct

201

for joint subluxations or dislocations. Remodeling potential also decreases as the child ages. Another common mistake is to assume that redisplacement is either unlikely or inconsequential in children. This study from Australia looking at redisplacement in distal radial or forearm fractures found that the overall redisplacement rate was 21%. Initial displacement of more than 50% was the biggest risk factor for redisplacement, with an odds ratio of 5.4 compared with less than 50% initial displacement. Seventy percent of the fractures that redisplaced were more than 50% displaced initially. Failure to achieve an anatomic reduction was also a significant factor in redisplacement. Of all the radiographic parameters that were measured, only the cast index was significantly associated with redisplacement. Therefore, fractures of the distal forearm that are initially displaced beyond acceptable parameters and do not reduce anatomically should be followed up closely. At the minimum, a good cast index and proper plaster technique should be used as the best chance to hold a reduction. For fractures that involve the physes, follow-up radiographs should be obtained within 1 week of the reduction. If there is any redisplacement, the fracture should be re-reduced and fixed with smooth pins that avoid crossing the physis whenever possible. For extraphyseal fractures, weekly follow-up radiographs are required until union.

D. A. Zlotolow, MD

Hand Fractures in Children: Epidemiology and Misdiagnosis in a Tertiary Referral Hospital

Chew EM, Chong AKS (Singapore General Hosp; Natl Univ Hosp, Singapore; et al)
J Hand Surg 37:1684-1688, 2012

Purpose.—To determine the local epidemiology of pediatric hand fractures and the rate of misdiagnosis.

Methods.—A retrospective study was performed on children aged 17 years and younger who were referred for actual or suspected metacarpal and phalangeal fractures. Medical records were reviewed for age at the time of injury, sex, fracture pattern, venue where the injury was sustained, injury mechanism, and diagnoses made by the referring doctor and hand surgeon. Differing diagnoses were considered misdiagnoses. The misdiagnosis rate was calculated as the percentage of misdiagnoses over the number of referrals.

Results.—Of 204 cases reviewed, emergency physicians referred 146 cases (72%), and primary health care physicians referred the rest. There were 193 cases of actual fractures in 181 patients and 16 cases of misdiagnosis. The fracture incidence peaked at 14 and 15 years. The median ages of children sustaining fractures of the distal phalanges, proximal phalanges, and metacarpals were 9, 12, and 15 years, respectively. The proximal phalanx was most commonly fractured (95 cases, 49%), as was the fifth ray (78 cases, 40%). Most fractures occurred at school (79 cases, 44%). Sports-related injury was the leading cause of fractures (70 cases, 39%). The misdiagnosis rate was 8% (16 of 204). The leading cause of misdiagnosis was misinterpretation of epiphyses (6 of 16), followed by missing multiple fractures (3 of 16).

Conclusions.—The higher fracture incidence in teenagers is likely related to sports participation. Sports accounted for proximal fractures in older children, whereas young children sustained distal fractures through crushing injuries. Although the misdiagnosis rate seemed low, it might reflect that emergency physicians, who referred most of the cases, were adept at diagnosing fractures. To improve diagnostic accuracy, doctors should familiarize themselves with the location of epiphyses and look carefully for multiple fractures.

Type of Study/Level of Evidence.—Economic and Decision Analysis IV.

▶ As children engage in higher-impact sports at earlier ages, the risks of injury increase. This study out of a major referral center in Singapore shows that the trends we are seeing in the United States are likely happening worldwide. Boys were more likely to sustain hand fractures than girls, and the incidence increased as children became older. More interesting was the authors' analysis of misdiagnosed or underdiagnosed cases. Eight percent of their cases were diagnosed incorrectly, which seems quite low for a busy emergency department. Of the cases that had been incorrectly diagnosed as fracture, nearly half were the result of misinterpretation of the physes. Missed fractures were less common and were often the result of a distracting injury. The number of overcalls was more than twice the number of missed fractures, which seems appropriate for this population.

D. A. Zlotolow, MD

Displaced Humeral Lateral Condyle Fractures in Children: Should We Bury the Pins?

Das De S, Bae DS, Waters PM (Children's Hosp Boston, MA)
J Pediatr Orthop 32:573-578, 2012

Background.—The purpose of this investigation was to determine if leaving Kirschner wires exposed is more cost-effective than burying them subcutaneously after open reduction and internal fixation (ORIF) of humeral lateral condyle fractures.

Methods.—A retrospective cohort study of all lateral condyle fractures treated over a 10-year period at a single institution was performed. Data on surgical technique, fracture healing, and complications were analyzed, as well as treatment costs. A decision analysis model was then constructed to compare the strategies of leaving the pins exposed versus buried. Finally, sensitivity analyses were performed, assessing cost-effectiveness when infection rates and costs of treating deep infections were varied.

Results.—A total of 235 children with displaced fractures were treated with ORIF using Kirschner wires. Pins were left exposed in 41 cases (17.4%) and buried in 194 cases (82.6%); the age, sex, injury mechanisms, and fracture patterns were similar in both the groups. The median time to removal of implants was shorter with exposed versus buried pins (4 vs. 6 wk, $P < 0.001$), although there was no difference in fracture union or loss of reduction rates. The rate of superficial infection was higher with exposed pins (9.8% vs. 3.1%), but this was not statistically significant ($P = 0.076$). There were no deep infections with exposed pins, whereas the rate of deep infection was 0.5% with buried pins ($P = 1.00$). Buried pins were associated with additional complications, including symptomatic implants (7.2%); pins protruding through the skin (16%); internal pin migration necessitating additional surgery (1%); and skin necrosis (1%). The decision analysis revealed that leaving pins exposed resulted in an average cost savings of $3442 per patient. This strategy remained cost-effective even when infection rates with exposed pins approached 40%.

Conclusions.—Leaving the pins exposed after ORIF of lateral condyle fractures is safe and more cost-effective than burying the pins subcutaneously.

Level of Evidence.—Retrospective cohort study (level III).

▶ The authors address the question of the cost effectiveness of exposed vs buried pins in the treatment of displaced lateral condyle fractures in children utilizing a retrospective review, systemic review of literature, and a decision analysis model. Cost analyses are increasingly important to the practice of modern medicine. They reported a significant cost savings associated with leaving the pins exposed ($3442 per patient) taking into account the higher rate of complications associated with buried pins (deep infection, internal and external pin migration, and superficial skin necrosis). Although the cohort of patients with exposed pins in this study (41 cases) is relatively small compared with the buried pin group (194 cases), this discrepancy was addressed by the sensitivity analysis. This study shows that leaving pins exposed does not lead to an increased rate of superficial infection requiring removal of pins and jeopardizing fracture union. It is generally easier from a scheduling perspective, both for the surgeon and the patient, to undergo pin removal in the office. The results of this study can reasonably be applied to other pediatric fractures that are treated with internal fixation consisting of k-wires or smooth pins and, therefore, can help with decision making in future treatment of pediatric fractures.

F. Fishman, MD

Indirect Reduction of the Radial Head in Children With Chronic Monteggia Lesions
Song KS, Ramnani K, Bae KC, et al (Keimyung Univ, Daegu, Korea)
J Orthop Trauma 26:597-601, 2012

Objective.—The purpose of this study was to report the long-term follow-up results of chronic Monteggia fractures treated with angulation–translation osteotomy of ulna and closed reduction of the radial head.

Design.—Retrospective.

Setting.—Level 1 trauma center.

Patients.—We retrospectively reviewed 10 missed Monteggia fractures in children. The mean age of the patients was 7.5 years (range, 6—10 years), and there were 2 girls and 8 boys. The mean duration of time between initial injury and initial presentation was 1.7 years (range, 6 weeks to 5 years).

Intervention.—Closed reduction with ulna osteotomy or lengthening was performed in all 10 cases. Annular ligament reconstruction (ALR) was done in 2 cases. Final follow-up ranged from 3 to 20 years (mean 10 years).

Main Outcome Measurement.—We assessed preoperative and postoperative radiographs to evaluate the quality of the radial head reduction. Clinical results were assessed according to the functional elbow score devised by Kim et al.

Results.—Radial head reduction was achieved and maintained in 8 of 10 cases after primary or secondary surgery. The radial head was mildly subluxated in one case and dislocated in another case at final follow-up. ALR was performed in only 2 cases. Open reduction and ALR is not required in every case, and its need should depend on intraoperative stability of radial head.

▶ Chronic Monteggia lesions in children remain a challenging clinical problem. If addressed surgically, treatment generally consists of open reduction of the radio-capitellar joint and correction of any remaining ulnar deformity, with or without reconstruction of the annular ligament. The authors of this study propose treating chronic Monteggia lesions with an ulnar osteotomy and indirect reduction of the radial head. Although their final conclusion states that they feel their technique can achieve good functional results and maintenance of a reduced radial head, I did not feel their data truly supported this assertion. Three of 10 patients required revision surgery secondary to redislocation or subluxation of the radial head. Two of 10 patients underwent open reduction with annular ligament reconstruction at the time of initial surgery. One additional patient (case 2) was noted to have mild subluxation at the time of final follow-up. In total, 60% of their small patient population either failed to maintain a reduced radial head having undergone indirect reduction or underwent annular ligament reconstruction initially. Theoretically, avoiding opening the radiocapitellar joint at the time of surgery would likely lead to quicker recovery and better functional results of the elbow, but the data presented in this article do not convincingly demonstrate that an indirect reduction of the radial head and an ulnar osteotomy is adequate treatment for the chronic Monteggia lesion in children.

F. G. Fishman, MD

14 Congenital

The Fate of the Index Metacarpophalangeal Joint Following Pollicization
Lochner HV, Oishi S, Ezaki M, et al (Texas Scottish Rite Hosp for Children, Dallas, TX; Johns Hopkins Univ, Baltimore, MD)
J Hand Surg 37A:1672-1676, 2012

Purpose.—To characterize the complications that occur at the index metacarpophalangeal (MCP) joint following pollicization and to identify the blood supply of the index MCP joint.

Methods.—Eighty-five pollicized digits in 74 patients (1974–2007) were followed after surgery and had documented clinical examinations and radiographs to evaluate physeal arrest, nonunion at the pollicized digit base, and instability of the new carpometacarpal joint at a minimum of 2 years following surgery.

Results.—Proximal phalanx physeal arrest was the most common complication. Radiographic nonunion at the juncture of the index metacarpal head and base occurred with and without instability. Twenty-one of 85 pollicized digits showed radiographic evidence of physeal arrest, 12 of which were complete and 9 partial. No clinical factor was found to significantly correlate with a physeal arrest, although the 9 patients with the diagnosis of Holt-Oram syndrome trended toward a higher percentage, with 6 digits in 5 patients with Holt-Oram syndrome showing this complication. Twenty pollicized MCP joints did not have bony union to the base of the index metacarpal, but only 3 were clinically unstable and required surgical stabilization. Ten pollicized digits developed some degree of instability and subluxation at the new carpometacarpal joint, but only one required surgical intervention. In recent cases, a search for the blood supply to the MCP joint has demonstrated a consistent vessel deep to the interosseous muscles that arborizes on the volar metacarpal neck. Our surgical technique has evolved to preserve this vessel whenever possible.

Conclusions.—Our complications are most likely due to technical factors. Careful dissection of the index MCP joint during pollicization should help reduce physeal growth arrest. Patients with Holt-Oram syndrome might have an increased risk of growth arrest. However, the majority of patients did not require secondary surgery and have good function.

Type of Study/Level of Evidence.—Therapeutic IV.

▶ The technique of pollicization remains one of the crowning achievements of surgery. The index finger is shortened, rotated, and set in the position of a thumb attached briefly only by its tendons and neurovascular bundles. Success of the total operation rests on the success of all of its component steps, of which there are many. One critical step is the preservation of the metacarpophalangeal joint of the index finger to fashion a new thumb basal joint. Nonunion or avascular necrosis of the metacarpal head can lead to basal joint instability, compromising effective use of the new thumb. Of 85 pollicizations, this study found 21 growth arrests (25%) and 20 nonunions (24%) circa the index metacarpophalangeal joint. The authors identified a feeder vessel of the deep anterior metacarpal artery that was the vascular supply to the metacarpophalangeal joint in 10 consecutive cases of pollicization. Preservation of this vascular supply during dissection of the joint may help prevent these complications.

D. A. Zlotolow, MD

Complex Syndactyly: Aesthetic and Objective Outcomes
Goldfarb CA, Steffen JA, Stutz CM (Shriners Hosp for Children, St Louis, MO; Washington Univ School of Medicine, St Louis, MO)
J Hand Surg 37A:2068-2073, 2012

Purpose.—Outcome data after the treatment of complex syndactyly are lacking. The purpose of this investigation was to critically analyze and report our results after surgical reconstruction of complex syndactyly.

Methods.—We included 13 patients and 21 hands (25 webspaces) in this retrospective call-back investigation. There were 17 middle/ring finger and 8 ring/little finger complex syndactylies, each with a defined, isolated osseous bridge between the distal phalanges. We excluded complicated and syndrome-associated syndactylies. Patients returned for clinical examination and subjective assessment at an average of 9 years (range, 2—27 y) after the most recent surgery. Of 21 hands, 6 had undergone a revision surgery.

Results.—The Vancouver Scar Scale scores averaged 3 (range, 0—6), web creep averaged 1.5 (range, 0—3), and total active motion averaged 148° for the affected fingers. In the middle/ring finger syndactylies, the middle finger was most commonly supinated (average, 13°) and ulnarly deviated (average, 9°), and the ring finger was either supinated or pronated and radially deviated (average, 13°). In the ring/little finger syndactylies, the ring finger was most commonly supinated (average, 8°) without deviation, and the little finger was most commonly pronated (average, 8°) and radially deviated (average, 24°). There was a notable nail wall deformity in most fingers. Surgeon visual analog scale scores (range, 0—10, where lower scores are better) averaged 2.8 (range, 0.8—5.0). Patient visual analog scale scores were 0.4 (range, 0—3) for pain, 1.9 (range, 0—10) for appearance, and 1.1 (range, 0—3) for function.

Conclusions.—Complex syndactyly reconstruction is challenging, and common postsurgical findings include rotational and angular deformity and nail deformity. When deformity was present, the fingers typically rotated away from and deviated toward the site of the previous complex syndactyly. We describe how we have altered our approach based on these findings.

Type of Study/Level of Evidence.—Therapeutic IV.

▶ Complex syndactyly reconstruction can be more challenging than simple syndactyly because of the presence of synostosis. The lack of soft tissue between the digits compromises reconstructive options. This study used patient-derived and surgeon-derived subjective criteria to evaluate their outcomes, but no cohort of simple syndactyly reconstructions was available for comparison. Lateral nail-fold reconstruction was cited as problematic, despite the use of Buck-Gramcko type flaps, which are commonly used. Rotational and angular deformities were common after digital separation. Their data were insufficient to recommend specific remedies to limit postoperative deformity, but the authors cite using their data to counsel patients on expectations after surgery.

D. A. Zlotolow, MD

Comparison of Splinting Versus Nonsplinting in the Treatment of Pediatric Trigger Finger

Shiozawa R, Uchiyama S, Sugimoto Y, et al (Shinshu Univ School of Medicine, Matsumoto, Japan; Hata General Hosp, Matsumoto, Japan; Yodakubo Hosp, Japan; et al)

J Hand Surg 37A:1211-1216, 2012

Purpose.—Because pediatric trigger finger is much less common than pediatric trigger thumb, there is no consensus on the efficacy of splinting, owing to both the rarity of the condition and a lack of natural history and comparative therapeutic data. We performed the present retrospective study on 47 fingers to compare pediatric trigger finger treatment by splinting and nonsplinting.

Methods.—We included 24 children with a total of 47 trigger fingers. Affected fingers included 4 index, 28 middle, 11 ring, and 4 little fingers. Patient age at initial examination ranged from 1 month to 9 years (mean, 2 y). We observed 24 fingers treated with a static splint and 23 fingers treated without it. The time from initial examination to follow-up ranged from 2 to 18 years.

Results.—In the splinting group, 16 fingers (67%) resolved, 4 fingers (17%) improved, and 4 fingers (17%) remained unchanged. Seven fingers (29%) ultimately required surgery. In the nonsplinting group, 7 fingers (30%) resolved spontaneously, 1 (4%) improved, and 15 (65%) remained unchanged. Fifteen fingers (65%) later underwent surgical release. The rate of resolution in the splinting group was significantly higher than that in the nonsplinting group. The proportion of fingers needing surgical treatment in the splinting group was significantly lower than that in the nonsplinting group.

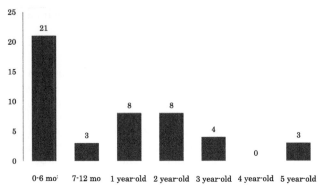

Patient age at presentation

FIGURE 1.—Number of fingers in different age groups, classified by onset of trigger symptoms. We noted 24 trigger fingers (51%) at less than 12 months of age, and 44 trigger fingers (94%) at 3 years of age or younger. (Reprinted from The Journal of Hand Surgery. Shiozawa R, Uchiyama S, Sugimoto Y, et al. Comparison of splinting versus nonsplinting in the treatment of pediatric trigger finger. *J Hand Surg.* 2012;37A:1211-1216, Copyright 2012, with permission from the American Society for Surgery of the Hand.)

Conclusions.—For treatment of pediatric trigger finger, it is advisable to fit a static splint at the first visit.
Type of Study/Level of Evidence.—Therapeutic IV (Fig 1).

► This Japanese report of pediatric trigger finger supports early splinting on presentation. Ten of the 17 references in this article come from Japanese (7), Korean (2), and Taiwanese (1) centers, suggesting an association with race, although little is known about the etiology and natural history given its rare presentation. The authors recommend night splinting for 6 months, based on the premise that complete resolution required a minimum of 5 months in their series. The authors admit the wide range of age presentation (Fig 1), the bias toward parental preference to attempt splinting, and the variable compliance with splinting all as limitations of the study. Nonetheless, they suggest that pediatric trigger finger behaves differently than trigger thumb and deserves an attempt of splinting. My limited experience with pediatric trigger finger supports this; I've seen it more commonly in older children, including one who had successful surgery of a ring finger and later was able to elicit triggering on the remaining digits by hyperextending the metacarpophalangeal joints in something of a party trick. This resolved with splinting and parental incentives.

A. Ladd, MD

Technique of Forearm Osteotomy for Pediatric Problems
Ezaki M, Oishi SN (Texas Scottish Rite Hosp for Children, Dallas)
J Hand Surg 37A:2400-2403, 2012

Correction of a rigid forearm deformity in children is often desired in congenital radioulnar synostosis, brachial plexus palsy, cerebral palsy, or posttraumatic torsional deformity. Osteotomies at the diaphyseal level present difficulties with maintenance of reduction, whether or not internal or pin fixation is used. The stabilizing and healing potential of the periosteum in these cases can be used to advantage in the correction of these deformities.

▶ The authors describe a unique technique for correction of rigid forearm deformities in children. This technique is applicable to a variety of etiologies, including congenital radioulnar synostosis, brachial plexus birth palsy, cerebral palsy, and posttraumatic rotational deformities. Because this technique relies on the integrity and particular strength of the pediatric periosteum, it is clearly only applicable to younger children and cannot be used for rotational deformities of the forearm in older children or adults. The technique proposed does not require internal fixation with pins or a plate and screw configuration, which eliminates the need for future hardware removal or the possibility of implant failure. However, there is a possibility that the patient will need to return to the operating room for adjustment of the position under anesthesia within the first 10 to 14 days. The authors note that complications can include compartment syndrome as well as a less-than-ideal forearm position; however, they do not specifically discuss the possible loss of maintenance of the new position. This appears to be an excellent surgical option for pediatric patients with rigid forearm deformities, but it would be helpful to review the follow-up data on maintenance of forearm position for these children before adopting this technique into one's practice.

F. G. Fishman, MD

15 Shoulder: Instability

Treatment of Bankart Lesions in Traumatic Anterior Instability of the Shoulder: A Randomized Controlled Trial Comparing Arthroscopy and Open Techniques

Netto NA, Tamaoki MJS, Lenza M, et al (Universidade Federal de São Paulo—Escola Paulista de Medicina, Brazil)

Arthroscopy 28:900-908, 2012

Purpose.—The objective of this study was to compare the functional assessments of arthroscopy and open repair for treating Bankart lesion in traumatic anterior shoulder instability.

Methods.—Fifty adult patients, aged less than 40 years, with traumatic anterior shoulder instability and the presence of an isolated Bankart lesion confirmed by diagnostic arthroscopy were included in the study. They were randomly assigned to receive open or arthroscopic treatment of an isolated Bankart lesion. In all cases of both groups, the lesion was repaired with metallic suture anchors. The primary outcomes included the Disabilities of the Arm, Shoulder and Hand (DASH) questionnaire.

Results.—After a mean follow-up period of 37.5 months, 42 patients were evaluated. On the DASH scale, there was a statistically significant difference favorable to the patients treated with the arthroscopic technique, but without clinical relevance. There was no difference in the assessments by University of California, Los Angeles and Rowe scales. There was no statistically significant difference regarding complications and failures, as well as range of motion, for the 2 techniques.

Conclusions.—On the basis of this study, the open and arthroscopic techniques were effective in the treatment of traumatic anterior shoulder instability. The arthroscopic technique showed a lower index of functional limitation of the upper limb, as assessed by the DASH questionnaire; this, however, was not clinically relevant.

▶ This study compared patients with traumatic instability who were randomly assigned into open vs arthroscopic Bankart repair. It is one more of the many studies that show there is no difference in recurrence rates or outcomes between these 2 repair techniques.[1,2]

J. P. Braman, MD

References

1. Fabbriciani C, Milano G, Demontis A, Fadda S, Ziranu F, Mulas PD. Arthroscopic versus open treatment of Bankart lesion of the shoulder: a prospective randomized study. *Arthroscopy.* 2004;20:456-462.
2. Bottoni CR, Smith EL, Berkowitz MJ, Towle RB, Moore JH. Arthroscopic versus open shoulder stabilization for recurrent anterior instability: a prospective randomized clinical trial. *Am J Sports Med.* 2006;34:1730-1737.

A Comparison of Glenoid Morphology and Glenohumeral Range of Motion Between Professional Baseball Pitchers With and Without a History of SLAP Repair

Sweitzer BA, Thigpen CA, Shanley E, et al (Albert Einstein Med Ctr, Philadelphia, PA; Proaxis Therapy, Greenville, SC; et al)
Arthroscopy 28:1206-1213, 2012

Purpose.—We sought to examine the relation among glenoid morphology, glenohumeral range of motion (ROM), and history of shoulder injury in professional baseball pitchers.

Methods.—We studied 58 professional baseball pitchers. Internal rotation (IR) and external rotation (ER) ROM was measured at 90° of abduction. Horizontal adduction (HAdd) ROM was also measured. Glenoid superior inclination and glenoid retroversion (GRV) were then measured radiographically. Separate mixed-model analyses of variance were used to compare dependent measures between the dominant and nondominant shoulders of pitchers with or without a history of SLAP repair. Significant interaction effects were interpreted by use of a test for simple main effects ($\alpha = .05$).

Results.—GRV was significantly greater on the dominant side (8.7° ± 5.6°) versus nondominant side (5.5° ± 5.2°) ($P = .001$), whereas glenoid superior inclination was equivalent (99.5° ± 4.3° for dominant side v 99.2° ± 4.4° for nondominant side, $P = .853$). Post hoc analysis indicated that pitchers with a history of SLAP repair did not display an adaptive increase in dominant GRV compared with nondominant GRV ($P = .016$). There were no statistical differences between groups for ER ($P = .29$), IR ($P = .39$), or HAdd ($P = .39$). The dominant shoulder displayed greater ER (mean increase, 6.2° ± 12.2°) with a complementary decrease in IR (mean decrease, 5.8° ± 13.2°) and HAdd (mean decrease, 8.9° ± 13.7°) compared with the nondominant side.

Conclusions.—Our findings suggest that the development of increased GRV in the dominant shoulder of professional baseball pitchers may be a protective adaptive change not reflected in glenohumeral ROM measures.

Level of Evidence.—Level IV, therapeutic case series.

▶ The authors must be congratulated on introducing the new thought of glenoid morphology contribution toward a pitcher's shoulder. They showed increased glenoid retroversion in the pitching arm compared with the nonpitching arm.

Unfortunately, they failed to show a causal relationship, an association, or a risk ratio between injury and glenoid retroversion. This could be because of inadequate sample size or significant bias from other contributing anatomy. I feel the authors should have discussed the proximal humeral anatomy, including humeral retroversion. Inclusion of a repaired superior labrum anterior-posterior (SLAP) may play a role in affecting the range of motion and cannot be counted toward reduction in motion. This could have been because of surgery itself or poor rehabilitation. Hence, I would have liked to see the comparison with preoperative SLAP lesions. I agree with the authors that the study has significant limitations, and further research is the need of the hour.

R. A. Habbu, MS, MBBS

Bony Adaptation of the Proximal Humerus and Glenoid Correlate Within the Throwing Shoulder of Professional Baseball Pitchers
Wyland DJ, Pill SG, Shanley E, et al (Colorado Rockies Baseball Club spring training facility, Scottsdale, AZ)
Am J Sports Med 40:1858-1862, 2012

Background.—Elite throwing athletes have increased proximal humeral retrotorsion (HRT) and glenoid retroversion (GRV) in their throwing shoulders compared with their nonthrowing shoulders. These adaptive morphologic changes are thought to be independently protective against shoulder injury; however, their relationship to each other is poorly understood.

Purpose.—To determine if an association exists between HRT and GRV within the same shoulders of professional pitchers.

Study Design.—Cross-sectional study; Level of evidence, 3.

Methods.—The HRT and GRV measurements were determined using published techniques in asymptomatic bilateral shoulders of 32 professional pitchers (mean age, 23 years). Three measurements for each variable were averaged, and the reliability of the techniques was verified. The relationship between HRT and GRV within the same shoulders was determined with Pearson correlation coefficients. Paired t tests were used to compare HRT and GRV between the throwing and nonthrowing shoulder. Simple ratios were calculated between HRT and GRV.

Results.—Humeral retrotorsion and GRV were both significantly greater on the throwing side compared with the nonthrowing side (HRT: throwing $= 9.0° \pm 11.4°$ and nonthrowing $= 22.1° \pm 10.7°$, $P < .001$; GRV: throwing $= 8.6° \pm 6.0°$ and nonthrowing $= 4.9° \pm 4.8°$, $P = .001$). Within the same shoulders, there was a statistically significant positive association between HRT and GRV on the throwing side ($r = 0.43$, $P = .016$) but not on the nonthrowing side ($r = -0.13$, $P = .50$). The HRT:GRV ratio was 2.3:1 for throwing shoulders and 7:1 for nonthrowing shoulders.

Conclusion.—The concurrent increases in dominant shoulder HRT and GRV were observed as a 2:1 "throwers ratio." As this relationship was not observed on the nondominant shoulder, it suggests that bony adaptation of the proximal humerus and glenoid are coupled during skeletal development in the throwing shoulder. Longitudinal studies are needed to confirm this hypothesis.

▶ The authors of this report evaluated professional baseball pitchers' throwing shoulders for bony adaption of the glenohumeral joint. They used 2 newer techniques to determine humeral retrotorsion (HRT) and glenoid retroversion (GRV) between the throwing and nonthrowing shoulders. HRT was measured using an ultrasound scan and had been previously validated in adolescent baseball pitchers.[1] GRV was measured from scapular external landmarks (coracoid and posterior acromion) using a standard axillary radiograph, a technique developed for intraoperative use during total shoulder arthroplasty.[2] In the original report, the glenoid measurement technique was developed to provide an internal operative control to place the glenoid implant in the correct version.

The study verified differences in bony architecture on both the glenoid and humeral side of a pitcher's shoulder. However, there were no longitudinal data to support a cause-and-effect relationship between the throwing and the osseous changes. Additionally, the authors proposed the recognition of osseous changes in a ratio of 2.3:1 for the throwing shoulder. The accuracy of this ratio is applicable only when using this GRV measurement technique, which is not universally accepted as the standard method to measure GRV. Finally, the authors confirmed osseous architecture differences in a professional pitcher's shoulder, with little clinical applicability to the general population treated by an orthopedic surgeon.

C. J. Tuohy, MD

References

1. Whitely RJ, Ginn K, Nicholson L, Adams R. Indirect ultrasound measurement of humeral torsion in adolescent baseball players and non-athletic adults: reliability and significance. *J Sci Med Sport.* 2006;9:310-318.
2. Braunstein V, Korner M, Brunner U, Mutschler W, Biberthaler P, Wiedmann E. The fulcrum axis: a new method for determining glenoid version. *J Shoulder Elbow Surg.* 2008;17:819-824.

16 Shoulder: Arthroplasty

Unconstrained Shoulder Arthroplasty for Treatment of Proximal Humeral Nonunions
Duquin TR, Jacobson JA, Sanchez-Sotelo J, et al (Mayo Clinic, Rochester, MN)
J Bone Joint Surg Am 94:1610-1617, 2012

Background.—Unconstrained shoulder arthroplasty is one of several methods for treatment of proximal humeral fracture nonunions. The goal of this study was to define the results and complications of this procedure.

Methods.—From 1976 to 2007, sixty-seven patients underwent unconstrained shoulder arthroplasty for proximal humeral nonunion and were followed for more than two years. There were forty-nine women and eighteen men with a mean age of sixty-four years and a mean duration of follow-up of nine years (range, two to thirty years). The fracture type according to the Neer classification was two-part in thirty-six patients, three-part in sixteen, and four-part in fifteen. Hemiarthroplasty was performed in fifty-four patients and total shoulder arthroplasty was done in the remaining thirteen.

Results.—There were thirty-three excellent or satisfactory results according to the modified Neer rating. Tuberosity healing about the prosthesis occurred in thirty-five shoulders. The mean pain score improved from 8.3 preoperatively to 4.1 at the time of follow-up ($p < 0.001$). The average active shoulder elevation and external rotation improved from 46° and 26° to 104° and 50° ($p < 0.001$). Shoulders with anatomic or nearly anatomic healing of the tuberosities had greater active elevation at the time of final follow-up ($p = 0.02$). There were fourteen complications in twelve patients, with twelve reoperations including five revisions. Kaplan-Meier survivorship with revision as the end point was 97% (95% confidence interval [CI]: 94.3, 100) at one year and 93% (95% CI: 88.0, 99.2) at five, ten, and twenty years.

Conclusions.—Shoulder arthroplasty decreases pain and improves function in patients with a proximal humeral nonunion. However, the overall results are satisfactory in less than half of the patients. Tuberosity healing is inconsistent and influences the functional outcome.

▶ The authors present a study on the outcome of 67 patients that underwent unconstrained shoulder arthroplasty for proximal humerus nonunion. The authors do report significant improvement in motion as well as pain with shoulder arthroplasty. However, the investigators also note that more than half of the patients had an unsatisfactory outcome at a mean follow-up of 9 years. The primary reason for an unsatisfactory outcome was due to restriction in shoulder motion. The authors note that a nonunion of the tuberosities at the time of the most recent follow-up was associated with poor results as well as a rotator cuff tear being present at the time of surgery. This is one of the largest published series to date to evaluate unconstrained shoulder arthroplasty for the treatment of proximal humerus nonunions. In the future, this will serve as an important article to compare the outcome of reverse arthroplasty, which is becoming more frequently employed for the treatment of proximal humerus nonunions.

J. Sperling, MD, MBA

Secondary Rotator Cuff Dysfunction Following Total Shoulder Arthroplasty for Primary Glenohumeral Osteoarthritis: Results of a Multicenter Study with More Than Five Years of Follow-up
Young AA, Walch G, Pape G, et al (Sydney Shoulder Specialists, New South Wales, Australia; Centre Orthopédique Santy, Lyon, France; Univ of Heidelberg, Germany; et al)
J Bone Joint Surg Am 94:685-693, 2012

Background.—Secondary rotator cuff dysfunction is a recognized complication following shoulder arthroplasty. We hypothesized that the rate of secondary rotator cuff dysfunction would increase with follow-up and result in less satisfactory clinical and radiographic outcomes. Our aim was to investigate the rate of secondary rotator cuff dysfunction following shoulder arthroplasty for primary osteoarthritis and identify factors associated with the dysfunction.

Methods.—Between 1991 and 2003, in ten European centers, 704 total shoulder arthroplasties were performed for primary glenohumeral osteoarthritis. Complete radiographic and clinical follow-up of more than five years was available for 518 shoulders. The diagnosis of secondary rotator cuff dysfunction was made when moderate or severe superior subluxation of the prosthetic humeral head was present on radiographs. Multivariate logistic regression identified factors associated with the development of rotator cuff dysfunction. Kaplan-Meier survivorship analysis was performed, with the end point being secondary rotator cuff failure. Clinical outcome was assessed with use of the Constant score, a subjective assessment of the shoulder, and an evaluation of shoulder motion.

Results.—At an average of 103.6 months (range, sixty to 219 months) after shoulder arthroplasty, the rate of secondary rotator cuff dysfunction was 16.8%. Survivorship free of secondary cuff dysfunction was 100% at five years, 84% at ten years, and 45% at fifteen years. Duration of follow-up ($p < 0.0001$), implantation of the glenoid implant with superior tilt ($p < 0.001$), and fatty infiltration of the infraspinatus muscle ($p < 0.05$) were risk factors for the development of secondary cuff dysfunction. Patients with secondary rotator cuff dysfunction had significantly worse clinical outcomes (Constant score, subjective assessment, and range of motion; $p < 0.0001$) and radiographic results (radiolucent line score, radiographic loosening, glenoid component migration; $p < 0.0001$).

Conclusions.—In this study, rates of secondary rotator cuff dysfunction with moderate or severe superior subluxation of the prosthetic humeral head increased with the duration of follow-up and significantly influenced the clinical and radiographic outcome of total shoulder arthroplasty performed for primary glenohumeral osteoarthritis. Preoperative fatty infiltration of the infraspinatus muscle and implantation of the glenoid component with superior tilt were prognostic factors.

▶ The authors present an important study on the outcome of 704 total shoulder arthroplasties that were originally performed for primary osteoarthritis. Of that cohort, 518 shoulders had a minimum 5-year clinical and radiographic follow-up. The authors note that the presence of fatty infiltration of the infraspinatus muscle and implanting a glenoid component with superior tilt were associated with the development of secondary rotator cuff dysfunction. The authors also noted that patients with rotator cuff dysfunction had worse clinical outcomes compared with those without dysfunction. This study raises important risk factors for the potential development of rotator cuff dysfunction following shoulder arthroplasty. This study will also be an important benchmark to compare with future studies on the potential use of reverse arthroplasty in the setting of an intact rotator cuff.

J. Sperling, MD, MBA

Unconstrained Shoulder Arthroplasty for Treatment of Proximal Humeral Nonunions

Duquin TR, Jacobson JA, Sanchez-Sotelo J, et al (Mayo Clinic, Rochester, MN)
J Bone Joint Surg Am 94:1610-1617, 2012

Background.—Unconstrained shoulder arthroplasty is one of several methods for treatment of proximal humeral fracture nonunions. The goal of this study was to define the results and complications of this procedure.

Methods.—From 1976 to 2007, sixty-seven patients underwent unconstrained shoulder arthroplasty for proximal humeral nonunion and were followed for more than two years. There were forty-nine women and eighteen men with a mean age of sixty-four years and a mean duration of follow-up of nine years (range, two to thirty years). The fracture type according to the Neer classification was two-part in thirty-six patients, three-part in sixteen, and four-part in fifteen. Hemiarthroplasty was performed in fifty-four patients and total shoulder arthroplasty was done in the remaining thirteen.

Results.—There were thirty-three excellent or satisfactory results according to the modified Neer rating. Tuberosity healing about the prosthesis occurred in thirty-five shoulders. The mean pain score improved from 8.3 preoperatively to 4.1 at the time of follow-up ($p < 0.001$). The average active shoulder elevation and external rotation improved from 46° and 26° to 104° and 50° ($p < 0.001$). Shoulders with anatomic or nearly anatomic healing of the tuberosities had greater active elevation at the time of final follow-up ($p = 0.02$). There were fourteen complications in twelve patients, with twelve reoperations including five revisions. Kaplan-Meier survivorship with revision as the end point was 97% (95% confidence interval [CI]: 94.3, 100) at one year and 93% (95% CI: 88.0, 99.2) at five, ten, and twenty years.

Conclusions.—Shoulder arthroplasty decreases pain and improves function in patients with a proximal humeral nonunion. However, the overall results are satisfactory in less than half of the patients. Tuberosity healing is inconsistent and influences the functional outcome.

▶ The authors retrospectively reviewed the results of unconstrained shoulder arthroplasty for the treatment of proximal humeral nonunion. Thirty-three patients had excellent outcomes. Pain improved reliably, and active shoulder motion improved as well. Better results were seen with those patients who had better healing of the tuberosities. This study shows that unconstrained arthroplasty can yield reliable pain relief and improve function in expert hands.

J. P. Braman, MD

Prognostic Factors for Bacterial Cultures Positive for *Propionibacterium acnes* and Other Organisms in a Large Series of Revision Shoulder Arthroplasties Performed for Stiffness, Pain, or Loosening
Pottinger P, Butler-Wu S, Neradilek MB, et al (Univ of Washington Med Ctr, Seattle; The Mountain-Whisper-Light Statistics, Seattle, WA)
J Bone Joint Surg Am 94:2075-2083, 2012

Background.—*Propionibacterium acnes* has been grown on culture in half of the reported cases of chronic infection associated with shoulder arthroplasty. The presence of this organism can be overlooked because its subtle presentation may not suggest the need for culture or because, in contrast to many orthopaedic infections, multiple tissue samples and weeks of culture incubation are often necessary to recover this organism. Surgical decisions regarding implant revision and antibiotic therapy must be made before the results of intraoperative cultures are known. In the present study, we sought clinically relevant prognostic evidence that could help to guide treatment decisions.

Methods.—We statistically correlated preoperative and intraoperative observations on 193 shoulder arthroplasty revisions that were performed because of pain, loosening, or stiffness with the results of a *Propionibacterium acnes*-specific culture protocol. Regression models were used to identify factors predictive of a positive culture for *Propionibacterium acnes*.

Results.—One hundred and eight of the 193 revision arthroplasties were associated with positive cultures; 70% of the positive cultures demonstrated growth of *Propionibacterium acnes*. The rate of positive cultures per shoulder increased with the number of culture specimens obtained from each shoulder. Fifty-five percent of the positive cultures required observation for more than one week. Male sex, humeral osteolysis, and cloudy fluid were each associated with significant increases of ≥600% in the likelihood of obtaining a positive *Propionibacterium acnes* culture. Humeral loosening, glenoid wear, and membrane formation were associated with significant increases of >300% in the likelihood of obtaining a positive *Propionibacterium acnes* culture.

Conclusions.—Preoperative and intraoperative factors can be used to help to predict the risk of a positive culture for *Propionibacterium acnes*. This evidence is clinically relevant to decisions regarding prosthesis removal or retention and the need for immediate antibiotic therapy at the time of revision shoulder arthroplasty before the culture results become available.

Level of Evidence.—Prognostic Level II. See Instructions for Authors for a complete description of levels of evidence.

▶ In a retrospective review of 193 revision arthroplasties, the authors found that 108 had positive intraoperative cultures. Of those, 70% were positive for *Propionibacterium acnes* (P. acnes). Patients were more likely to have cultures that were positive if there were more cultures taken intraoperatively. Fifty-five percent of the cultures required more than 1 week to demonstrate growth. Male sex, humeral osteolysis, and cloudy fluid seen at revision were all associated with increased likelihood of *P. acnes* growth on culture. These data show that *P. acnes* is common in revision shoulder arthroplasty surgery and that it requires different detection algorithms than standard staphylococcal and streptococcal infections.

J. P. Braman, MD

Patterns of Loosening of Polyethylene Keeled Glenoid Components After Shoulder Arthroplasty for Primary Osteoarthritis: Results of a Multicenter Study with More Than Five Years of Follow-up

Walch G, Young AA, Boileau P, et al (Centre Orthopédique Santy, Lyon, France; Sydney Shoulder Specialists, New South Wales, Australia; Med Univ of Nice-Sophia Antipolis, France; et al)

J Bone Joint Surg Am 94:145-150, 2012

Background.—The aim of this study was to radiographically analyze the long-term glenoid migration patterns following total shoulder arthroplasty to better understand the factors responsible for loosening.

Methods.—Complete radiographic follow-up of more than five years was available for 518 total shoulder arthroplasties performed for primary glenohumeral osteoarthritis with use of an anatomically designed prosthesis with a cemented, all-polyethylene, keeled glenoid component. Radiographs were assessed for humeral head subluxation, periprosthetic radiolucent lines, and shifting of the position of the glenoid component. The type of migration of the glenoid was defined according to the direction of tilt, or as subsidence in the case of medial migration.

Results.—Definite radiographic evidence of glenoid loosening was observed in 166 shoulders (32%) and was characterized by radiolucency of ≥ 2 mm over the entire bone-cement interface in thirty shoulders and by a migration of the glenoid component (shift or subsidence) in 136 shoulders. Three predominant patterns of migration of the glenoid component were observed: superior tilting in fifty-two shoulders (10%), subsidence in forty-one shoulders (7.9%), and posterior tilting in thirty-three shoulders (6.4%). Superior tilting of the glenoid was associated with three risk factors: low positioning of the glenoid component, superior tilt of the glenoid component on the immediate postoperative coronal plane radiographs, and superior subluxation of the humeral head ($p < 0.05$ for all). Subsidence of the glenoid component was associated with the use of reaming to optimize the seating and positioning of the glenoid component ($p < 0.001$). Posterior tilting of the glenoid component was associated with preoperative posterior subluxation (i.e., a Walch type-B glenoid) and with excessive reaming ($p < 0.01$ for both).

Conclusions.—The three patterns of migration observed in this study underscore the potential importance of the supporting bone beneath the glenoid component. In some shoulders, use of a keel or pegs to provide fixation of a polyethylene component in the absence of good support from subchondral bone may not be sufficient to resist compressive and eccentric forces, resulting in loosening. Preserving subchondral bone may be important for long-term longevity of the glenoid component.

▶ This is an important study, with useful clinical information. What stood out for this reviewer was that these expert shoulder surgeons had 32% glenoid loosening in a large cohort of shoulder arthroplasties at an average of 8.6 years out. Average age at implantation was 68 years. Possible loosening was noted in another 15%;

therefore, less than 53% of shoulders had no definite evidence of loosening at less than 9 years.

This study supports the concept of balancing the shoulder but also preserving the subchondral bone. These 2 issues can, at times, be at odds, although new-generation components, which are built up, can balance the shoulder while preserving the subchondral bone.

The glenoid continues to be the weak link in total shoulder arthroplasty. This study only serves to emphasize that we must continue to work to do better for our patients and provide better longevity for their arthroplasties.

R. F. Papandrea, MD

Secondary Rotator Cuff Dysfunction Following Total Shoulder Arthroplasty for Primary Glenohumeral Osteoarthritis: Results of a Multicenter Study With More Than Five Years of Follow-up
Young AA, Walch G, Pape G, et al (Centre Orthopédique Santy, Lyon, France)
J Bone Joint Surg Am 94:685-693, 2012

Background.—Secondary rotator cuff dysfunction is a recognized complication following shoulder arthroplasty. We hypothesized that the rate of secondary rotator cuff dysfunction would increase with follow-up and result in less satisfactory clinical and radiographic outcomes. Our aim was to investigate the rate of secondary rotator cuff dysfunction following shoulder arthroplasty for primary osteoarthritis and identify factors associated with the dysfunction.

Methods.—Between 1991 and 2003, in ten European centers, 704 total shoulder arthroplasties were performed for primary glenohumeral osteoarthritis. Complete radiographic and clinical follow-up of more than five years was available for 518 shoulders. The diagnosis of secondary rotator cuff dysfunction was made when moderate or severe superior subluxation of the prosthetic humeral head was present on radiographs. Multivariate logistic regression identified factors associated with the development of rotator cuff dysfunction. Kaplan-Meier survivorship analysis was performed, with the end point being secondary rotator cuff failure. Clinical outcome was assessed with use of the Constant score, a subjective assessment of the shoulder, and an evaluation of shoulder motion.

Results.—At an average of 103.6 months (range, sixty to 219 months) after shoulder arthroplasty, the rate of secondary rotator cuff dysfunction was 16.8%. Survivorship free of secondary cuff dysfunction was 100% at five years, 84% at ten years, and 45% at fifteen years. Duration of follow-up ($p < 0.0001$), implantation of the glenoid implant with superior tilt ($p < 0.001$), and fatty infiltration of the infraspinatus muscle ($p < 0.05$) were risk factors for the development of secondary cuff dysfunction. Patients with secondary rotator cuff dysfunction had significantly worse clinical outcomes (Constant score, subjective assessment, and range of motion; $p < 0.0001$) and radiographic results (radiolucent line score, radiographic loosening, glenoid component migration; $p < 0.0001$).

Conclusions.—In this study, rates of secondary rotator cuff dysfunction with moderate or severe superior subluxation of the prosthetic humeral head increased with the duration of follow-up and significantly influenced the clinical and radiographic outcome of total shoulder arthroplasty performed for primary glenohumeral osteoarthritis. Preoperative fatty infiltration of the infraspinatus muscle and implantation of the glenoid component with superior tilt were prognostic factors.

▶ The authors of this study provided important long-term results regarding total shoulder arthroplasty with serial radiographs and Constant scores of 518 patients (average follow-up of about 9 years) related to secondary rotator cuff dysfunction and its effects on implant survivorship. Interestingly, the authors found no difference in revision surgery between groups with glenoid loosening/rotator cuff dysfunction and those with an intact rotator cuff. Furthermore, they concluded age was not a risk factor for rotator cuff dysfunction. These observations should be tempered because of the underpowered nature of the study.

Another limitation was the determination of rotator cuff dysfunction by radiographs that showed moderate or severe superior subluxation. Another limitation was the universal applicability of the conclusions, because all study patients received cemented keel glenoids. Previous studies have found increased lucency around these implants compared with peg glenoids over time. The use of this glenoid type and rotator cuff dysfunction may have led to the need for revision of the glenoid components.

Most importantly in this study, the survivorship curves for normal rotator cuff function showed a slow decline to 45% at 15 years. This result should be another important long-term topic for the surgeon to discuss with patients before surgery. Because magnetic resonance imaging is not routinely obtained for preoperative planning for shoulder arthroplasty, and when obtained often shows significant tendonosis in primary osteoarthritis patients, future studies are needed to look at the relationship between preoperative rotator cuff tendonosis and postoperative rotator cuff function after total shoulder arthroplasty.

C. J. Tuohy, MD

The Rationale for an Arthroscopic Approach to Shoulder Stabilization
Tjoumakaris FP, Bradley JP (Thomas Jefferson Univ, Philadelphia, PA; Univ of Pittsburgh Med Ctr, PA)
Arthroscopy 27:1422-1433, 2011

The gold standard of treatment for glenohumeral instability has traditionally been viewed as open shoulder stabilization. With the increased awareness of complex instability patterns and the ability to preoperatively detect concomitant pathology with advanced imaging modalities, an evidence-based shift to an all-arthroscopic approach to shoulder stabilization surgery is occurring. Current data suggest that patients who meet eligibility criteria for arthroscopic stabilization (those without significant bony lesions or significant deformity) can expect equivalent rates of recurrence, better functional outcomes, and less morbidity. Modern arthroscopic techniques using suture anchors and capsular plication have resulted in a significant improvement over previous reports in the orthopaedic literature. An argument is put forth on the benefits of an all-arthroscopic approach to shoulder stabilization in athletes and nonathletes alike based on a review of the current orthopaedic literature comparing the evolved arthroscopic technique with more traditional open methods.

▶ The authors make a convincing argument that the preferred approach to shoulder instability should be arthroscopic. They support their argument by summarizing current literature, with care to examine the type of arthroscopic repair reviewed. Older studies, with inferior results, were done with now outdated techniques.

Improved understanding of the pathology and newer implants, devices, and approaches has made arthroscopic techniques equal to or superior to open techniques. More recent literature outlined in this report supports this. Preservation of the subscapularis and better outcomes for motion are rationale presented to make an argument for an arthroscopic approach to treat instability.

Some pathology, most notably humeral avulsion of the glenohumeral ligament lesions, are such that arthroscopic intervention has not evolved to the point to make this the preferred technique. Much like other pathologies in shoulder instability, this will most likely change as our techniques advance.

R. F. Papandrea, MD

Long-Term Results After SLAP Repair: A 5-Year Follow-up Study of 107 Patients With Comparison of Patients Aged Over and Under 40 Years

Schrøder CP, Skare Ø, Gjengedal E, et al (Lovisenberg Deaconal Hosp, Oslo, Norway; et al)
Arthroscopy 28:1601-1607, 2012

Purpose.—The aims of this prospective cohort study were to assess the long-term results after isolated superior labral repair and to determine whether the results were associated with age.

Methods.—One hundred seven patients underwent repair of isolated SLAP tears. There were 36 women and 71 men with a mean age of 43.8 years (range, 20 to 68 years). Mean follow-up was 5.3 years (range, 4 to 8 years). Of the patients, 62 (57.9%) were aged 40 years or older. Follow-up examinations were performed by an independent examiner; 102 patients (95.3%) had a 5-year follow-up.

Results.—The Rowe score improved from 62.8 (SD, 11.4) preoperatively to 92.1 (SD, 13.5) at follow-up (*P* < .001). Satisfaction was rated excellent/ good for 90 patients (88%) at 5 years. There was no significant difference in the results for patients aged 40 years or older and those aged under 40 years. Difficulty with postoperative stiffness and pain was reported by 14 patients (13.1%).

Conclusions.—Our results suggest that long-term outcomes after isolated labral repair for SLAP lesions are good and independent of age. Postoperative stiffness was registered in 13.1% of the patients.
Level of Evidence.—Level IV, therapeutic case series.

▶ The authors of this prospective study evaluated a cohort of patients that underwent isolated arthroscopic superior labrum anterior-posterior (SLAP) repairs. They provided an average 5-year follow-up to determine if there was a difference in outcome between patients under and over the age of 40. The patient groups were compared using a modified Rowe score and evaluated for complications, including stiffness and reoperations. The authors concluded that age was not an independent risk factor for outcomes or complications after a SLAP repair.

Limitations of the study were the use of the modified Rowe score, an instrument for assessing instability. Specifically, the instrument attributes 15 points to instability and another 10 points to a qualitative strength scale. Consequently, this instrument may not have provided adequate sensitivity to detect a difference in the groups. The authors had even published a previous study that raised these concerns about this instrument, stating, "Moreover, the agreement and reliability for the different domains and validity of the Rowe score are not acceptable. Results using the 1988 version of the Rowe score should be critically interpreted."[1]

One other concern in this study was the lack of a power analysis. This weakened the authors' conclusions that there was no statistical difference in the postoperative stiffness group (average age, 47.9) compared with those without stiffness. Closer analysis of the stiffness group found 11 of those 14 patients were older than 40 years. Consequently, the conclusion that long-term outcomes from SLAP repairs were independent of age should be taken with caution in light of these methodologic flaws. Further studies randomly assigning these age cohorts to biceps tenodesis or nonoperative treatment with a more appropriate shoulder outcome instrument are needed for stronger validated conclusions.

C. J. Tuohy, MD

Reference

1. Skare Ø, Schrøder CP, Mowinckel P, Reikerås O, Brox JI. Reliability, agreement and validity of the 1988 version of the Rowe score. *J Shoulder Elbow Surg.* 2011;20:1041-1049.

Arthroscopic Management of Selective Loss of External Rotation After Surgical Stabilization of Traumatic Anterior Glenohumeral Instability: Arthroscopic Restoration of Anterior Transverse Sliding Procedure
Ando A, Sugaya H, Takahashi N, et al (Funabashi Orthopaedic Sports Medicine Ctr, Japan; et al)
Arthroscopy 28:749-753, 2012

Purpose.—The purpose of this study was to clarify the effectiveness of an arthroscopic procedure for restoration of anterior transverse sliding (RATS) mechanism of the subscapularis tendon in patients with loss of external rotation after surgical stabilization of anterior glenohumeral instability.

Methods.—Seven patients who underwent an arthroscopic RATS procedure for loss of external rotation after surgical stabilization of anterior glenohumeral instability were retrospectively reviewed. There were 4 male and 3 female patients with a mean age of 30.7 years. The original procedure was arthroscopic Bankart repair and rotator interval closure in 5 patients, open Bankart repair in 1, and an open Bristow procedure in 1. The arthroscopic RATS procedure was performed as follows: (1) removal of the fibrous tissue in the rotator interval; (2) release of the subscapularis tendon from the glenoid neck; and (3) incision of the superior part of the inferior glenohumeral ligament until a sufficient external rotation angle was obtained without causing anterior instability. We evaluated the mean forward flexion and external and internal rotation angles, Constant score, and University of California, Los Angeles score before the arthroscopic RATS procedure and at final follow-up (mean, 24 months).

Results.—The mean forward flexion and external and internal rotation angles improved from $162.1° \pm 9.5°$ to $171.4° \pm 3.8°$ ($P < .05$), from $2.9° \pm 4.9°$ to $47.9° \pm 9.1°$ ($P < .005$), and from T10 to T8 ($P < .05$), respectively. The mean Constant and University of California, Los Angeles scores improved from 81.0 ± 13.6 points to 95.1 ± 4.0 points and from 24.0 ± 3.7 points to 33.9 ± 2.0 points, respectively ($P < .005$).

Conclusions.—The arthroscopic RATS mechanism procedure is a useful treatment option with minimum morbidity in patients with loss of external rotation after surgical stabilization of traumatic anterior glenohumeral instability.

Level of Evidence.—Level IV, therapeutic case series.

▶ This study reviewed the results of arthroscopic surgery to improve external rotation loss after anterior stabilization procedures. The authors provided a simple and concise arthroscopic surgical technique to improve external rotation less than 10°. The technique involved debridement of the rotator interval and, most importantly, freeing the subscapularis from the anterior glenoid neck. If these interventions resulted in less than 20° of external rotation, then a partial superior release of the inferior glenohumeral ligament was performed, gaining 25° to 40° and resulting in full motion at the final outcome.

The authors' technique demonstrated statistically significant improvement in range of motion, Constant scores, and University of California Los Angeles scores. The main strength of this study was that there were no complications and, most specifically, no recurrence of instability. Limitations of the study included its retrospective nature, the use of nonvalidated outcome instruments, and the use of instruments not designed to evaluate shoulder instability. Although the study has limited applicability (hence making a randomized study most likely unfeasible), the authors' simple arthroscopic technique provides another reasonable method to manage external rotation loss in the postsurgical instability patient.

C. J. Tuohy, MD

Return to High-Level Throwing After Combination Infraspinatus Repair, SLAP Repair, and Release of Glenohumeral Internal Rotation Deficit

Van Kleunen JP, Tucker SA, Field LD, et al (Mississippi Sports Medicine and Orthopaedic Ctr, Jackson; Tulane Univ School of Medicine, New Orleans, LA)
Am J Sports Med 40:2536-2541, 2012

Background.—The overhead-throwing athlete is a unique patient, requiring an elite, precise functional ability. Superior labral tears are quite common, and the percentage of athletes who return to play after superior labrum anterior-posterior (SLAP) repair has been variable. A tear of the infraspinatus caused by either internal impingement or tension overload may compromise this return.

Hypothesis.—The rate of return to a level of play similar to or greater than the preinjury level after repair of combined SLAP and infraspinatus injuries will be lower than in previous reports of SLAP repair alone.

Study Design.—Case series; Level of evidence, 4.

Methods.—In the current study, we examined a series of overhead-throwing athletes with diagnoses of both a SLAP tear and a significant (>50%) tear of the infraspinatus tendon who underwent surgical repair of both injuries. We identified 17 high-level baseball players younger than 25 years who underwent simultaneous arthroscopic repairs of a SLAP tear with a standard suture anchor technique and of an infraspinatus tear with either a free polydioxanone (PDS) suture or suture anchor between 2005 and 2008. The postoperative records of all patients were reviewed to determine their ability to return to play and their postoperative level of performance. All patients were then contacted to determine their Kerlan-Jobe Orthopaedic Clinic Overhead Athlete Shoulder and Elbow score and their current sport participation level.

Results.—All 17 patients in the series attempted to return to their prior sport after completion of postoperative rehabilitation. Only 6 patients (35%) were able to return to the same or a superior preinjury level of performance. Five of the remaining 11 patients returned to play at a lower level, either playing the same position or else forced to switch to another position of play because of a decline in throwing velocity. Six patients were unable to return to play. No complications or reoperations occurred in any of the patients following surgery.

Conclusion.—A significant (>50%) tear of the infraspinatus in combination with glenohumeral internal rotation deficit (GIRD) and SLAP tears in the throwing athlete results in a guarded prognosis in return to play at the same level. While the rates of return to play in overhead-throwing athletes with an isolated SLAP tear have historically been encouraging, the prognosis for an athlete with both a SLAP and infraspinatus tear is more guarded. These patients are not likely to return to their preinjury level of play.

▶ The authors present a retrospective (level 4 evidence) study evaluating results of return to sports of overhead athletes treated with a combination of superior labrum anterior-posterior (SLAP) repair and infraspinatus repair. They describe their technique and indications for the 2 procedures. Previous studies have found that presence of cuff injury along with a SLAP lesion is a negative prognostic factor for return to play. This study supports the conclusion. It reports poor outcomes after a combination of SLAP and cuff repairs. This allows me and other surgeons to counsel the athlete about the expected outcomes with regard to his or her return to play so that he or she can make an informed decision. However, I fail to understand the role of limited capsular release. If it was done for improving the range of motion, the authors should discuss any improvement in range at follow-up. If it was done to prevent any cuff impingement, the authors did not find any significant difference. Hence, in my practice, I would hesitate to add this to the procedures. Another problem with the study was its small sample size (n=17). Owing to this, any conclusion may not reach statistical significance. The authors do talk about statistical trend with *P* value just over .05. However, this should be used with caution because it still does not reach significance. Nevertheless, cuff repair and SLAP repair should be done provided there are adequate indications. Cuff anchors provide better hold and pullout strength than other types of repairs. Hence, it is surprising that the anchor subset of athletes had poorer scores than those with suture repairs. A reason for this could be the type of cuff tear and quality of tissue. Additionally, the sample size makes this variable difficult to compare. I agree with the authors that return to play for these athletes is poor, especially in baseball pitchers and at competitive levels.

R. A. Habbu, MS, MBBS

17 Shoulder: Rotator Cuff

American Academy of Orthopaedic Surgeons Clinical Practice Guideline on: Optimizing the Management of Rotator Cuff Problems
Pedowitz RA, Yamaguchi K, Ahmad CS, et al
J Bone Joint Surg Am 94:163-167, 2012

Background.—The American Academy of Orthopaedic Surgeons (AAOS) has published a clinical practice guideline on optimizing the management of rotator cuff problems. The recommendations were summarized, with the caveat that treatment decisions be based on consideration of all circumstances presented by the patient and mutual communication between patient and physician.

Treatment Options.—Surgery is not recommended for asymptomatic, full-thickness rotator cuffs, but rotator cuff repair is an option for patients with chronic, symptomatic full-thickness tears. Patients who have rotator cuff-n-related symptoms but no full-thickness tear can be initially treated nonoperatively using exercise and/or nonsteroidal anti-inflammatory drugs (NSAIDs). For patients with rotator cuff tears who are managed nonoperatively, no clear guidelines support or refute the benefits of exercise programs (supervised or not), subacromial injections, NSAIDS, activity modification, ice, heat, iontophoresis, massage, transcutaneous electrical nerve stimulation (TENS), pulsed electromagnetic field (PEMF), or phonophoresis (ultrasound). For patients with symptoms but no full-thickness tear, no clear guidelines were developed for the use of subacromial corticosteroid injection, PEMF, iontophoresis, phonophoresis, TENS, ice, heat, massage, or activity modification. Acute traumatic rotator cuff tears may benefit from early surgical repair. Perioperatively, neither subacromial corticosteroid injections nor NSAIDs show a clear benefit for patients having rotator cuff surgery. Less favorable outcomes after rotator cuff surgery may be related to increasing age, magnetic resonance imaging (MRI), tear characteristics, and worker's compensation status. Factors that confound outcomes include the presence of diabetes, comorbidities, smoking, previous shoulder infection, and cervical disease.

Surgical Recommendations.—For patients having surgery, routine acromioplasty is not required. Options include partial rotator cuff repair, debridement, or muscle transfers for irreparable rotator cuff tears. Surgeons may attempt tendon-to-bone healing of the cuff in all patients. The preferential use of suture anchors rather than bone tunnels to repair full-thickness rotator cuff tears is not clearly supported. Although it is suggested that surgeons not use a non-crosslinked, porcine small intestine submucosal xenograft patch for rotator cuff tears, no clear evidence indicates which specific technique should be used and whether soft tissue allografts or other xenografts should be used.

Postoperative Considerations.—The opinion of the work group is that local cold therapy is beneficial for pain relief after surgery. However, whether an abduction pillow is better than a standard sling or how long shoulder immobilization without range of motion exercises should be observed remain to be determined. Similarly, decisions regarding the length of time before initiating active resistance exercises, the use of home-based versus facility-based rehabilitation efforts, and the use of an indwelling subacromial infusion catheter for pain management are lacking clear supportive evidence.

▶ Any attempt to summarize orthopedic treatment utilizing only scientific data will have voids for consensus or support. This article is yet another summary developed by the American Academy of Orthopaedic Surgeons for clinical practice guidelines. Like the other efforts, it leaves something to be desired, but that is not the fault of the group of experts; rather, it highlights the lack of sound scientific data for much of how surgeons treat even common pathologies like rotator cuff problems.

The findings of the group will not be a surprise to those who keep abreast of the current literature but may be enlightening to those who follow the lead of industry or only a select few leaders. Currently, the approach to rotator cuff repair (open vs arthroscopic) as well as the method of fixation (bone tunnel vs anchors) has no superior method. Because of this, no recommendation for repair type/method is made by the group.

One of the few moderate recommendations made was against routine acromioplasty at the time of rotator cuff repair. There is current literature to support their conclusion but not longer follow-up to support this practice. On the contrary, there is a study reported by Björnsson[1] that found lower rates of rotator cuff tearing (when compared with historical controls) after acromioplasty.

Instead of focusing on what is missing in such a report, it is more useful to understand the current status of evidence for what is done in clinical practice as well as give a framework for more sound recommendations once better data are available.

R. F. Papandrea, MD

Reference

1. Björnsson H, Norlin R, Knutsson A, Adolfsson L. Fewer rotator cuff tears fifteen years after arthroscopic subacromial decompression. *J Shoulder Elbow Surg.* 2010;19:111-115.

Long-Term Longitudinal Follow-up of Mini-Open Rotator Cuff Repair

Bell S, Lim Y-J, Coghlan J (Melbourne Shoulder and Elbow Centre, Brighton, Victoria, Australia; General Hosp, Singapore; Monash Univ, Brighton, Victoria, Australia)

J Bone Joint Surg Am 95:151-157, 2013

Background.—Rotator cuff tears are a common clinical problem, and few long-term studies concerning the outcomes of rotator cuff repairs have been performed. The purpose of this study was to report the fifteen-year outcomes of arthroscopic subacromial decompression with mini-open rotator cuff repair.

Methods.—The study included seventy-nine patients who had undergone arthroscopic subacromial decompression with mini-open rotator cuff repair from 1993 to 1996. Outcomes were reviewed in 1997, 2002, and 2010. At the final review, forty-nine patients (forty-nine shoulders) were available or were suitable for evaluation. There were eight large tears, forty medium tears, and one small tear. The patients were assessed with the University of California, Los Angeles (UCLA) score at each evaluation. The mean age of the patients at the time of follow-up was 70.1 years, and the mean follow-up period was 15.6 years.

Results.—At the time of final follow-up, the outcome was good or excellent in thirty-four patients (69%), fair in seven, and poor in eight. Three patients required a reoperation. Between the two and fifteen-year evaluations, twenty-nine patients (59%) had maintained their good or excellent result; the overall raw scores had deteriorated for fifteen patients (31%), and they had improved for twenty-four (49%). Forty-one patients (84%) were satisfied with the final outcome of the shoulder surgery.

Conclusions.—This study shows that arthroscopic subacromial decompression with mini-open rotator cuff repair can provide a lasting, durable, and satisfactory outcome for a large proportion of patients fifteen years after surgery. Patient satisfaction at the final evaluation did not necessarily correspond with a good or an excellent UCLA score.

▶ This study evaluated the long-term effect of performing mini-open rotator cuff repair. The authors compared the clinical outcomes at 15 years with those in the same cohort of patients at 2 years postoperatively. Nearly half of the patients were better at 15 years than they were at 2 years. Additionally, there was a high rate of satisfaction with the procedure (84% patient satisfaction). This study shows that arthroscopic subacromial decompression with associated mini-open rotator cuff repair provides durable improvement to patient outcomes and long-lasting patient satisfaction to 15 years.

J. P. Braman, MD

The Cost-Effectiveness of Single-Row Compared with Double-Row Arthroscopic Rotator Cuff Repair

Genuario JW, Donegan RP, Hamman D, et al (The Steadman Hawkins Clinic-Denver, Lone Tree, CO; Dartmouth-Hitchcock Med Ctr, Lebanon, NH; et al)

J Bone Joint Surg Am 94:1369-1377, 2012

Background.—Interest in double-row techniques for arthroscopic rotator cuff repair has increased over the last several years, presumably because of a combination of literature demonstrating superior biomechanical characteristics and recent improvements in instrumentation and technique. As a result of the increasing focus on value-based health-care delivery, orthopaedic surgeons must understand the cost implications of this practice. The purpose of this study was to examine the cost-effectiveness of double-row arthroscopic rotator cuff repair compared with traditional single-row repair.

Methods.—A decision-analytic model was constructed to assess the cost-effectiveness of double-row arthroscopic rotator cuff repair compared with single-row repair on the basis of the cost per quality-adjusted life year gained. Two cohorts of patients (one with a tear of <3 cm and the other with a tear of ≥3 cm) were evaluated. Probabilities for retear and persistent symptoms, health utilities for the particular health states, and the direct costs for rotator cuff repair were derived from the orthopaedic literature and institutional data.

Results.—The incremental cost-effectiveness ratio for double-row compared with single-row arthroscopic rotator cuff repair was $571,500 for rotator cuff tears of <3 cm and $460,200 for rotator cuff tears of ≥3 cm. The rate of radiographic or symptomatic retear alone did not influence cost-effectiveness results. If the increase in the cost of double-row repair was less than $287 for small or moderate tears and less than $352 for large or massive tears compared with the cost of single-row repair, then double-row repair would represent a cost-effective surgical alternative.

Conclusions.—On the basis of currently available data, double-row rotator cuff repair is not cost-effective for any size rotator cuff tears. However, variability in the values for costs and probability of retear can have a profound effect on the results of the model and may create an environment in which double-row repair becomes the more cost-effective surgical option. The identification of the threshold values in this study may help surgeons to determine the most cost-effective treatment.

▶ Using a decision-analytic model that varied different parameters, the authors sought to determine the cost utility of double-row rotator cuff repair compared with single-row rotator cuff repair. In their model, retear rates had little implication on the cost utility, likely because patients who have retear often do not seek additional care. Consequently, the authors state that only in the setting in which additional costs can be limited to less than $287 for small tears and $352 for larger tears would double-row repair be considered cost effective. In the current environment, there is little chance that the increased operating room time as well as the increased implant cost would fall under this benchmark. Addressing increasing implant costs and other operating room expenses represents one opportunity for improving the cost utility of this type of intervention.

J. P. Braman, MD

Use of Platelet-Leukocyte Membrane in Arthroscopic Repair of Large Rotator Cuff Tears: A Prospective Randomized Study

Gumina S, Campagna V, Ferrazza G, et al (Univ of Rome "Sapienza," Italy; Military Hosp "Celio," Rome, Italy; et al)
J Bone Joint Surg Am 94.1345-1352, 2012

Background —Arthroscopic rotator cuff repair generally provides satisfactory results including decreased shoulder pain and improved shoulder motion. Unfortunately, imaging studies demonstrate that the retear rate associated with the available arthroscopic techniques may be high. The purpose of this study was to evaluate the clinical and magnetic resonance imaging (MRI) results of arthroscopic rotator cuff repair with and without the use of platelet-leukocyte membrane in patients with a large posterosuperior rotator cuff tear.

Methods.—Eighty consecutive patients with a large full-thickness posterosuperior rotator cuff tear were enrolled. All tears were repaired using an arthroscopic single-row technique. Patients were randomized to treatment either with or without a platelet-leukocyte membrane inserted between the rotator cuff tendon and its footprint. In patients treated with this membrane, one membrane was utilized for each suture anchor. The primary outcomes were the difference between the preoperative and postoperative Constant scores and the repair integrity assessed by MRI according to the Sugaya classification. The secondary outcome was the difference between the preoperative and postoperative Simple Shoulder Test (SST) scores.

Results.—The only significant differences between the two groups involved the patient age and the preoperative and postoperative Constant scores; the differences in the Constant score were due to differences in the shoulder pain subscore. At a mean of thirteen months of follow-up, rotator cuff retears were observed only in the group of patients in whom the membrane had not been used, and a thin but intact tendon was observed more frequently in this group as well. The use of the membrane was associated with significantly better repair integrity ($p = 0.04$).

Conclusions.—The use of the platelet-leukocyte membrane in the treatment of rotator cuff tears improved repair integrity compared with repair without membrane. However, the improvement in repair integrity was not associated with greater improvement in the functional outcome. In fact, the Constant scores of the two groups would have been similar if the shoulder pain component (which had differed preoperatively) had been excluded.

▶ The authors conducted a randomized trial of 39 patients with and 37 patients without a platelet-leukocyte membrane inserted between the cuff and the greater tuberosity at the time of arthroscopic rotator cuff repair. They analyzed outcomes and retear rates. They had a 0% retear rate in their treated group after single-row repair and had an 8% (3 of 37) retear rate in the untreated group. The outcomes were better in the membrane group as measured by the constant score. The retear rates in this study are very low compared with historical controls, and if the results could be duplicated, it would represent an advance in the treatment of rotator cuff tears arthroscopically.

J. P. Braman, MD

Optimizing Pressurized Contact Area in Rotator Cuff Repair: The Diamondback Repair

Burkhart SS, Denard PJ, Obopilwe E, et al (Univ of Texas Health Science Ctr at San Antonio; The San Antonio Orthopaedic Group, TX; Univ of Connecticut, Farmington)
Arthroscopy 28:188-195, 2012

Purpose.—The purpose of this study was to compare tendon-bone footprint contact area over time under physiologic loads for 4 different rotator cuff repair techniques: single row (SR), triangle double row (DR), chainlink double row (CL), and diamondback double row (DBK).

Methods.—A supraspinatus tear was created in 28 human cadavers. Tears were fixed with 1 of 4 constructs: SR, DR, CL, or DBK. Immediate post-repair measurements of pressurized contact area were taken in neutral rotation and 0° of abduction. After a static tensile load, pressurized contact area was observed over a 160-minute period after repair. Cyclic loading was then performed.

Results.—The DBK repair had the highest pressurized contact area initially, as well as the highest pressurized contact area and lowest percentage decrease in pressurized contact area after 160 minutes of testing. The DBK repair had significantly larger initial pressurized contact than CL ($P = .003$) and SR ($P = .004$) but not DR ($P = .06$). The DBK technique was the only technique that produced a pressurized contact area that exceeded the native footprint both at initial repair ($P = .01$) and after 160 minutes of testing ($P = .01$). DBK had a significantly larger mean pressurized contact area than all the repairs after 160 minutes of testing ($P = .01$). DBK had a significantly larger post–cyclic loading pressurized contact area than CL ($P = .01$) and SR ($P = .004$) but not DR ($P = .07$).

Conclusions.—This study showed that a diamondback repair (a modification of the transosseous repair) can significantly increase the rotator cuff pressurized contact area in comparison with other standard rotator cuff repair constructs when there is sufficient tendon mobility to perform a double-row repair without excessive tension on the repair site.

Clinical Relevance.—The persistent pressurized contact area of a DBK repair may be desirable to enhance healing potential when there is sufficient tendon mobility to perform a double-row repair, particularly for large or massive rotator cuff tears where it is important to optimize footprint area and contact to encourage biologic healing.

▶ This comparison study of arthroscopic rotator repair technique is well done in that it not only measures initial contact area of repair but also looks at the sustained area over time at rest and after cycling.

Four techniques were used to repair an isolated full-thickness supraspinatus tear: A single-row repair with 3 anchors, a double-row repair with 3 anchors, a chain-link repair with 4 anchors, and a diamondback repair with 5 anchors. The diamond back repair outperformed at time zero as well as at 160 minutes and after cyclic loading. It was the only repair to exceed native footprint contact area at all 3 times.

This study suffers from the same issues as most pure biomechanical studies in that it is uncertain as to how much is enough (contact pressure in this study) and if there could be unexpected consequences of exceeding normal. Likewise, there is always the concern that excessive pressure or suture could alter the microcirculation during healing.

Lastly, comparison of cost of the methods, especially if bone tunnel repairs were included, would be helpful in today's economic environment. This reviewer wonders if any medical system could support the use of 5 anchors to repair every isolated supraspinatus tear.

R. F. Papandrea, MD

Retraction of Supraspinatus Muscle and Tendon as Predictors of Success of Rotator Cuff Repair
Meyer DC, Wieser K, Farshad M, et al (Balgrist Univ Hosp, Zurich, Switzerland)
Am J Sports Med 40:2242-2247, 2012

Background.—The structural failure rate of rotator cuff repair can exceed 50%. Important predictors for repair failure are preoperative fatty muscle infiltration and myotendinous retraction.

Purpose.—To quantitatively assess the prognostic value of preoperative retraction of both the supraspinatus muscle and tendon for the outcome of supraspinatus repair.

Study Design.—Cohort study; Level of evidence, 3.

Methods.—In 33 shoulders with complete supraspinatus tendon ruptures subjected to arthroscopic repair, magnetic resonance imaging (MRI) scans taken preoperatively and after a mean follow-up of 24 months were studied. The exact position of the lateral extension of the supraspinatus muscle and of the tendon end was evaluated and correlated with the preoperative stage of fatty infiltration (Goutallier) and the failure rate of tendon repair.

Results.—The mean lengthening of the muscle and tendon end was −3 mm and 4 mm in the failed repairs (n = 19) and 14 mm and 8 mm in the successful repairs (n = 14). If the supraspinatus had preoperative Goutallier stages 2 to 3 and a tendon length of less than 15 mm, the failure rate was 92%, but if the tendon length was greater than 15 mm, the failure rate was only 33%. With Goutallier stages 0 to 1, the corresponding failure rates were 57% and 25%, respectively.

Conclusion.—Rotator cuff repair lengthens the tendon, even if the repair fails. The possibility to lengthen the myotendinous unit is related to the preoperative length of the tendon. The combination of Goutallier grading and preoperative tendon length appears to be a more powerful predictor for the reparability of a tendon tear than Goutallier grading alone.

▶ The authors compared preoperative and postoperative lengths of rotator cuff muscle and tendon in magnetic resonance imaging (MRI) of patients who had undergone arthroscopic cuff repair. They found shorter tendon length and higher Goutallier grading to be predictors of failure of repair. Previous literature has shown similar findings with musculotendinous retraction considered the main factor behind failures. I feel that the authors of this study have done a great job of describing the MRI sequences in detail along with the planes for measurements. I would be eager to use these sequences and look for the specific measurements before having a discussion with the patient. I think this allows for standardization and comparison of variables across the board in the future. However, I am concerned about the intraobserver and interobserver variability that might affect these small and specific measurements. The need for good MRI images cannot be understated. This study included personnel who were familiar with the measurements. I would assume the MRI technicians in this center were also familiar with the process. Problems may arise if the personnel are not routinely doing the sequences and measurements. Hence, I would hesitate to base my conclusions on every film measured. Nevertheless, this study is one of a kind, although a longer follow-up in all cases would have contributed toward the strength of the study. It shows the importance of a good MRI assessment before cuff repair.

R. A. Habbu, MS, MBBS

A Multicenter Randomized Controlled Trial Comparing Single-Row with Double-Row Fixation in Arthroscopic Rotator Cuff Repair
Lapner PLC, Sabri E, Rakhra K, et al (The Ottawa Hosp, Ontario, Canada; Ottawa Hosp Res Inst, Ontario, Canada; et al)
J Bone Joint Surg Am 94:1249-1257, 2012

Background.—Controversy exists regarding the optimal technique for arthroscopic rotator cuff repair. The purpose of this multicenter, randomized, double-blind controlled study was to compare the functional outcomes and healing rates after use of single-row and double-row suture techniques for repair of the rotator cuff.

Methods.—Ninety patients undergoing arthroscopic rotator cuff repair were randomized to receive either a single-row or a double-row repair. The primary objective was to compare the Western Ontario rotator cuff index (WORC) score at twenty-four months. Secondary objectives included comparison of the Constant and American Shoulder and Elbow Surgeons (ASES) scores and strength between groups. Anatomical outcomes were assessed with magnetic resonance imaging (MRI) or ultrasonography to determine the postoperative healing rates.

Results.—Baseline demographic data including age ($p = 0.29$), sex ($p = 0.68$), affected side ($p = 0.39$), and rotator cuff tear size ($p = 0.28$) did not differ between groups. The WORC score did not differ significantly between groups at any time point ($p = 0.48$ at baseline, $p = 0.089$ at three months, $p = 0.52$ at six months, $p = 0.83$ at twelve months, and $p = 0.60$ at twenty-four months). The WORC score at each postoperative time point was significantly better than the baseline value. The Constant score, ASES score, and strength did not differ significantly between groups at any time point. Logistic regression analysis demonstrated that a smaller initial tear size and double-row fixation were associated with higher healing rates.

Conclusions.—No significant differences in functional or quality-of-life outcomes were identified between single-row and double-row fixation techniques. A smaller initial tear size and a double-row fixation technique were associated with higher healing rates as assessed with ultrasonography or MRI.

Level of Evidence.—Therapeutic Level I. See Instructions for Authors for a complete description of levels of evidence.

▶ Arthroscopic double-row repairs of the rotator cuff tendon are becoming more common despite a minimal amount of evidence regarding its clinical superiority. This multicenter, randomized trial compares the functional outcome of arthroscopic single- and double-row repairs of the rotator cuff.

The benefits of this study are its large numbers (90 patients total), its randomized design, and its use of primary and secondary outcome measures. No differences were noted by the authors for Western Ontario Rotator Cuff Index, Constant and American Shoulder and Elbow Surgeons scores, or manual strength testing. Magnetic resonance imaging or ultrasound analysis did suggest that double-row repairs had a higher level of healing than single-row repairs; however, this difference was not duplicated in the functional scores assessed. It is worth noting that a priori power analysis suggests that an adequate sample size was used for this study.

This study is not without limitations. It reports on data generated during the first 2 years following surgery. Certainly, longer term follow-up will be necessary. Further, a variety of single- and double-row techniques have become popular. Each of these techniques was not tested in this study and may be associated with better or worse functional outcomes.

This study does suggest that improved function is noted with both single- and double-row rotator cuff repairs at 2 years. Although no functional differences were noted between the 2 techniques in this study, a higher rate of healing was seen in the double-row cohort, suggesting future research is necessary on this topic.

J. Macalena, MD

Rotator Cuff Tear Arthropathy: Evaluation, Diagnosis, and Treatment: AAOS Exhibit Selection
Nam D, Maak TG, Raphael BS, et al (Hosp for Special Surgery, NY)
J Bone Joint Surg Am 94:e34.1-e34.11, 2012

Rotator cuff tear arthropathy encompasses a broad spectrum of pathology, but it involves at least three critical features: rotator cuff insufficiency, degenerative changes of the glenohumeral joint, and superior migration of the humeral head. Although many patients possess altered biomechanics of the glenohumeral joint secondary to rotator cuff pathology, not all patients develop rotator cuff tear arthropathy, and thus the exact etiology of rotator cuff tear arthropathy remains unclear. The objectives of this manuscript are to (1) review the biomechanical properties of the rotator cuff and the glenohumeral joint, (2) discuss the proposed causes of rotator cuff tear arthropathy, (3) provide a brief review of the historically used surgical options to treat rotator cuff tear arthropathy, and (4) present a treatment algorithm for rotator cuff tear arthropathy based on a patient's clinical presentation, functional goals, and anatomic integrity (Figs 2A and 7).

▶ The authors offer a thorough review of the evaluation, diagnosis, and treatment of rotator cuff arthropathy. This was presented as an American Academy of

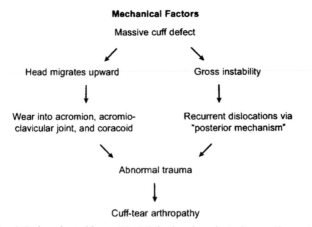

FIGURE 2.—A. Both mechanical factors (**Fig. 2-A**) has been hypothesized to contribute to joint destruction in rotator cuff tear arthropathy. (Reproduced, with modification, from: Neer CS 2nd, Craig EV, Fukuda H. Cuff-tear arthropathy. *J Bone Joint Surg Am.* 1983;65:1232-44.) (Reprinted from Nam D, Maak TG, Raphael BS, et al. Rotator cuff tear arthropathy: evaluation, diagnosis, and treatment: AAOS exhibit selection. *J Bone Joint Surg Am.* 2012;94:e34.1-e34.11, with permission from the Journal of Bone and Joint Surgery, Incorporated. http://jbjs.org/.)

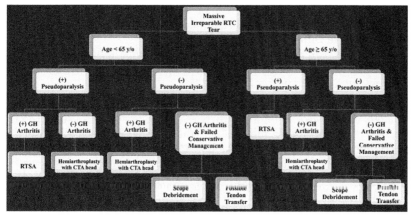

FIGURE 7.—A proposed treatment algorithm for the management of a massive, irreparable rotator cuff tear. RTC = rotator cuff, GH = glenohumeral, RTSA = reverse total shoulder arthroplasty, and CTA = cuff tear arthropathy. (Reprinted from Nam D, Maak TG, Raphael BS, et al. Rotator cuff tear arthropathy: evaluation, diagnosis, and treatment: AAOS exhibit selection. *J Bone Joint Surg Am.* 2012;94:e34.1-e34.11, with permission from the Journal of Bone and Joint Surgery, Incorporated. http://jbjs.org/.)

Orthopedic Surgeons exhibit selection. Coined by Charles Neer in 1983, rotator cuff arthropathy encompasses a multitude of changes. However, it always includes rotator cuff insufficiency, superior migration of the humeral head, and degeneration of the glenohumeral joint. In Fig 2A, the authors highlight a series of mechanical and nutritional factors that occur with the ultimate endpoint of rotator cuff arthropathy. The authors concede that it is unclear why only a portion of patients with longstanding massive rotator cuff tears go on to end-stage rotator cuff arthropathy.

The diagnosis of rotator cuff arthropathy is made clinically and confirmed radiographically. Visual inspection for atrophy of the rotator cuff muscles is frequently present. Decreased motion profile, both actively and passively, as well as decreased strength, can manifest clinically as a positive hornblower's sign. The radiographic changes of rotator cuff arthropathy include acetabularization of the acromion, loss of the acromial humeral distance, and glenohumeral joint space narrowing.

In Fig 7, the authors propose a treatment algorithm for massive irreparable rotator cuff tears. Patient age, presence of pseudoparalysis, and presence of glenohumeral arthritis provide decision points in this algorithm with available surgical options spanning from arthroscopic debridement, tendon transfer, hemiarthroplasty, and reverse total shoulder arthroplasty.

This excellent review of rotator cuff arthropathy provides a well-rounded and critical evaluation of the diagnosis and treatment of this difficult clinical problem.

J. Macalena, MD

Injection of the Subacromial Bursa in Patients With Rotator Cuff Syndrome: A Prospective, Randomized Study Comparing the Effectiveness of Different Routes

Marder RA, Kim SH, Labson JD, et al (Univ of California-Davis Health System, Sacramento)

J Bone Joint Surg Am 94:1442-1447, 2012

Background.—Rotator cuff syndrome is often treated with subacromial injection of corticosteroid and local anesthetic. It has not been established if the common injection routes of the bursa are equally accurate.

Methods.—We conducted a prospective clinical trial involving seventy-five shoulders in seventy-five patients who were randomly assigned to receive a subacromial injection through an anterior, lateral, or posterior route with respect to the acromion. An experienced physician performed the injections, which contained radiopaque contrast medium, corticosteroid, and local anesthetic. After the injection, a musculoskeletal radiologist, blinded to the injection route, interpreted all of the radiographs.

Results.—The rate of accuracy varied with the route of injection, with a rate of 56% for the posterior route, 84% for the anterior route, and 92% for the lateral route ($p = 0.006$; chi-square test). The accuracy of injection through the posterior route was significantly lower than that through either the anterior or the lateral route ($p < 0.05$ for both comparisons; Poisson regression). In addition, the accuracy of injection was significantly lower in females than in males ($p < 0.006$; chisquare test). Among males, no differences between the routes were noted (with accuracy rates of 89% for the posterior route, 92% for the anterior route, and 93% for the lateral route). Among females, however, the accuracy of injection was lower for the posterior route than for either the anterior or the lateral route (with accuracy rates of 38% for the posterior route, 77% for the anterior route, and 91% for the lateral route) ($p < 0.05$).

Conclusions.—The anterior and lateral routes of subacromial bursal injection were more accurate than the posterior route. The accuracy of subacromial bursal injection was significantly different between males and females, mainly because of a lower accuracy of bursal injection with use of the posterior route in females. The present study suggests that the posterior route is the least accurate method for injection of the subacromial bursa in females (Fig 2).

▶ The effectiveness of 3 commonly used techniques for injections to the subacromial bursa were studied in this report. The authors found a high degree of success with both anterior and laterally based techniques of approaching the subacromial space (84% and 92%, respectively). The posterior approach was considerably less reliable with only 56% of subjects injected successfully from this technique.

A lower success rate, as seen in Fig 2, was noted in women undergoing injection via a posterior route (38%) and anterior route (77%) when compared with the lateral route (92%).

% of accurate injections

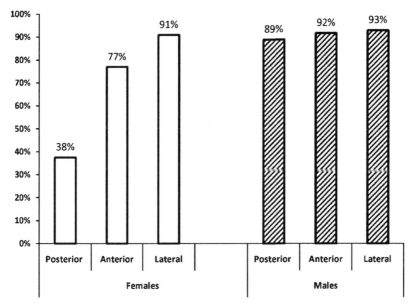

FIGURE 2.—Bar graph showing the rate of accuracy of subacromial injection in males and females according to the route of injection. (Reprinted from Marder RA, Kim SH, Labson JD, et al. Injection of the subacromial bursa in patients with rotator cuff syndrome: a prospective, randomized study comparing the effectiveness of different routes. *J Bone Joint Surg Am*. 2012;94:1442-1447, with permission from the Journal of Bone and Joint Surgery, Incorporated. http://jbjs.org/.)

The different techniques were not affected by body mass index.

The authors suggest using either a lateral or anterior technique when performing subacromial injections, as these techniques have a higher rate of success entering the subacromial bursa.

J. Macalena, MD

18 Rehabilitation

Mobilization with movement and kinesiotaping compared with a supervised exercise program for painful shoulder: results of a clinical trial
Djordjevic OC, Vukicevic D, Katunac L, et al (Clinic for Rehabilitation "Dr Miroslav Zotovic," Belgrade, Serbia)
J Manipulative Physiol Ther 35:454-463, 2012

Objective.—The purpose of this study was to compare the efficacy of Mobilization with Movement (MWM) and kinesiotaping (KT) techniques with a supervised exercise program in participants with patients with shoulder pain.

Methods.—Twenty subjects with shoulder pain were included if subjects were diagnosed by the referring physician with either rotator cuff lesion with impingement syndrome or impingement shoulder syndrome. Participants were randomly assigned to 1 of 2 groups after clinical and radiologic assessment: group 1 was treated with MWM and KT techniques, whereas group 2 was treated with a supervised exercise program. The main outcome measures were active pain-free shoulder abduction and flexion tested on days 0, 5, and 10.

Results.—Improvement in active pain-free shoulder range of motion was significantly higher in the group treated with MWM and KT. Repeated-measures analysis of variance indicated significant effects of treatment, time, and treatment × time interaction.

Conclusion.—This study suggests that MWM and KT may be an effective and useful treatment in range of motion augmentation of subjects with rotator cuff lesion and impingement syndrome or impingement shoulder syndrome.

▶ This is the first study to look at the effect on shoulder pain of both a mobilization technique and textile taping compared with traditional supervised shoulder exercises. The aim of this double-blind, randomized cross-sectional study was to investigate whether the joint mobilization technique named *Mobilization with Movement* (MWM) combined with kinesio taping (KT) is better in the initial phase of rehabilitation than supervised exercise for shoulder pain related to the diagnoses of rotator cuff (RTC) lesion or impingement syndrome. Twenty participants, 34 to 79 years of age, with shoulder pain or painful arc of shoulder range of motion (ROM) were included. Exclusion criteria were shoulder girdle fractures, dislocations, shoulder surgery in the previous 12 months, diagnosis of adhesive capsulitis, full-thickness RTC tear, cervicobrachial pain secondary to cervical spine pathology, neuromuscular disorders of the upper extremities, or use of corticosteroid or nonsteroidal anti-inflammatory therapy within 10 days before the first ROM measures.

Each participant went through the full battery of shoulder clinical assessments and radiologic and ultrasound imaging. Group 1 received MWM and KT treatment, whereas group 2 received supervised exercises, described as the "usual initial exercise program for shoulder impingement syndrome." Both groups received 10 sessions of therapy, 24 hours between each therapy session. Outcomes were pain-free ROM of active shoulder abduction and flexion, measured at days 0, 5, and 10. All subjects completed the study. There were no significant differences between the groups in age, sex, duration of shoulder pain, or of the pain present in the dominant or nondominant arm, or of radiologic or ultrasound imaging of the shoulder pathology. There was no significant difference between the groups in ROM at day 0. Using repeated-measures analysis of variance, a significant treatment × time effect was found for both ROM of abduction and flexion; the effect of treatment between the groups and the effect of time within subjects was found to be significant. Both groups showed ROM improvement; however, there was a greater effect in group 1, and this effect occurred quicker in this group than that of the supervised exercise group.

This short-term study was limited by the lack of a second experimental group that received only KT. However, this randomized, controlled trial found significant effects in pain-free shoulder ROM within 10 days, which helps to establish a positive effect of the combination of both these therapeutic effects. The limitation is the lack of long-term follow-up, but the study still gives the basis for further clinical research into this realm of MWM and taping for the painful shoulder.

V. H. O'Brien, OTD, OTR/L, CHT

Validation of the Brief International Classification of Functioning, Disability, and Health (ICF) Core Set for Hand Conditions

Kus S, Oberhauser C, Cieza A (Ludwig-Maximilians-Univ, Munich, Germany)
J Hand Ther 25:274-287, 2012

Study Design.—Cross-sectional multi-centre study.

Introduction.—The ICF Core Sets for Hand Conditions (HC) have been developed to describe functioning of patients with HC.

Purpose of the Study.—To study the content validity of the Brief ICF Core Set for HC.

Methods.—Patients with HC were interviewed using the Comprehensive ICF Core Set for HC. ICF categories that best explained variation in patients' general health were identified using multiple regression methods.

Results.—Overall, 12 of the 23 ICF categories of the Brief ICF Core Set could be validated. Our analyzes further revealed that the categories "b134 Sleep functions", "s830 Structure of nails", "e225 Climate" as well as categories referring to "e4 Attitudes" also deserve consideration when assessing functioning in patients with HC.

Assessment	ICF Qualifier				
Body functions, Body structures, Activities and Participation	0	1	2	3	4
b152 Emotional functions					
b265 Touch function					
b280 Sensation of pain					
b710 Mobility of joint functions					
b730 Muscle power functions					
s720 Structure of shoulder region					
s730 Structure of upper extremity					
d230 Carrying out daily routine					
d440 Fine hand use					
d445 Hand and arm use					
d7 Interpersonal interactions and relationships					
d840 - d859 Work and employment					

FIGURE 2.—Extract of a categorical profile using the Brief ICF Core Set for hand condition and the ICF qualifier (0 = no impairment/restriction or 0–4%; 1 = mild impairment/restriction or 5–24%; 2 = moderate impairment/restriction or 25–49%; 3 = severe impairment/restriction or 50–95%, and 4 = complete impairment/restriction or 96–100%). ICF = International Classification of Functioning, Disability, and Health. (Reprinted from Journal of Hand Therapy. Kus S, Oberhauser C, Cieza A. Validation of the brief international classification of functioning, disability, and health (ICF) core set for hand conditions. *J Hand Ther.* 2012;25:274-287, Copyright 2012, with permission from the American Society of Hand Therapists.)

Conclusions.—Clinicians are encouraged to complement the Brief ICF Core Set for HC by adding sleep functions, structure of nails, climate and attitudes, especially when following patients over time.

Level of Evidence.—Level 3 (Fig 2, Table 3).

▶ To fully grasp the relevance of this reported research, one must have a basic understanding of the International Classification of Functioning, Disability and Health (ICF), which was developed by the World Health Organization in 2001. The ICF classifies health and disability in a way that determines function of the individual. It provides a framework for measuring disability along with providing a common language for interdisciplinary teams of health care practitioners to communicate patient needs and the effectiveness of treatments. The ICF core sets have been developed to allow the ICF to be used in clinical practice, including core sets for hand conditions (HC). There are 2 core sets for HC: the Comprehensive ICF Core Set, which consists of 117 categories, and the Brief ICF Core Set for HC (BCS-HC). These core sets take into account impairments in body functions and body structures as well as psychological aspects, difficulties with activities of daily living, and environmental factors (Fig 2).

The ICF has the potential to become an international standard in providing a profile that would then guide the planning, implementation, outcomes, and reporting of health care interventions. Therefore, the ICF core sets, and in this study the BCS-HC, must be validated for content. The authors completed a cross-sectional multicenter study that included 260 patients. All patients were interviewed using the ICF Core Set for HC along with the Disabilities of the Arm, Shoulder, and Hand Questionnaire, the EuroQol, and the visual analog scale. The full 117 core set categories were reduced to 110 because 7 of the categories had a consistent prevalence of problems including high and low frequency when used in the interview. A BCS-HC category was validated if the category remained in 1 of the final sets of the 110 ICF categories that were analyzed. Of

TABLE 3.—ICF Categories of the Brief ICF Core Set for HCs ($n = 23$) along with the Respective Final Set Categories That Validated 12 Categories of the BCS-HC

The 23 Brief ICF Core Set Categories		Final Set Categories Validating the BCS-HC	
ICF Code	Title	ICF Code	Title
Body functions			
b152	**Emotional functions**	b152	Emotional functions
b265	Touch function		
b270	Sensory functions related to temperature and other stimuli		
b280	Sensation of pain		
b710	Mobility of joint functions		
b715	Stability of joint functions		
b730	Power of muscles functions		
b760	**Control of voluntary movement functions**	b760	Control of voluntary movement functions
b810	Protective functions of the skin		
Body structures			
s120	Spinal cord and related structures		
s720	Structure of shoulder region		
s730	**Structure of upper extremity**	s7300	Structure of upper arm
		s7301	Structure of forearm
		s7302*	Structure of the hand
Activities and participation			
d230	**Carrying out daily routine**	d230	Carrying out daily routine
d430	Lifting and carrying objects		
d440	**Fine hand use**	d4408	Fine hand use, other specified —pinch grip
d445	**Hand and arm use**	d4450	Pulling
d5	**Self-care**	d520	Caring for body parts
d6	**Domestic life**	d620	Acquisition of goods and services
d7	Interpersonal interactions and relationships		
d840–d859	**Work and employment**	d840–d859	Work and employment
Environmental factors			
e1	**Products and technology**	e115	Products and technology for personal use in daily living
		e135	Products and technology for employment
		e140	Products and technology for culture, recreation, and sport
		e150	Design, construction, and building products, and technology of buildings for public use
		e155	Design, construction, and building products, and technology of buildings for private use
e3	**Support and relationships**	e310*	Immediate family
		e325	Acquaintances, peers, colleagues, neighbors, and community members
		e330	People in positions of authority
		e335	People in subordinate positions
		e345	Strangers
		e355*	Health professionals
		e360	Other professionals

(Continued)

TABLE 3.—(*Continued*)

The 23 Brief ICF Core Set Categories		Final Set Categories Validating the BCS-HC	
ICF Code	Title	ICF Code	Title
e5	Services, systems, and policies	e525	Housing services, systems, and policies
		e540	Transportation services, systems, and policies
		e550	Legal services, systems, and policies
		e575	General social support services, systems, and policies
		e580	Health services, systems, and policies
		e585	Education and training services, systems, and policies

ICF = International Classification of Functioning, Disability, and Health; HC = hand condition.
Note: The 12 BCS-HC categories that have been validated by our analyses are printed in bold.
*These categories were not part of the analyses, however, were considered as essential because of prevalence of ≥90% among the study population.

the 23 ICF categories that form the BCS-HC, 12 could be validated by this research, confirming the overall content validity of the BCS-HC (Table 3). The researchers conclude that in clinical practice the health practitioner should highly consider the BCS-HC as a basic tool for classifying function in the hand-injured population. They also suggest that categories including sleep functions, structure of nails, climate, and attitudes be included when evaluating functional levels, as these assist in determining the patient's overall health.

The authors clearly state the limitations of this study because the research was conducted solely in Germany, with a large proportion of those studied having severely injured hands and with patients in various states of health. They propose ongoing research analysis in other countries and in different settings. Because the ICF is not yet widely used in the United States, this important research may not seem as relevant to the hand therapist practicing in the US. However, change is always on the horizon, and should the US begin using the ICF more frequently, hand therapists everywhere should be aware of the BCS-HC and its validity.

S. J. Clark, OTR/L, CHT

19 Miscellaneous

Steroid Injection Versus NSAID Injection for Trigger Finger: A Comparative Study of Early Outcomes
Shakeel H, Ahmad TS (Univ of Malaya, Kuala Lumpur, Malaysia)
J Hand Surg 37A:1319-1323, 2012

Purpose.—Stenosing tenosynovitis of the flexor tendon sheath of the digits of the hand results from a discrepancy between the diameter of the flexor tendon and its sheath at the A1 pulley. The treatment options for trigger digits include oral nonsteroidal anti-inflammatory drugs (NSAIDs) and local NSAID applications, splintage, steroid injection, and percutaneous and open release of the A1 pulley. Injectable NSAID is used intramuscularly and locally in other sites. The hypothesis is that an injectable NSAID is as effective as the traditionally used steroid injection in the treatment of trigger digit, based on Quinnell grading, and that the treatment works as well in patients with diabetes as in those without diabetes.

Methods.—In this prospective, randomized, double-blinded controlled study for trigger digits, we injected diclofenac sodium locally in one group (NSAID group) and triamcinolone acetonide in another (corticosteroid group). A total of 100 patients (50 patients in each group) were followed up and assessed 3 weeks and 3 months after the injection.

Results.—At the end of the follow-up, 35 patients (70%) in the corticosteroid group and 28 patients (53%) in the NSAID group had complete symptomatic resolution. There was no difference between the response of patients with and without diabetes. There was no significant difference found in Quinnell score between treatments at 3 months, although at 3 weeks, the patients who received steroid had significantly better Quinnell scores.

Conclusions.—We concluded that, although steroids gave quicker relief, NSAID injections are equally effective at 3 months in the treatment of trigger digits. We were unable to detect a statistically significant difference in the response of patients with and without diabetes to either treatment.

▶ The purpose of this study is comparison of efficacy of injection of a nonsteroidal anti-inflammatory drug (NSAID) (diclofenac sodium) with that of a steroid (triamcinolone acetonide) into the flexor tendon sheath for treatment of stenosing tenosynovitis. The strengths of the study include its prospective, randomized, double-blinded, controlled design and its high follow-up rate (100%).

The weaknesses of this study include small cohorts, a short-term follow-up, and insufficient statistical analysis. The 3-month follow-up is too short to evaluate the efficacy of the steroid injection for trigger finger. A long-term follow-up might have elicited significant differences in Quinnell scoring grades between the NSAID and steroid groups. Significant differences might not have been found between the 2 groups because of the small cohorts. The authors should have performed a power analysis when no significant difference was found in the statistical analysis. They should have considered seriously the difference of the recurrent rates of snapping fingers between the groups (NSAID group 18%, steroid group 2%).

R. Kakinoki, MD

Is Antibiotic Prophylaxis Necessary in Elective Soft Tissue Hand Surgery?
Tosti R, Fowler J, Dwyer J, et al (Temple Univ School of Medicine, Philadelphia, PA; et al)
Orthopedics 35:e829-e833, 2012

Antibiotic prophylaxis for clean soft tissue hand surgery is not yet defined. Current literature focuses on overall orthopedic procedures, traumatic hand surgery, and carpal tunnel release. However, a paucity of data exists regarding the role of antibiotic prophylaxis in a broader variety of soft tissue hand procedures. The goal of the current study was to evaluate the rates of surgical site infection following elective soft tissue hand surgery with respect to administration of prophylactic antibiotics.

A multicenter, retrospective review was performed on 600 consecutive elective soft tissue hand procedures. Procedures with concomitant implant or incomplete records were excluded. Antibiotic delivery was given at the discretion of the attending surgeon. Patient comorbidities were recorded. Outcomes were measured by the presence of deep or superficial infections within 30 days postoperatively. The 4 most common procedures were carpal tunnel release, trigger finger release, mass excision, and first dorsal compartment release. The overall infection rate was 0.66%. All infections were considered superficial, and none required surgical management. In patients who received antibiotic prophylaxis (n = 212), the infection rate was 0.47%. In those who did not receive prophylaxis (n = 388), the infection rate was 0.77%. These differences were not statistically significant ($P = 1.00$) (Table 4).

▶ This is a retrospective study showing no statistically significant difference ($P = 1.00$) in infection rates when preoperative antibiotics were given for straightforward soft tissue procedures. Diabetes, sex, and smoking status were not shown to be predictors of surgical site infections. If this were a prospective study, a power analysis to indicate the number of patients necessary to determine a difference would have been essential as the infection rate in this study and others is extremely low.

Although this is not a randomized clinical trial, it does provide additional evidence that antibiotic prophylaxis is not necessary for elective, soft tissue

TABLE 4.—Infection Rates by Procedure

Procedure	No. (%) Superficial Infection	Deep Infection
Carpal tunnel release (n = 300)	3 (1.00)	0
Trigger finger release (n = 173)	1 (0.58)	0
DeQuervain release (n = 44)	0	0
Mass excision (n = 81)	0	0
Total (N = 600)	4 (0.66)	0

procedures in the hand and distal forearm. The authors have nicely broken this down into infection rates by procedure as described in Table 4.

W. C. Hammert, DDS, MD

A National Survey of Program Director Opinions of Core Competencies and Structure of Hand Surgery Fellowship Training

Sears ED, Larson BP, Chung KC (Univ of Michigan Health System, Ann Arbor)
J Hand Surg 37A:1971-1977.e7, 2012

Purpose.—We assessed hand surgery program directors' opinions of essential components of hand surgery training and potential changes in the structure of hand surgery programs.

Methods.—We recruited all 74 program directors of Accreditation Council of Graduate Medical Education—accredited hand surgery fellowship programs to participate. We designed a web based survey to assess program directors' support for changes in the structure of training programs and to assess opinions of components that are essential for graduates to be proficient. Respondents were asked to rate 9 general areas of practice, 97 knowledge topics, and 172 procedures. Each component was considered essential if 50% or more of respondents thought that graduates must be fully knowledgeable of the topic and be able to perform the procedure at the end of training.

Results.—The response rate was 84% (n = 62). A minority of program directors (n = 15; 24%) supported creation of additional pathways for hand surgery training, and nearly three-quarters (n = 46; 74%) preferred a fellowship model to an integrated residency model. Most program directors (n = 40; 65%) thought that a 1-year fellowship was sufficient to train a competent hand surgeon. Wrist, distal radius/ulna, forearm, and peripheral nerve conditions were rated as essential areas of practice. Of the detailed components, 76 of 97 knowledge topics and 98 of 172 procedures were rated as essential. Only 48% respondents (n = 30) rated microsurgery as it relates to free tissue transfer as essential. However, small and large vessel laceration repairs were rated as essential by 92% (n = 57) and 77% (n = 48) of respondents, respectively.

Conclusions.—This study found resistance to prolonging the length of fellowship training and introduction of an integrated residency pathway. To train all hand surgeons in essential components of hand surgery, programs must individually evaluate exposure provided and find innovative ways to augment training when necessary.

Clinical Relevance.—Studies of curriculum content in hand surgery affect the future scope of hand surgery practice and highlight areas in need of reform and enhancement.

▶ Hand surgery training has been a topic of significant interest; consideration has been given to extending the period of training or establishing a subspecialty residency to replace the current fellowship system. This study surveyed the 2011-year program directors for their opinions on a longer period of training and on the essential topics of hand surgery training. A sizable majority (84%) of current fellowship directors responded. Nearly three-quarters prefer a fellowship model to a residency model, and 65% felt a 1-year program is sufficient. This study also investigated whether fellowship directors feel individual areas of practice and procedures are essential for hand training. There is a high degree of consensus about the necessity of experience in many topics and procedures. Topics and procedures proximal to the forearm, not surprisingly, were usually not rated as essential. This study asserts that the movement to replace the current 1-year fellowship program is not supported by most hand fellowship directors. It also provides fellowship directors an opportunity to review their program content and contrast it with the topics and procedures their peers feel are essential.

P. E. Blazar, MD

The Influence of Job Satisfaction, Burnout, Pain, and Worker's Compensation Status on Disability After Finger Injuries

Kadzielski JJ, Bot AGJ, Ring D (Massachusetts General Hosp, Boston)
J Hand Surg 37A:1812-1819, 2012

Purpose.—Motivation, job satisfaction, burnout, and secondary gain are factors that can influence return to work and disability after orthopedic injuries. The current study evaluated the separate effects of job satisfaction, burnout, and secondary gain on arm-specific disability after a finger injury.

Methods.—Ninety-three employed patients with finger injuries were enrolled in this prospective study, and 51 completed the follow-up. Burnout (measured with Shirom-Melamed's Burnout Measure), job satisfaction (measured with the Job Descriptive Index questionnaire), and demographics were assessed at the initial visit. After 6 months, arm-specific disability was measured with the Disabilities of the Arm, Shoulder, and Hand (DASH) questionnaire, and general health status was measured with the Short Form-36 (SF-36) survey, mental component summary (MCS) and physical component summary (PCS).

Results.—In the 51 patients with complete follow-up, the mean DASH score was 12, the mean SF-36 PCS was 48, the mean SF-36 MCS was 49, and the mean pain rating was 2.1. In multivariable analysis, pain and worker's compensation status explained 52% of the variability in DASH scores (pain alone accounted for 49%); pain accounted for 14% of the variability in SF-36 PCS scores; and worker's compensation accounted for 11% of the variation in the SF-36 MCS scores.

Conclusions.—The majority of variation in the SF-36 PCS and MCS scores remained unaccounted for by the models, but pain and worker's compensation were more important than job burnout or job satisfaction. Pain and worker's compensation were also significant predictors of the DASH.

Clinical Relevance.—Worker's compensation and pain were more important than job satisfaction and burnout in explaining variations in arm-specific disability in patients with finger injuries.

▶ This interesting level II study by Ring et al evaluated the influence of job satisfaction, burnout, pain, and workers' compensation status on disability after various finger injuries. Although 93 patients were initially enrolled in the study and completed the initial surveys, only 51 completed the follow-up surveys at 6 months. Work-related injuries occurred in 28 of 51 individuals, with a wide variety of injuries ranging from a skin laceration to an amputation. Of the 51 patients, 34 required no surgery, whereas 17 required 1 or more procedures. Four different rating scales were employed to evaluate job satisfaction (Job Description Index), burnout (Shirom-Melamed Burnout Measure), arm-specific disability (Disabilities of the Arm, Shoulder, and Hand [DASH]), and general health status (Short Form-36). Complex statistical analysis was then performed The most significant findings demonstrated a correlation between DASH scores with pain and workers' compensation status. Burnout and job satisfaction did not correlate with pain or arm-specific disability. The authors are to be commended for attempting to apply science to these psychosocial issues. My experience echoes that of the authors: After injuries sustained at work, workers' compensation patients have a higher perceived pain level than non-workers' compensation patients, and return-to-work issues remain problematic, particularly with those in litigation.

D. Zelouf, MD

Enchondromas of the Hand: Factors Affecting Recurrence, Healing, Motion, and Malignant Transformation
Sassoon AA, Fitz-Gibbon PD, Harmsen WS, et al (Mayo Clinic, Rochester, MN)
J Hand Surg 37A:1229-1234, 2012

Purpose.—Enchondromas represent the most common primary bone tumor in the hand. Despite their frequency, a standardized treatment protocol is lacking. This study examines the outcome of surgically treated enchondromas of the hand with regard to tumor location, graft choice, and presence or absence of fracture.

Methods.—We retrospectively reviewed 102 enchondromas in 80 patients, identified between 1991 and 2008, with a mean clinical follow-up of 38 months. We assessed the effects of age, tumor location, and graft choice on outcomes for all lesions. Patients presenting with Ollier disease, Maffucci syndrome, pathologic fractures, or recurrent disease were separated for additional analysis.

Results.—Of the 102 lesions, 62 (61%) achieved complete radiographic healing in a median time of 6 months. Full range of motion was achieved following treatment of 68 lesions (67%) in a median time of 3 months. A total of 95 lesions (93%) remained recurrence free following surgery. One case of malignant transformation occurred in a patient with Maffucci syndrome. Tumor location and graft choice did not affect healing grade, time to healing, range of motion, or recurrence rate. Age at presentation greater than 30 was associated with more rapid healing. Monocentric, non-expanding lesions were associated with improved postoperative range of motion. Patients with a diagnosis of multiple enchondromas had a higher rate of recurrence following surgery, and patients presenting with a recurrent lesion had a higher rate of complications. Following pathologic fracture, no differences in outcomes were observed when enchondromas were treated primarily or following fracture healing.

Conclusions.—Following surgical treatment of enchondromas in the hand, the majority of patients achieve complete bony healing and full range of motion, regardless of the graft material used. Malignant transformation is rare, and aggressive follow-up measures should be reserved for patients with a diagnosis of multiple enchondromas.

Type of Study/Level of Evidence.—Therapeutic IV.

▶ The study represents a single center review of 102 enchondromas of the hand treated surgically. The outcomes reported were favorable, and the article addresses a number of questions raised in the care of enchondromas of the hand. Malignant transformation is in the range of 1% in this series; one intraoperative chondrosarcoma was found, which required immediate amputation. This would lead the reader to consider an intraoperative biopsy of all lesions that required curettage. Graft choice does not make a difference, and use of allograft is supported to minimize donor morbidity. Timing of surgical care related to fracture did not affect outcome other than requiring 7 weeks of immobilization. Age older than 30 years and recurrent tumors led to more potential for complication. This article is an excellent guide for the care of this problem. Although it was a retrospective review, the authors offer good advice to the reader. In the future, it appears that we can fix pathologic fractures or treat them until healing and then curette them knowing that the outcomes will be unchanged. Patient factors should determine the timing. Autograft can be used, as can allograft, without concern when it comes to healing and function. This large series does not answer the question as to whether graft is even needed, but the nature of the level IV study precludes answering that question. The findings match my observations in practice. This article warrants consideration by all who treat this common problem in hand surgery.

C. Carroll, MD

Anatomy of the Thumb Metacarpophalangeal Ulnar and Radial Collateral Ligaments

Carlson MG, Warner KK, Meyers KN, et al (Hosp for Special Surgery, NY; Mayo Clinic, Rochester, MN)
J Hand Surg 37A:2021-2026, 2012

Purpose.—To describe the origin and insertion of the ulnar (UCL) and radial collateral ligaments (RCL) of the thumb metacarpophalangeal (MCP) joint.

Methods.—We dissected 18 UCLs and 18 RCLs from fresh-frozen human cadaveric thumbs. We removed all soft tissue overlying the MCP joint, isolating the proper collateral ligaments. We detached the collateral ligaments from the bone while marking their origin and insertion points and measured these attachment sites in relation to bony landmarks by digital photo analysis.

Results.—The center of the UCL origin at the metacarpal was 4.2 mm from the dorsal surface and 5.3 mm from the articular surface. The dorsal aspect of the metacarpal origin site was 2.1 mm from the dorsal edge of the metacarpal. The center of the phalangeal insertion was 2.8 mm from the volar surface and 3.4 mm from the articular surface. The volar aspect of the phalangeal insertion site was 0.7 mm from the volar edge of the phalanx. The center of the RCL origin at the metacarpal was 3.5 mm from the dorsal surface and 3.3 mm from the articular surface. The dorsal aspect of the metacarpal origin site was 1.5 mm from the dorsal edge of the metacarpal. The center of the phalangeal insertion was 2.8 mm from the volar surface and 2.6 mm from the articular surface. The volar aspect of the phalangeal insertion site was 0.5 mm from the volar edge of the phalanx.

Conclusions.—Our study accurately defined the origin and insertion sites of the UCL and RCL of the thumb MCP joint.

Clinical Relevance.—An accurate definition of the anatomical origin and insertion points of the thumb MCP UCL and RCL may allow for more successful surgical repair and reconstruction.

▶ This is an excellent anatomic study examining the origins and insertions of the thumb collateral ligaments. The concept is simple, but the implications may be significant. The authors found that the insertions of both radial and ulnar collateral ligaments are consistently volar and proximal to the tubercles at the base of the proximal phalanx. These findings run counter to the often-used technique of repairing ulnar collateral ligaments at the medial tubercle and radial collateral ligaments at the lateral tubercle when addressing tears at the proximal phalanx insertion sites. The authors suggest that an accurate definition of the anatomical origin and insertion points of the thumb collateral ligaments "may allow for more successful surgical repair and reconstruction." Although this claim is not substantiated in a clinical sense, the data provided should certainly aid surgeons in achieving anatomic repairs of these important structures.

E. Shin, MD

Hand Education for Emergency Medicine Residents: Results of a Pilot Program

Lifchez SD (Johns Hopkins Univ, Baltimore, MD)
J Hand Surg 37A:1245-1248.e12, 2012

Purpose.—Multiple studies have demonstrated the lack of knowledge of hand anatomy and pathology among those who first see patients with hand disorders. The goal of this study was to determine whether a hand surgery rotation for emergency medicine residents would improve this group's knowledge of the hand and its disorders as assessed at the end of their residency training.

Methods.—Seven postgraduate year (PGY) 2 emergency medicine residents completed a 4-week hand surgery rotation. Hand knowledge was assessed at the start, at the end, and 1 year after this rotation (end of PGY 3). Knowledge of a control group of 7 PGY 3 emergency medicine residents who did not have this rotation was also assessed.

Results.—Hand knowledge in the residents who completed the rotation was significantly improved. This was true for overall test performance (88% vs 70% correct responses), as well as for each of the anatomy and function (89% vs 57%), diagnosis (96% vs 86%), and treatment (79% vs 51%) categories. Overall test performance (78% vs 66%) and anatomy and function category performance (75% vs 43%) were significantly better at the end of PGY 3 for the residents who completed the rotation as compared to the control residents.

Conclusions.—A hand surgery rotation during an emergency medicine residency program improved the knowledge of hand anatomy and disorders. This knowledge was retained 1 year later and was greater than the knowledge of matched emergency medicine residents who did not have this rotation. Better knowledge of hand anatomy and disorders among emergency physicians might improve their ability to initially evaluate and treat patients with these conditions. Such knowledge might allow emergency department physicians to play a more important role in the management of hand emergencies. A hand surgery rotation has been incorporated into the PGY 2 curriculum for all emergency medicine residents at my institution.

▶ Several studies have found knowledge deficiencies in the care of hand problems among primary and emergency physicians. This study responded to these findings by designing an educational intervention to improve the knowledge of emergency medicine residents on the care of the hand. The intervention was a 4-week clinical hand rotation for second-year emergency medicine residents. The rotation and didactics were tailored to meet their needs. The program was evaluated through knowledge tests given before and after rotation and compared with a control group of residents. In the end, the hand rotation improved knowledge on care among the participating residents.

This study takes the next step of trying to design a solution to a well-documented problem. However, the study is limited significantly by its small sample size (only 7 residents completed the rotation), which limits the generalizability of this pilot program.

Emergency physicians are required to know a wide array of clinical fields, and their educational time is pulled by many competing demands. Thus, the most impressive outcome of this study is that after this pilot program, the hand surgery rotation was subsequently adopted as a standard emergency resident rotation. This tells us that the residents and emergency department physicians valued the knowledge gained from a hand rotation and were willing to devote some of their limited time to this endeavor.

C. Curtin, MD

Contribution of Flexor Pollicis Longus to Pinch Strength: An *In Vivo* Study
Goetz TJ, Costa JA, Slobogean G, et al (Univ of British Columbia, Vancouver)
J Hand Surg 37A:2304-2309, 2012

Purpose.—To estimate the contribution of the flexor pollicis longus (FPL) to key pinch strength. Secondary outcomes include tip pinch, 3-point chuck pinch, and grip strength.

Methods.—Eleven healthy volunteers consented to participate in the study. We recorded baseline measures for key, 3-point chuck, and tip pinch and for grip strength. In order to control for instability of the interphalangeal (IP) joint after FPL paralysis, pinch measurements were repeated after immobilizing the thumb IP joint. Measures were repeated after subjects underwent electromyography-guided lidocaine blockade of the FPL muscle. Nerve conduction studies and clinical examinations were used to confirm FPL blockade and to rule out median nerve blockade. Paired *t*-tests were used to compare pre- and postblock means for both unsplinted and splinted measures. The difference in means was used to estimate the contribution of FPL to pinch strength.

Results.—All 3 types of pinch strength showed a significant decrease between pre- and postblock measurements. The relative contribution of FPL for each pinch type was 56%, 44%, and 43% for key, chuck, and tip pinch, respectively. Mean grip strength did not decrease significantly. Splinting of the IP joint had no significant effect on pinch measurements.

Conclusions.—FPL paralysis resulted in a statistically significant decrease in pinch strength. IP joint immobilization to simulate IP joint fusion did not affect results.

Clinical Relevance.—Reconstruction after acute or chronic loss of FPL function should be considered when restoration of pinch strength is important.

▶ Of equal interest is how important it is to force the activity of the thenar cone of intrinsic muscles. These, working in concert, supply more than 50% of the force for most thumb postures, with the ulnar innervated intrinsics performing the yeoman's part of the job. In the circumstance of low ulnar nerve palsy, our concern should be directed more at restoring pinch force and balance than digital balance to prevent a claw-type deformity. The authors correctly point out the not totally controllable variables in such a study, particularly the crafty way that patients and subjects learn to get around the deficit; for example, by changing how they position digits during pinch activities, particularly those where they are asked to exert maximal force.

One concern is the author's interpretation or the study of Kozin[1] in which median and ulnar nerve blocks were performed to paralyze the intrinsic muscles so that their contribution to pinch could be judged. The authors, in their discussion, mention the importance of joint positioning and stability, but they fail to mention what is probably the key difference in their study and that of Kozin. The hands of Kozin's volunteers lost sensation and proprioception and, therefore, they lost the ability of their hands to tell their brains what was happening. As Moberg long ago demonstrated, sensation is a key element in voluntary force generation.

V. R. Hentz, MD

Reference

1. Kozin SH, Porter S, Clark P, Thoder JJ. The contribution of the intrinsic muscles to grip and pinch strength. *J Hand Surg Am.* 1999;24:64-72.

Determinants of Grip Strength in Healthy Subjects Compared to That in Patients Recovering From a Distal Radius Fracture
Bot AGJ, Mulders MAM, Fostvedt S, et al (Massachusetts General Hosp, Boston)
J Hand Surg 37A:1874-1880, 2012

Purpose.—Grip strength is influenced primarily by body mass index, sex, and age. It is also partly voluntary and correlates with symptoms of depression. This study examined whether psychological factors influence grip more in the setting of injury than in healthy volunteers.

Methods.—Grip strength was evaluated in one hundred subjects, 50 healthy individuals and 50 patients 6 weeks after a nonsurgically treated fracture of the distal radius. Grip strength was measured as the mean of 3 attempts, and patients completed questionnaires for arm-specific disability (Disabilities of the Arm, Shoulder, and Hand), depression, pain anxiety, catastrophic thinking, and negative thoughts in response to pain.

Results.—The mean grip strength in the injured group was 55% of the uninjured side. Pain anxiety accounted for 9% of the variability in grip strength in injured wrists. Among healthy patients, sex was the only correlate of dominant-side grip strength, and body mass index accounted for 8% of the variation in the grip strength of the nondominant side divided by the dominant side.

Conclusions.—The majority of the variation in grip strength remains unaccounted for, but physical factors correlate best with grip strength and percent grip strength of the nondominant side divided by the dominant side in healthy patients, and psychological factors correlate best with absolute grip in patients recovering from distal radius fractures.

Clinical Relevance.—The influences on grip strength are complex, but the differences among recovering and healthy patients demonstrate a role for nonphysical factors in grip strength during recovery.

▶ The study by Bot et al is an excellent foray into a difficult subject in orthopedics and hand surgery. It is well known that there is significant loss of grip power after injury. It also well known that early rehabilitation of an injured extremity is not able to deter all of the atrophy seen in an injured extremity. In an effort to get to the bottom of whether this difference is caused by psychological factors, the authors have taken a well-structured and vigorous analytical study of 2 cohorts—one injured and one uninjured—and looked at differences in grip strength. The results are that the influences on grip strength are complex, and neither the physical factors nor the psychological factors make up for most unexplained variations in grip strength. Their findings are important and well supported. The indication is that there is still some undetermined factor-causing weakness after injury in patients with distal radius fractures. This finding correlates well with findings in the sports medicine literature indicating that quadriceps weakness after anterior cruciate ligament reconstruction is not able to be explained simply by disuse atrophy.

The study does have some weaknesses, including some decisions in statistical analysis that could have an effect on the data set. They also discarded several variables based on judgment calls that also could have significantly impacted the outcomes of their analysis. Additionally, there could be a significant alteration in the power caused by changes in the architecture of the radius and the fracture group. These findings are important for the future of treatment—not just of distal radius fractures but musculoskeletal injury in general. As we attempt to return patients to functional status more quickly, we will need to ascertain what biomechanical and potentially neuromuscular factors are negatively affecting their function and return to activity.

In our own experience, postinjury weakness is a significant problem as we try to return patients to functional status. Efforts to return functional status to an injured limb in the early postoperative period have only met with marginal success. There are still significant problems with weakness and functional disability in patients over and above what would be expected by the injury with early return to function.

D. Mastella, MD

Survey of Hand Surgeons Regarding Their Perceived Needs for an Expanded Upper Extremity Fellowship

Kakar S, Bakri K, Shin AY (Mayo Clinic, Rochester, MN)
J Hand Surg 37A:2374-2380, 2012

Purpose.—To survey practicing hand surgeons regarding their perceived need for an expanded upper extremity fellowship.

Methods.—Electronic surveys were sent to 248 surgeons who had completed a hand surgery fellowship between 2008 and 2010. The survey was structured to ascertain whether there was a need for expanded education encompassing the entire upper extremity. Four separate mailings were made. Of the 248 surgeons who were sent the survey, 131 (53%) responded. Of the respondents, 74% (97) were trained in orthopedics, 16% (21) in plastic surgery, and 10% (13) in general surgery.

Results.—Of the 131 respondents, 7% (9) felt that 1 year of specialty training was insufficient, 48% (63) had sought shoulder and elbow training in their fellowship, and 52% (68) did not have dedicated plastic surgery rotations. Microsurgical experience was variable: 8% (10) of respondents had not been exposed to replantation, 23% (30) had not been exposed to free flap surgery, 32% (42) had not participated in brachial plexus surgery, and 17% (22) had not done a vascularized bone graft. Fifty-six percent (73) of respondents had not had dedicated time for research during their fellowship. Eleven percent (15) had obtained additional training after their fellowship, including shoulder and elbow, microsurgery, pediatrics, and peripheral nerve surgery. When asked if they would have applied to a 2-year hand and upper extremity fellowship, 60% (79) of respondents would have applied.

Conclusions.—Based on the results of this survey, 1 year of hand fellowship training has been perceived as inadequate by 7% (9) of respondents, with exposure insufficient in shoulder and elbow, microsurgery, pediatrics, and clinical research. Further critical review of hand fellowship education should be considered, with the availability of extended fellowship tracks for those requesting an increased breadth of upper extremity surgical training.

Type of Study/Level of Evidence.—Economic/Decision Analysis II.

▶ In recent years, there has been renewed interest in reassessing the education of hand surgeons in the United States. Ideas and options have included expanding to 2-year fellowships, additional training in shoulder and elbow surgery, and even the concept of integrating hand surgery training in residency leading to hand surgery board certification. What has become evident is that every trainee and every hand surgeon has unique experiences and ideas related to optimal training.

In this study by Kakar et al from the Mayo Clinic, recent graduates from hand surgery fellowship programs were surveyed regarding their training and education. Of the respondents, 7% felt that 1 year of specialty training was insufficient. There is likely some respondent bias in this result. By nature, most people who have completed a program would feel that it was adequate for their continued performance. Rarely do individuals feel that they are not well trained.

The additional data are more telling: 48% of respondents felt that shoulder and elbow training in their fellowship was important, and 52% of respondents did not have a dedicated plastic surgery rotation. Furthermore, microsurgery experience was extremely variable, with 23% not having been exposed to free flap surgery. Finally, when asked if they would have applied to a 2-year hand and upper extremity fellowship program, 60% of respondents would have applied. However, this does not mean they would actually choose this as their top option.

What these data tell us is that program directors and educators in hand surgery must reevaluate the curriculum of hand fellowship programs. There continues to be deficiencies in shoulder and elbow surgery, replantation, brachial plexus surgery, congenital surgery, and flap surgery. Recently, the American Society for Surgery of the Hand has developed several unique 2-year fellowship programs that will offer additional experiences in these areas. It is hoped that these pilot programs will allow all hand fellowship programs to better assess their needs in offering important educational opportunities.

J. Chang, MD

The value of provocative tests for the wrist and elbow: A literature review
Valdes K, Lastayo P (Hand Works Therapy, Sarasota, FL; Univ of Utah, Salt Lake City)
J Hand Ther 26:32-43, 2013

To describe and determine the usefulness of provocative tests for the wrist and elbow a literature search was performed. A total of 31 diagnostic studies were identified, assessed, and ranked. The highest ranking tests had a mean positive likelihood ratio of ≥2.0, or a mean negative likelihood ratio of ≤0.5, from more than one study. The highly recommended tests were found to be the Phalen's, Tinel's test for carpal tunnel and cubital tunnel, and modified compression test, scaphoid shift test, and elbow flexion test. A total of 14 tests met our requirements to be considered a recommended test. A greater number of provocative tests either do not have adequate data to support their usefulness or their clinical utility has not been assessed. This information may assist hand therapists in choosing which provocative tests are considered clinically useful in improving the probability of the presence or absence of pathology in the hand, wrist, and elbow.

Level of Evidence.—NA (Tables 1-3).

▶ This interesting article is a meta-analysis of the available literature on the value of provocative testing for hand evaluation. Perhaps the most interesting finding is that a high number of commonly used provocative maneuvers have little or no data to support their use.

TABLE 1.—Highly Recommended Provocative Tests for the Wrist & Elbow

Test	Author, Year	MacDermid[5] Study Score	+LR	−LR
Wrist neuropathy testing				
Phalen's	LaJoie, 2005[14]	8/12	7.6	0.09
	Boland, 2009[15]	9/12	2.54	0.49
	Wainner, 2005[16]	10/12	1.3	0.50
	Amerifeyz, 2005[17]	8/12	0.98	0.85
	Tekeoglu, 2007[11]	10/12	1.0	0.77
	Mean		**2.68**	**0.54**
Tinel's	LaJoie, 2005[14]	8/12	10.77	0.03
	Wainner, 2005[16]	10/12	1.4	0.78
	Cheng, 2008[13]	9/12	0.96	0.59
	Amerifeyz, 2005[17]	8/12	0.64	0.71
	Tekeoglu, 2007[11]	10/12	1.0	0.75
	Mean		**2.95**	**0.57**
Modified compression test	Boland, 2009[15]	9/12	3.64	0.89
	Tekeoglu, 2007[11]	10/12	0.92	0.93
	Mean		**2.28**	**0.91**
Wrist musculoskeletal pathology testing				
Scaphoid shift	Wolfe, 1994[18]	8/12	4.7	0.17
	Wolfe, 1997[19]	9/12	1.68	0
	Prosser, 2011[20]	10/12	2.88	0.28
	LaStayo, 1995[21]	10/12	1.78	0.55
	Mean		**2.76**	**0.25**
Elbow neuropathology testing				
Tinel	Cheng, 2008[13]	8/12	53.99	0.46
	Beekman, 2009[22]	9/12	1.3	0.72
	Mean		**27.65**	**0.59**
Elbow flexion	Beekman, 2009[22]	9/12	1.0	0.99
	Ochi, 2011[23]	8/12	Infinity	0.64
	Cheng, 2008[13]	9/12	45.99	0.54
	Mean		**27.66**	**0.72**

Editor's Note: Please refer to original journal article for full references.
Bold numerical values are the resultant mean likelihood ratios.

TABLE 2.—Reasonable Provocative Tests for the Hand, Wrist & Elbow

Test	Author, Year	MacDermid[5] Study Score	+LR	−LR
Wrist neuropathy testing				
Symptom relief maneuver	Gok, 2008[24]	9/12	3.3	0.39
Flick	Gok, 2008[24]	9/12	5.9	0.22
Wrist musculoskeletal pathology testing				
Ulnar fovea	Tay, 2007[27]	11/12	7.06	0.05
Press test	Lester, 1995[26]	7/12	Infinity	0
Series of 3 tests	Christodoulou, 1999[28]	8/12	16.22	0.24
CMC grind	Merritt, 2010[25]	12/12	4.45	0.60
ECU synergy	Ruland, 2008[29]	9/12	2.9	0
Midcarpal	Prosser, 2011[20]	10/12	2.67	Not calculated
DRUJ	Prosser, 2011[20]	10/12	1.79	0.30
Elbow neuropathy testing				
Scratch collapse	Cheng, 2008[13]	9/12	68.99	0.31
Ulnar nerve thickening	Beekman, 2009[22]	9/12	2.2	0.82
Shoulder IR	Ochi, 2011[23]	8/12	Infinity	0.19
Crossed fingers	Earle, 1980[31]	8/12	Infinity	0.36
Elbow musculoskeletal pathology testing				
Moving valgus stress test	O'Driscoll, 2005[30]	9/12	Infinity	0.05

Editor's Note: Please refer to original journal article for full references.
+LR = positive likelihood ratio; −LR = negative likelihood ratio; DRUJ = distal radioulnar joint; CMC = carpometacarpal; IR = internal rotation.

TABLE 3.—Neutral/No Recommendation Provocative Tests for the Wrist & Elbow

Test	Author, Year	MacDermid[5] Study Score	+LR	−LR
Wrist neuropathology testing				
Carpal compression	Amirfeyz, 2011[40]	7/12	0.80	0.83
test	Goloborod'ko, 2004[32]	7/12	0.88	0.90
	Wainner, 2005[16]	10/12	0.91	1.2
	El Miedany, 2008[41]	7/12	0.61	2.16
	Mean		**0.80**	**1.27**
Tourniquet test	Amirfeyz, 2011[40]	7/12	0.72	0.90
	Goloborod'ko, 2004[32]	7/12	0.95	0.87
	Mean		**0.83**	**0.89**
Hand elevation test	Amirfeyz, 2011[40]	7/12	0.92	0.99
	Amirfeyz, 2005[17]	8/12	0.98	0.88
	Mean		**0.95**	**0.94**
Phalen's wrist	Goloborod'ko, 2004[32]	7/12	0.92	0.88
extension	El Miedany, 2008[41]	7/12	0.64	1.65
	Yoshida, 2010[34]	7/12	1	Unable to calculate
	Mean		**0.85**	**1.27**
Tanzer's	Goloborod'ko, 2004[32]	7/12	0.91	0.79
Postural provocation	Goloborod'ko, 2004[32]	7/12	0.98	0.98
Constant pressure on lunate	Goloborod'ko, 2004[32]	7/12	0.98	0.98
Pneumatic compression test	Tekeoglu, 2007[11]	10/12	0.98	0.83
Okutsu	Yoshida, 2010[34]	7/12	1.0	Unable to calculate
Upper limb tension test Part A	Wainner, 2005[16]	10/12	0.91	1.2
Upper limb tension test Part B	Wainner, 2005[16]	10/12	0.86	1.9
Upper limb neurodynamic test	Vanti, 2011[35]	9/12	1.81	0.65
Combined wrist flexion & carpal compression	Cheng, 2008[13]	9/12	0.98	0.65
Scratch collapse test	Cheng, 2008[13]	9/12	0.99	0.73
Phalen's combined with sensory testing	Bilkis, 2011[36]	6/12	1.0	0.74
Wrist musculoskeletal pathology testing				
Ulnomenisco-triquetral dorsal glide	LaStayo, 1995[21]	10/12	1.2	0.77
Ballottement	LaStayo, 1995[21]	10/12	1.12	0.83
Lunotriquetral test	Prosser, 2011[20]	10/12	1.03	0.80
GRIT	Prosser, 2011[20]	10/12	1.12	0.83
Ulnocarpal stress test	Nakamura, 1997[37]	7/12	1.0	Unable to calculate
Elbow neuropathology testing				
Ulnar nerve tenderness	Beekman, 2009[22]	9/12	1.6	0.85
Elbow musculoskeletal pathology testing				
Chair sign	Regan, 2006[38]	4/10	0.87	Unable to calculate
Push-up sign	Regan, 2006[38]	4/10	0.87	Unable to calculate
Tabletop relocation	Arvind, 2006[39]	4/10	1.0	Unable to calculate

Editor's Note: Please refer to original journal article for full references.
Bold numerical values are the resultant mean likelihood ratios.
+LR = positive likelihood ratio; −LR = negative likelihood ratio; GRIT = gripping rotatory impaction test.

The "highly recommended" tests (Table 1) include the carpal tunnel Tinel, modified carpal compression test, Phalen's maneuver, scaphoid shift test, cubital tunnel Tinel, and elbow flexion tests. "Recommended tests" are listed in Table 2, while a surprisingly high number of tests fit the "neutral/no recommendation" category (Table 3). This highlights the lack of evidence for many provocative maneuvers we rely upon.

J. E. Adams, MD

Article Index

Chapter 1: Hand and Wrist Arthritis

Chapter 2: Wrist Arthroscopy

Chapter 3: Carpus

Chapter 4: Dupuytren's Contracture

Chapter 5: Compressive Neuropathies

Chapter 6: Nerve

Chapter 7: Brachial Plexus

Chapter 8: Microsurgery

Chapter 9: Tendon

Chapter 10: Trauma

Chapter 11: Distal Radius Fractures

Chapter 12: Elbow: Trauma

Chapter 13: Pediatric Trauma

Chapter 14: Congenital

Chapter 15: Shoulder: Instability

Chapter 16: Shoulder: Arthroplasty

Chapter 17: Shoulder: Rotator Cuff

Chapter 18: Rehabilitation

Chapter 19: Miscellaneous

Author Index

Printed and bound by CPI Group (UK) Ltd, Croydon, CR0 4YY

08/05/2025

01864755-0005